Numerical Reasoning in Judgments and Decision Making about Health

Every day thousands of individuals need to make critical decisions about their health based on numerical information, yet recent surveys have found that over half the population of the USA is unable to complete basic math problems. How does this lack of numerical ability (also referred to as low numeracy, quantitative illiteracy, or statistical illiteracy) impact healthcare? What can be done to help people with low numeracy skills? *Numerical Reasoning in Judgments and Decision Making about Health* addresses these questions by examining and explaining the impact of quantitative illiteracy on healthcare and in specific healthcare contexts, and discussing what can be done to reduce these healthcare disparities. This book will be a useful resource for professionals in many health fields including academics, policy makers, physicians, and other healthcare providers.

Britta L. Anderson is a Research Associate at the American College of Obstetricians and Gynecologists.

Jay Schulkin is the Senior Director of Research in the Division of Practice at the American College of Obstetricians and Gynecologists. He is also a Research Professor of Neuroscience at Georgetown University and Research Professor in the Department of Obstetrics and Gynecology at the University of Washington.

Numerical Reasoning in Judgments and Decision Making about Health

Edited by
Britta L. Anderson & Jay Schulkin

CAMBRIDGE
UNIVERSITY PRESS

CAMBRIDGE
UNIVERSITY PRESS

University Printing House, Cambridge CB2 8BS, United Kingdom

Cambridge University Press is part of the University of Cambridge.

It furthers the University's mission by disseminating knowledge in the pursuit of education, learning and research at the highest international levels of excellence.

www.cambridge.org
Information on this title: www.cambridge.org/9781107040946

First published 2014

Printed in the United Kingdom by Clays, St Ives plc

A catalog record for this publication is available from the British Library

Library of Congress Cataloging in Publication data
Numerical reasoning in judgments and decision making about health / [edited by] Britta L. Anderson & Jay Schulkin.
p. ; cm.
Includes bibliographical references.
ISBN 978-1-107-04094-6 (hardback)
I. Anderson, Britta L., editor of compilation. II. Schulkin, Jay, editor of compilation.
[DNLM: 1. Health Literacy – United States. 2. Decision Making – United States. 3. Judgment – United States. 4. Mathematical Concepts – United States. WA 590]
RA427
362.1–dc23

2013043959

ISBN 978-1-107-04094-6 Hardback

Britta L. Anderson would like to dedicate this book to Bo Peery and to her grandparents.

Jay Schulkin would like to dedicate this book to Jonathan Baron and George Loewenstein.

Contents

Figures

Tables

Contributors

BRITTA L. ANDERSON, Department of Research, American College of Obstetricians and Gynecologists.

JILLIAN BERKMAN, Department of Medicine, Division of Nephrology, Vanderbilt University Medical Center.

PRISCILA G. BRUST-RENCK, Department of Human Development, Cornell University.

KERRI L. CAVANAUGH, Department of Medicine, Division of Nephrology, Vanderbilt University Medical Center.

EDWARD T. COKELY, Department of Cognitive and Learning Sciences, Michigan Technological University; Center for Adaptive Behavior and Cognition, Max Planck Institute for Human Development.

STEPHANIE DUKHOVNY, Maternal Fetal Medicine, Brigham and Women's Hospital.

ANGELA FAGERLIN, Center for Bioethics and Social Sciences in Medicine; Internal Medicine, University of Michigan; VA Ann Arbor Center for Clinical Management Research.

WOLFGANG GAISSMAIER, Department of Psychology, University of Konstanz.

ROCIO GARCIA-RETAMERO, Department of Experimental Psychology, University of Granada; Center for Adaptive Behavior and Cognition, Max Planck Institute for Human Development.

SAIMA GHAZAL, Department of Cognitive and Learning Sciences, Michigan Technological University, MI, USA.

GILLIAN MAYMAN, Center for Managing Chronic Disease, School of Public Health, University of Michigan.

JAN MULTMEIER, Harding Center for Risk Literacy and Center for Adaptive Behavior and Cognition, Max Planck Institute for Human Development.

RONALD PAULUS, Mission Health System.

ELLEN PETERS, Department of Psychology, The Ohio State University.

VALERIE F. REYNA, Department of Human Development and Psychology, Cornell University; Cornell University Magnetic Resonance Imaging Facility; Center for Behavioral Economics and Decision Research, Cornell University.

JAY SCHULKIN, Department of Research, American College of Obstetricians and Gynecologists; Department of Neuroscience, Georgetown University; Department of Obstetrics and Gynecology, University of Washington School of Medicine.

PETER H. SCHWARTZ, Indiana University Center for Bioethics; Division of General Internal Medicine and Geriatrics, Indiana University School of Medicine; Philosophy Department, Indiana University – Purdue University, Indianapolis.

WALTER F. STEWART, Sutter Health.

ODETTE WEGWARTH, Harding Center for Risk Literacy and Center for Adaptive Behavior and Cognition, Max Planck Institute for Human Development.

LOUISE WILKINS-HAUG, Maternal Fetal Medicine and Reproductive Genetics, Brigham and Women's Hospital; Harvard Medical School.

BRIAN J. ZIKMUND-FISHER, Health Behavior and Health Education, School of Public Health, University of Michigan; Internal Medicine, University of Michigan.

Acknowledgments

The life of the mind is a social event and we could not have done this without the help and support of our colleagues and friends.

Many of the issues that appear in this book were discussed in a small conference held at the Center for Advanced Study in the Behavioral Sciences at Stanford. We thank Stephen Kosslyn, Director of the Center, for his generous hospitality and to Hal Pashler, Ron Paulus, Ellen Peters, and Louise Wilkins-Haug who gave presentations.

Finally, we thank our granting agency, the US Department of Health and Human Services, Health Resources and Services Administration, Maternal and Child Health Research Program for their support for our research (UA6MC19010).

Introduction

Britta L. Anderson & Jay Schulkin

The research discussed in this volume stems, in part, from work on health literacy. Health literacy is "the degree to which individuals have the capacity to obtain, process, and understand basic health information and services needed to make appropriate health decisions" (nnlm.gov). When people hear the term health literacy, they may think of a patient's ability to read medical information and understand medical terminology; however, health literacy not only includes literacy, but also *numeracy*.

A broad and basic definition of numeracy is *the ability to use and understand numbers*. Terms related to, and often used synonymously with, numeracy include quantitative literacy, health numeracy, and statistical literacy. Table I.1 highlights several examples of how these terms have been defined in previous research and throughout this book.

As shown in Table I.1, the terms used to describe numerical reasoning refer to a range of abilities, from the very basic (knowing which number is larger than another) to advanced (statistical terminology). We provide these examples to demonstrate the breadth of the concept at hand and encourage the reader to be mindful of the use of these terms throughout this book.

Large national samples have found that there is a significant proportion of the population who have only basic numeracy skills or less (meaning partial mastery or no mastery of grade-level skills). For example, 47% of adults who completed the National Adult Literacy Survey (NALS) were in the lowest two (of five) levels of performance (Kirsch et al., 2002). A more recent national survey of adults found that 36% are at or below basic levels (Kutner et al., 2006). Deficits in basic numeric ability are not only found in the general population, but also in subgroups of highly educated individuals (e.g., Lipkus et al., 2001; Anderson et al., 2014).

Along with basic numeracy, statistics is an essential part of the numeric language of medicine. However, unlike basic numeric abilities, statistics have not always had such a central role in medicine. The rise of statistical reasoning occurred due to the need to establish state records as well as catalog diseases, viruses, and plague events that impacted human and

Table I.1. *Definitions for numeracy and related terms.*

Term	Definition	Source
Numeracy	The term numeracy describes the aggregate of skills, knowledge, beliefs, dispositions, and habits of mind – as well as the general communicative and problem-solving skills – that is needed in order to effectively handle real-world situations or interpretative tasks with embedded mathematical or quantifiable elements.	Gal (1995, para. 9)
Numeracy	Numeracy, in the sense of knowledge and mastery of systems for quantification, measurement and calculation, is a practice-driven competence rather than abstract academic knowledge of "mathematics." Proficiency in numeracy varies with people's backgrounds and experience.	Adelsward and Sachs (1996, p. 1186)
Numeracy	The specific aspect of literacy that involves solving problems requiring understanding and use of quantitative information is sometimes called numeracy. Numeracy skills include understanding basic calculations, time and money, measurement, estimation, logic, and performing multistep operations. Most importantly, numeracy also involves the ability to infer what mathematical concepts need to be applied when interpreting specific situations.	Montori and Rothman (2005, p. 1071)
Quantitative literacy	The knowledge and skills required to apply arithmetic operations, either alone or sequentially, using numbers embedded in printed materials.	Kirsch et al. (2002, pp. 3–4)
Health numeracy	The degree to which individuals have the capacity to access, process, interpret, communicate, and act on numerical, quantitative, graphical, biostatistical, and probabilistic health information needed to make effective health decisions.	Golbeck et al. (2005, p. 375)
Health numeracy	The individual-level skills needed to understand and use quantitative health information, including basic computation skills, ability to use information in documents and non-text formats such as graphs, and ability to communicate orally.	Ancker and Kaufman (2007, p. 713)
Physician numeracy	Understanding the statistical aspects of and terminology associated with the design, analysis, and results of original research.	Rao and Kanter (2010)
Patient numeracy	The ability of patients to understand and use quantitative health data.	Chapter 2 in this volume
Statistical literacy	The ability to use and understand health statistics.	Chapter 4 in this volume

Adapted from Reyna et al., 2009.

animal populations. In the world of Newtonian certainty, statistics was looked down upon because it was concerned with probabilities. Although statistics were seen as a lesser science, "taming chance" became essential for critical and epidemiological thinking (Hacking 1964, 1975, 1999).

Only in the late nineteenth and early twentieth centuries did science and statistical methods merge and become a currency for genetics, economics, physics, medicine, etc. (Hacking 1964, 1975, 1999). Around this time the Flexner report was published (1910), which emphasized the importance of integrating research findings into medical education and decision making. The ability to use and understand statistical information is not only important for physicians and policy makers, but also for patients as they are increasingly involved in their health and healthcare.

The focus of this book is not only about individuals' numeracy and ability to use statistics, but how these abilities are associated with judgments and decision making about health. The next section introduces the study of judgments and decision making.

Judgments and decision making

The decision sciences investigate judgments and decision making using a scientific approach. The study of the decision sciences expanded during the cognitive revolution with the development of Herbert Simon's theory of bounded rationality (Simon 1955, 1978), which states that decision making is limited to the information we have, the amount of time we have to make a decision, and the limitations of our cognition. From Simon's seminal work, Kahneman and Tversky (1979), Gerd Gigerenzer and his colleagues (e.g., Gigerenzer & Goldstein, 1996), and too many others to mention, have made significant contributions to our understanding of judgment and decision making. Shortly after the decision sciences began, a subfield focused on decisions in medical contexts was established (Chapman & Sonnenberg, 2003; Elstein, 2004; Elstein et al., 1978).

Research on decision making generally takes one of three approaches: descriptive, normative, and prescriptive (Baron, 2000). Descriptive approaches describe how decisions are typically made, normative approaches describe ideal decision making, and prescriptive approaches focus on improving decision making, by prescribing how decisions ought to be made. Each approach contributes to our understanding of decision making, and examples of each perspective can be found throughout this book. All of the chapters discuss the descriptive approach, such as describing patient decision making in Chapter 4 and describing decision making about genetic testing in Chapter 6. The ideal that decisions can be made using systematic reviews of the latest evidence (evidence-based medicine) could be considered as a normative approach discussed throughout this book. Though examples of the prescriptive approach can be found throughout the book, it is especially prevalent in the last five chapters, which focus on improving decision making.

Intersection of numerical reasoning and judgments and decision making

The focus of this book is the intersection of the study of numerical reasoning and the study of judgment and decision making in the health context. Research examining how individuals' numeracy level is associated with decision making took hold in the late 1990s and early 2000s with publications by Schwartz and colleagues (1997), Lipkus and colleagues (2001), and others. For example, Schwartz and colleagues (1997) found that 40% of women with high numeracy scores had accurate breast cancer risk estimates compared to 5.8% of women with low numeracy scores. Many studies since have added to this growing field. The chapters of this volume provide further examples on a range of health topics.

Research on numeracy and decision making is especially important in light of how clinical medicine has evolved. For example, there is now a greater emphasis on collaborative decision making between patients and physicians. Rather than physicians making decisions *for* the patients, they are making decisions *with* the patients. With patients having a more active role in their healthcare, their knowledge and understanding about numeric information is becoming more relevant. There is also a greater emphasis on making decisions based on research findings (evidence-based medicine), which requires that doctors and patients understand the statistics used to describe study results. These and other aspects of clinical medicine as related to numeracy and decision making will be discussed in more detail throughout this book.

The organization of this book

The chapters in this book discuss how numerical reasoning skills impact healthcare and how these skills are associated with individuals' decision making. Importantly, the book also examines how we might improve numerical reasoning and judgments and decision making about health, and directions for future research.

We begin with a chapter that introduces the concept of numeracy and the tools used to measure numeracy, which is central to all of the chapters in this volume. While the original numeracy measures assessed performance on basic math tasks, such as converting between percentages and frequencies, new scales have been developed in recent years that offer unique advantages over the original measures. In Chapter 1, Cokely and colleagues provide a useful resource for those who wish to conduct research on numeracy by providing descriptions of different numeracy measures. These include the early measures by Schwartz and colleagues and Lipkus and colleagues, the Numeracy Understanding in Medicine Instrument (NUMi), the Abbreviated Numeracy Scale, and the adaptive Berlin numeracy test. Along with the history of numeracy measures, the advantages and disadvantages of the measures are discussed and suggestions for improving numeracy measurement are given.

Society, physicians, and patients

Chapter 2 by Multmeier, Gaissmaier, and Wegwarth, examines numeracy and society. The authors explain "collective statistical illiteracy," which refers to how society, including journalists, politicians, policy makers, and other professionals, all perpetuate misunderstandings about quantitative health information. While the following two chapters focus more on the individual, this chapter examines the impact of numeracy on a societal level, such as how our understanding of numeric information is shaped by public health messages, media, and advertising.

Changes in clinical medicine, such as increased reliance on evidence-based medicine and collaborative decision making, requires that physicians be able to use and understand numeric information and statistics. However, the statistics used in clinical medicine are becoming more advanced and studies assessing physicians' abilities to use numbers and statistics suggest that their abilities could be improved. Chapter 3 reviews physicians' numeracy and statistical literacy skills and discusses statistical literacy training during medical school. The authors also discuss what could be done to better prepare physicians for the statistical tasks that are relevant to providing the highest quality of care.

In Chapter 4, Zikmund-Fisher, Mayman, and Fagerlin describe how numeracy should help patients have more accurate risk perceptions, help them better use numeric information, and complete numeric tasks needed to manage a disease. They also describe how numeracy ability has been found to be associated with health outcomes, such as frequency of emergency department visits and ability to quit smoking. This chapter focuses on how numeracy is associated with health actions and health outcomes more than previous discussions of patient numeracy.

Applied contexts

Though numeric ability is relevant to an abundance of healthcare situations, two contexts are discussed in depth in this book. Chapter 5, which is on numeracy and diabetes care and management, provides an example of how numeracy has been applied to the care and management of a specific disease in order to improve heath and health outcomes. A considerable amount of work has been done to understand the problems that low numerate patients have with managing diabetes, as well as to develop tools to measure, predict, prevent, and assist diabetic patients. Berkman and Cavanaugh explain how low numeracy has been associated with knowledge about diabetes, self-efficacy for managing diabetes, self-care behaviors, and glycemic control. Current and future research on the impact of numeracy on diabetes care, including the development of tools and interventions, are also reviewed.

The other chapter in this section provides an example of how numeracy challenges must be considered and reconsidered as healthcare evolves. Medical advances bring about new numeracy challenges for patients and physicians. In the case of genetic screening, recent technological advances have increased the amount of numeric information that is available to patients about their screening test results. These advances in technology are only helpful in so far as patients and healthcare providers are able to correctly interpret the test results and appropriately apply the information to their decision making. In Chapter 6, Dukhovny and Wilkins-Haug discuss the numeracy skills that are important to the various types of genetic screening tests and suggest directions for future research in light of the advancements in genetic screening.

Improving healthcare for individuals with low numeracy

The final five chapters focus on helping individuals who have low numeracy skills. In Chapter 7, Garcia-Retamero and Cokely describe how visual aids such as line plots, bar charts, pies, and icon arrays can be used to improve people's ability to use and understand numeric information. Individuals who have low numeracy skills but have high graph literacy (i.e., ability to understand information in graph form) show significant improvements in understanding quantitative information when visual aids are used to communicate numeric information. They further show that visual aids can help to reduce or eliminate number-related biases and heuristics, and that they can be used in behavioral interventions to improve the clarity of information provided.

By addressing problems with communication, misunderstandings about numeric information can be corrected rather than perpetuated. The communication of numeric information takes place on many levels such as from a doctor to a patient, a television advertisement to the public, a government announcement to a patient, and so on. In Chapter 8, Peters discusses the communication barriers of the communicator, the consumer, and system.

Chapter 9 addresses healthcare systems. Paulus and Stewart discuss how the Geisinger healthcare system has been nationally recognized for providing high-quality healthcare at below average costs (www.geisinger.org/about/healthier). The Geisinger system values rigorous data collection through the use of health technology (e.g., electronic health records) in order to implement evidence-based practices and quality improvement. The authors discuss how numeracy research might be incorporated into these quality improvement efforts to improve performance and quality of care.

Another approach is to better understand the theoretical framework that explains how people understand numbers and how that understanding is associated with decision making. In Chapter 10, Reyna and Brust-Renck discuss the strengths and weaknesses of four theoretical frameworks and suggest directions for further theory development. The four approaches are: (1) our perception and distortion of numbers, as well as use of cognitive and neuropsychological data, (2) cognitive effort, memory, and the various ways that information can be organized, (3) examining the performance of two cognitive systems, fast and slow, and (4) how individuals utilize numbers by focusing on the meaning, or gist, of the numeric information.

In Chapter 11 Schwartz challenges whether it is beneficial to provide numeric information to all patients. Using research on numeracy and medical decision making, Schwartz discusses practical and ethical problems with providing numeric information to patients and addresses the challenging but important question about what information to provide patients. He ends the chapter with a discussion about how to study the impact of providing numeric information on the quality of patient decision making, and how these findings would inform the ethical concerns of limited disclosure.

Conclusion

This volume, which is the first to be published on numerical reasoning and decision making in health, examines the numeracy research from the perspectives of society, physicians, and patients. It also discusses the theoretical and methodological aspects of numeracy research, and provides insights and advice from the leading experts on how to improve the problems caused by low numeracy.

This book will be a useful resource for professionals in diverse health-related fields including academics, policy makers, physicians, and other healthcare providers. For example, medical educators and healthcare administrators may find Chapters 2, 3, 4, 9, and 11 useful when developing hospital policies and adapting the healthcare environment to help patients with low numeracy skills. Healthcare providers may especially benefit from reading Chapters 2, 3, 4, 7, 8, and 11 when trying to better understand the impact of low numeracy skills and how they can help patients. Researchers working to apply numeracy research to specific areas of healthcare can utilize Chapters 5 and 6 as models for their work and Chapter 1 to choose a numeracy measure. The book is written for individuals at a wide range of knowledge levels. Those who are not familiar with the concept of numeracy will be provided with an up-to-date overview of numeracy research with Chapters 1–4. Those who are familiar with research on numeracy will enjoy the fresh insights into theory, policy, and approaches to helping low numerate patients that can be found in all chapters, but particularly Chapters 5–11.

Over the past decade there has been growing interest in how individuals' numeric ability impacts healthcare. This is because low numeric ability has been found to be a widespread problem, and because researchers are describing ways in which numeric ability is associated with medical decision making. This book is written for researchers, clinicians, patients, academics, students, health policy makers, and those interested in health disparities. It is aimed at the larger culture of scholarship with regard to the relationships between numerical reasoning and judgments and decisions about health and healthcare. In diverse ways the authors discuss how to improve numerical reasoning in health contexts, and gathering ideas about future research directions are primary goals of this book.

References

Adelsward, V., & Sachs, L. (1996). The meaning of 6.8: Numeracy and normality in health information talks. *Social Science and Medicine*, 43, 1179–1187.

Ancker, J. S., & Kaufman, D. (2007). Rethinking health numeracy: A multidisciplinary literature review. *Journal of the American Medical Informatics Association*, 14, 713–721.

Anderson, B. L., Gigerenzer, G., Parker, S., & Schulkin, J. (2014). Statistical literacy in obstetricians and gynecologists. *Journal for Healthcare Quality*, 36(1), 5–17.

Baron, J. (2000). *Thinking and Deciding*. Cambridge, UK: Cambridge University Press.

Chapman, G. B., & Sonnenberg, F. A. (Eds.). (2003). *Decision Making in Health Care: Theory, Psychology, and Applications*. Cambridge, UK: Cambridge University Press.

Elstein, A. S. (2004). On the origins and development of evidence-based medicine and medical decision making. *Inflammation Research*, 53(2), S184–S189.

Elstein, A. S., Shulman, L. S., Sprafka, S. A., & Allal, L. (1978). *Medical Problem Solving: An Analysis of Clinical Reasoning* (Vol. 2). Cambridge, MA: Harvard University Press.

Flexner, A. (1910). Medical education in the United States and Canada: a report to the Carnegie Foundation for the Advancement of Teaching (No. 4). Carnegie Foundation for the Advancement of Teaching.

Gal, I. (1995). Big picture: What does "numeracy" mean? *GED Items*, 12(4/5). Retrieved from mathforum.org/teachers/adult.ed/articles/gal.html

Geisinger. *Geisinger and Healthcare Reform*, www.geisinger.org/about/healthier/, accessed 4/3/2013.

Gigerenzer, G., & Goldstein, D. G. (1996). Reasoning the fast and frugal way: Models of bounded rationality. *Psychological Review*, 103, 650–669.

Golbeck, A. L., Ahlers-Schmidt, C. R., Paschal, A. M., & Dismuke, S. E. (2005). A definition and operational framework for health numeracy. *American Journal of Preventive Medicine*, 29(4), 375–376.

Hacking, I. (1964). *Logic of Statistical Inference*. Cambridge, UK: Cambridge University Press.

Hacking, I. (1975). *The Emergence of Probability*. Cambridge, UK: Cambridge University Press.

Hacking, I. (1999). *The Taming of Chance*. Cambridge, UK: Cambridge University Press.

Kahneman, D., & Tversky, A. (1979). Prospect Theory: An analysis of decision under risk. *Econometrica*, 47(2), 263–291.

Kirsch, I. S., Jungeblut, A., Jenkins, L., & Kolstad, A. (2002). *Adult Literacy in America: A First Look at the Findings of the National Adult Literacy Survey* (NCES Report No. 1993–275; 3rd edn.). Washington, DC: US Department of Education, National Center for Education Statistics.

Kutner, M., Greenberg, E., Jin, Y., & Paulsen, C. (2006). *The Health Literacy of America's Adults: Results from the 2003 National Assessment of Adult Literacy* (NCES Report No. 2006–483). Washington, DC: Government Printing Office.

Lipkus, I. M., Samsa, G., & Rimer, B. K. (2001). General performance on a numeracy scale among highly educated samples. *Medical Decision Making*, 21, 37–44.

Montori, V. M., & Rothman, R. L. (2005). Weakness in numbers: The challenge of numeracy in health care. *Journal of General Internal Medicine*, 20(11), 1071–1072.

Rao, G., & Kanter, S. L. (2010). Physician numeracy as the basis for an evidence-based medicine curriculum. *Academic Medicine*, 85(11), 1794–1799.

Reyna, V. F., Nelson, W., Han, P., & Dieckmann, N. F. (2009). How numeracy influences risk comprehension and medical decision making. *Psychological Bulletin*, 135, 943–973.

Schwartz, L. M., Woloshin, S., Black, W. C., & Welch, H. G. (1997). The role of numeracy in understanding the benefit of screening mammography. *Annals of Internal Medicine*, 127(11), 966–972.

Simon, H. A. (1955). A behavioral model of rational choice. *The Quarterly Journal of Economics*, 69(1), 99–118.

Simon, H. A. (1978). Rationality as process and as product of thought. *The American Economic Review: Papers and Proceedings*, 68, 1–16.

1 Measuring numeracy

Edward T. Cokely, Saima Ghazal, &
Rocio Garcia-Retamero

Introduction

A century ago, the science fiction writer H. G. Wells predicted that statistical thinking would one day be as necessary for efficient citizenship as the ability to read and write. This day has come. Modern societies make sense of our world with information about risks and benefits presented in probabilities, percentages, and other ratio-type data. This information is then used to inform decision making by professionals, policy makers, and the public across a wide range of topics (e.g., medical, health, financial, environmental, political, legal, etc.). As can be seen in many of the chapters of this handbook, despite decades of steady progress, many questions about numeracy and decision making remain. Among the most fundamental questions are those concerning the *measurement of numeracy* and its implications. What *is* numeracy and how do we know? How can we be sure that our numeracy tests are reliable, valid, and unbiased? What types of tests are available and what do various test scores actually *mean*? These are the questions addressed in this chapter.

Numeracy in context

Researchers and philosophers have found it difficult to agree on an exact and uncontroversial theoretical definition of mathematics – which is ironic for a field otherwise characterized by its emphasis on elegance and precision. Thankfully, quantitative skills are easier to operationalize and measure, and there is a long history of research aimed at understanding and assessing the causes and consequences of *numeracy* (Huff & Geis, 1954; Paulos, 1988), including extensive longitudinal studies conducted in large adult and student samples such as the National Assessment of Adult Literacy

This review was supported in part by grants from the National Science Foundation (SES–1253263) and The Spanish Ministry of Economy (PSI2008–02019 and PSI2011–22954).

(NAAL; Kutner et al., 2006) and the Programme for International Student Assessment (www.oecd.org/pisa). Researchers and educators do widely agree that the term "numeracy" is not necessarily synonymous with pure mathematical skill but instead refers to mathematical or quantitative literacy (Steen, 1990; see also Reyna et al., 2009). Similar educational trends focusing on "mathematics in context" can also be seen in major national initiatives like the *Common Core State Standards Initiatives.* Specifically, the construct "numeracy" is said to reflect the "array of mathematically related proficiencies that are evident in adults' lives… including a connection to context, purpose, or use… for active participation in the democratic process and… in the global economy" (Ginsburg et al., 2006). At the more basic levels, numeracy is said to involve the "real number line, time, measurement, and estimation" whereas higher levels focus on an "understanding of ratio concepts, notably fractions, proportions, percentages, and probabilities" (Reyna et al., 2009). These and other conceptual distinctions have been subject to change over time with advances in knowledge and with shifts in lifestyles, technology, and educational practices. Although there are *many* carefully articulated models and frameworks, there is as yet no single unifying theory systematically linking numeracy, mathematics, and cognition.

Efforts to understand and measure individual differences in numeracy come primarily via performance tests, although there have been some notable recent advances involving the use of subjective instruments. For example, one reliable and validated subjective assessment of numeracy that has been applied in health and medical domains asks participants eight subjective questions in which they estimate their personal levels of numeracy (e.g., "How good are you at working with fractions?," Fagerlin et al., 2007; Zikmund-Fisher et al., 2007; and for subjective graph literacy see Garcia-Retamero, Cokely, & Ghazal, unpublished data). Several studies have reported moderate-to-high correlations between objective and subjective measures (Fagerlin et al., 2007; Zikmund-Fisher et al., 2007; Liberali et al., 2011; Weller et al., 2013); however, other recent studies such as the one conducted by Liberali et al. (2011) have found that objective and subjective numeracy scales can load on separate factors. Research also shows that people can be highly overconfident in reporting their subjective numerical ability. For example, Sheridan et al. (2003) showed that 70% of subjects reported that they consider themselves to be "good with numbers," while only 2% of those respondents answered the three Schwartz et al. (1997) questions correctly. This is not to say that these subjective instruments should be avoided. Just the opposite, they can be quite useful so long as researchers are aware of the appropriate range of uses as well as their limitations (e.g., subjective numeracy tests are well-suited for rapid, rough assessment including among people who have some math anxiety). The same can also be said for the objective performance measures of numeracy, which are the focus of this review – i.e., psychometric numeracy performance tests (Schwartz et al., 1997; Lipkus et al., 2001; Peters et al., 2006; Reyna et al., 2009; Galesic & Garcia-Retamero, 2010; Cokely et al., 2012; Schapira et al., 2012; Weller et al., 2013).

In what follows, we review the recent history numeracy assessment, with emphasis on available research instruments and their implications. The review is designed to provide a representative and relatively comprehensive (but not quite exhaustive) picture of the state-of-the-science, including a map for researchers who are interested in using numeracy assessments in their research. We start with a review of the evolution of popular numeracy research instruments used in medical decision making research. We illustrate differences in measurement approaches along with the costs and benefits of using different scales (e.g., Classical Testing, IRT (item response theory) and Rasch, Adaptive Testing and Hybrid Models), and provide details on key properties of various measurement instruments (e.g., difficulty levels, time required, skills assessed, sensitivity, reliability, validity) (for a computerized test recommendation system see www.RiskLiteracy.org). We close by briefly considering some frontiers, open questions, and emerging applications.

Approaches to measuring numeracy

Classical testing theory

Beyond the previously discussed national and international literacy assessments, and outside of quantitative skills tests in standardized intelligence assessments (e.g., Woodcock Johnson Test of Cognitive Abilities), the longest standing and most widely used assessments of numeracy come from a *classical testing theory* tradition (Novick, 1966). This robust approach requires relatively few theoretical assumptions about a test taker's ability or the implications of a test, instead focusing largely on one's relative standing. The essential theoretical assumption is simply that each individual has a "true" test score that can be inferred from the assessed score, which is the true score plus error. This has led the approach to focus extensively on issues related to test *reliability* (e.g., test–retest reliability: how much do test scores vary when the test is given across different locations, times, and samples). In theory, the emphasis on improving test reliability is a means of eliminating variance owing to error and thus improving the test's ability to assess one's "true" score. In practice, development of instruments tends to focus on accuracy of response rates of groups of participants across various items (i.e., test-wise accuracy) along with the internal consistency of those response rates (e.g., split-half reliability; Cronbach's alpha). To provide concrete examples of standard practices we turn to the influential work of Schwartz et al. (1997) and Lipkus et al. (2001).

In 1997, Schwartz and colleagues conducted a seminal randomized cross-sectional numeracy study investigating the relations between numeracy and relative risk perceptions. Five hundred women were initially mailed the study stimuli and asked to participate. Respondents included 287 mostly older adult women (mean age 68 years) who were veterans with modest incomes (e.g., less than $25 000 per year). The majority of participants had also completed high school (96%) and about a third had completed at least some college. Numeracy was assessed with three items that were similar to items used in the NAAL survey (see previous section). Once scored, these items were used to predict the women's understanding of data presented in one of four formats (e.g., relative risk reduction versus absolute risk reduction with baseline). Specifically, the women were asked to interpret the material provided and to report on the risks/benefits of mammography screening (e.g., "Imagine 1000 women exactly like you. Of these women what is your best guess about how many will die from breast cancer during the next 10 years if they are not screened every year for breast cancer?"). Results indicated that about half of the women (i.e., 54%) accurately answered two questions, while only 20% accurately answered all three (i.e., most could not convert 1 in 1000 to 0.1). As expected, results further revealed a moderate positive correlation between participants' final score and their relative risk reduction interpretations, indicating that the brief assessment had some criterion validity providing a basis for further refinement via standard practices in classical test theory.

In 2001, Lipkus et al. (2001) published the numeracy test for highly educated samples, as an extension of previous work by Schwartz et al. (1997). Lipkus et al. (2001) conducted a series of four studies (N = 463) on community samples of well-educated adult participants (at least 40 years of age) in North Carolina. Among other tasks, all participants answered 11 total numeracy questions including the three numeracy questions taken from Schwartz et al. (1997). A factor analysis showed that a one factor solution was appropriate, suggesting that the refined test by Lipkus et al. (2001) was a reliable and internally consistent measure of high school and college educated individuals' statistical numeracy, as is required by classical testing theory.

The results from Schwartz et al. (1997) and the Lipkus et al. (2001) tests were interesting for a number of reasons. First, the results provided additional evidence that even among educated US community samples some sizable proportion of individuals were likely to be statistically innumerate (e.g., 20% failed questions dealing with risk magnitude). Such findings were and continue to be important as many efforts designed to support informed and shared decision making rest on an erroneous assumption that decision makers are numerate (or at least sufficiently statistically numerate; see also Guadagnoli & Ward, 1998). Second, results indicated that domain framing (e.g., medical, financial, or abstract gambles) did not necessarily differentially affect test performance or comprehension. This finding indicates that various domain specific items (e.g., items framed in terms of financial or medical or gambling risks) can provide a reasonable basis for the assessment of general numeracy skills that will have predictive power across diverse domains, in the absence of domain-specific expertise.

Despite their many successes and their influential role in advancing research across the allied decision sciences, as anticipated by Lipkus et al. (2001), a growing body of data suggests some ways the current numeracy instruments need to be improved (for an item response theory based analysis see Schapira et al., 2009; see also Cokely et al., 2012; Weller et al., 2013; Schapira et al., 2012 in the next section). For example, one major concern is that the Lipkus et al. test is not hard enough to adequately differentiate among the higher-performing, highly educated individuals who are often studied (e.g., convenience samples from universities). To illustrate, in one study of college students at the Florida State University, data indicated that although the Lipkus et al. (2001) test was a significant predictor of risky decisions it showed extensive negative skew with scores approaching the measurement ceiling (e.g., most participants answered more than 80% of items correctly; Cokely & Kelley, 2009; for similar results see Peters et al., 2006, 2007b, 2008; Schapira et al., 2009; and for similar patterns from physicians-in-training see Hanoch et al., 2010). Another recent study using large probabilistically representative samples of the whole populations of two countries (i.e., the USA and Germany) revealed negative skew in numeracy scores even among participants from the general population (Galesic & Garcia-Retamero, 2010). Although most people are not college educated, most people in these two countries are likely to get the majority of questions right (please note however that roughly 25% of people are likely to get very few items correct, suggesting that a large proportion of the population is essentially innumerate and lacks any basic risk literacy). These data suggest that most individuals tend to produce distributions of scores that are negatively skewed and are subject to measurement ceiling effects. Although more recent classical testing theory based research has managed to address some of these concerns by adding four more complex numerical items to improve the distributional properties of the scale (Peters et al., 2007b), subsequent work indicates the distributional improvement is limited. Specifically, Weller et al. (2013) observed highly skewed distributional values for the Lipkus et al. (2001) 11 item measure (median = 9) along with moderate skew in the Peters et al. (2007a) extended 15 items measure (median = 11), indicating a need for better discriminability among average to more highly numerate individuals.

A second psychometric concern is that there is relatively little known about the relations between either the Lipkus et al. (2001) or Schwartz et al. (1997) numeracy test and other individual differences, such as basic cognitive abilities (Liberali et al., 2011). To illustrate, one might argue that statistical numeracy is a useful predictor of risky choice simply because it is correlated with measures of fluid intelligence. It is well known that tests of general intelligence, including those designed to measure fluid intelligence, are valid and reliable predictors of a wide variety of socially desirable cognitive, behavioral, occupational, and health-related outcomes (note that the underlying cognitive mechanisms that give rise to these effects are debated and remain unclear; Neisser et al., 1996; see also Cokely et al., 2006; Ericsson et al., 2007; Fox et al., 2009). Fluid intelligence tests such as Raven's Standard or Advanced Progressive Matrices tend to be more time consuming yet also confer considerable benefits in terms of psychometric rigor and cross-cultural fairness (Raven, 2000). To date, however, there are few tests that have investigated the extent to which the Lipkus et al. (2001) or Schwartz et al. (1997) instruments, or other second generation instruments like the NUMi (Schapira et al., 2012) or Weller et al. (2013) instrument, provide unique predictive power beyond other cognitive ability instruments either within or across cultures (but see Cokely et al., 2012; Cokely & Kelley, 2009; Galesic & Garcia-Retamero, 2010; Garcia-Retamero & Galesic, 2010a, 2010b; Liberali et al., 2011; Okan et al., 2013).

A third psychometric issue is that even if numeracy is compared with other abilities the observed measurement skew and ceiling effects will complicate comparative evaluations (e.g., intelligence versus statistical numeracy). Consider a recent study designed to investigate the extent to which each of several individual differences (e.g., executive functioning, cognitive impulsivity, and numeracy) influenced decision-making competence (Del Missier et al., 2012; but see also Del Missier et al., 2010). The study found that numeracy was less related to some decision-making competencies as compared to measures of executive functioning or cognitive impulsivity, measured by the cognitive reflection test (Frederick, 2005). It is however possible that, at least in part, some measurement ceiling effects in numeracy scores among the college student sample could have limited differentiation of those individuals with the highest levels of numeracy. In contrast, both executive functioning and the cognitive reflection tests are known to provide discrimination among highly educated individuals (i.e., high measurement sensitivity). To be clear, our reading of the individual differences study by Del Missier et al. (2012) is that it represents precise and sophisticated research using many of the best available methods and tools. However, the potential psychometric limits inherent in the now decade old Schwartz et al. (1997) and Lipkus et al. (2001) numeracy tests leave open important questions. To the extent that a numeracy instrument does not adequately or accurately estimate variation in the subpopulations of interest it is not an efficient basis for theory development or policy evaluations.

Item response theory and Rasch approaches to numeracy assessment

In contrast to classical testing theory, item response theory (IRT) requires considerably more complex modeling of probabilistic distributions over test taker's responses to specific items. The focus of test development is on the item rather than on the pooled responses to items as in classical testing theory (e.g., an item-level versus test-level analysis). A full description of the theory is beyond the scope of this chapter (see Lord, 1980; Van der Linden & Hambleton, 1997), nevertheless, it is valuable to note that the increased performance of IRT tests comes as a result of additional assumptions plus sophisticated response modeling (e.g., the item response function). Two of the key assumptions are that each item is measuring some unidimensional trait and that there is local independence of test items. Local independence roughly means that two items are assumed to be related only by the shared variance owed to the underlying trait that is being assessed. Accordingly, IRT test models improve predictive performance by eliminating item redundancy with estimated parameters such as item difficulty (e.g., how hard is any particular item for a given trait level), discrimination (e.g., how sharply and consistently does an item distinguish individuals at higher versus lower trait levels), and a guessing parameter (e.g., true/false items will be guessed correctly 50% of the time). The IRT family of approaches includes many variants such as the Rasch approaches, which can be seen as specific instantiations of IRT models that limit parameters and/or make use of alternative scaling.

The Numeracy Understanding in Medicine Instrument

The Numeracy Understanding in Medicine Instrument (NUMi) is the most comprehensive assessment of health numeracy designed for use with participants who have low levels of numeracy, such as inner-city and other underrepresented and minority individuals (Schapira et al., 2012). The pioneering work by Schapira and colleagues used a two parameter IRT analysis to design a test of health numeracy, defined as: "The ability to understand and apply information conveyed with numbers, tables, and graphs, probability and statistics to effectively communicate with health-care providers, take care of one's health, and participate in medical decisions." In the test development phase, Schapira et al. collected data on 110 different numeracy questions covering a wide range of health numeracy content drawn from four theoretically grounded categories of skill including (1) assessment of general number sense, (2) ability to understand tables and graphs, (3) understanding of probability, and (4) understanding of statistics. Schapira and colleagues began by testing 1000 participants in phase one of a multi-phase development study. All participants were English-speaking adults (21 years of age or older; 56% women; 29% Hispanic; 44% Black) drawn from community and clinical samples in Milwaukee and Chicago, and were tested in groups. Data collection included demographic information, a health literacy reading comprehension test (S-TOFHLA – Test of Functional Health Literacy in Adults) and an intelligence test (the Wonderlic). Following this phase, the two parameter IRT based scale was created including 20 items (5 from each theoretical category) optimized for discrimination (>0.80) and difficulty, and re-examined for content validity by subject matter experts. A random subset of 20% of the original participant sample was called back for further test validation assessment, in which the new 20 item "NUMi" test was further compared with an arithmetic test (WRAT-A), the Lipkus et al. (2001) test, and a medical data interpretation test (see Schapira et al., 2012 for details and references).

Schapira et al.'s (2012) results revealed many desirable psychometric properties including very high internal consistency coefficients (i.e., reliability) and considerable evidence of convergent validity when compared to other health literacy and numeracy instruments. For example, the NUMi test showed relatively high Pearson correlation coefficients across all benchmark tests including the Wonderlic intelligence test ($r = 0.82$), the health literacy reading comprehension test ($r = 0.43$), the Lipkus et al. test ($r = 0.69$), the medical data interpretation test ($r = 0.75$), and the arithmetic test ($r = 0.73$). Confirmatory dimensionality assessment further indicated that all 20 items were unidimensional (i.e., all items assessed a single underlying ability trait). Non-parametric estimates of sub-sample test-bias (e.g., race/ethnicity, education) showed that although there were significant between group differences, a series of 2-step DIF analyses failed to detect bias in any of the 20 single items. Although IRT based analyses can produce scoring matrices in which different items have different weights, additional analyses of the NUMi indicated that the NUMi items could be scored using a simple tally method.

Beyond the many strengths and benefits of the NUMi, as with any test, there are a number of limits and boundary conditions that should be considered before selecting this test for use in research. As Schapira and colleagues (2012) note, the test is most suitable and has maximum measurement sensitivity for individuals who are considerably below average in their level of numeracy. This likely follows from the fact that the test was normed on a sample of individuals with below average levels of intelligence, including a high proportion of people without additional education beyond high school. One potential benefit is that this suggests the test may be ideally suited for assessment of the large portion of the population who are most likely to be at risk of misunderstanding numerical information. However, this means the test is best suited to measure the same range of abilities that are captured by the Lipkus et al. (2001) and the Schwartz et al. (1997) tests. Yet because the Schapira et al. (2012) test involves 20 items, it will take longer (ca. 8–12 minutes estimated) to complete as compared to using the Lipkus et al. (2001; ca. 5 minutes) or the Schwartz et al. (1997; ca. 2 minutes) test. These results also mean the NUMi is not likely suitable for assessment of numeracy among average-to-highly educated individuals.

Schapira et al.'s (2012) test validation study provided considerable evidence of convergent validity (i.e., correlated with other instruments known to predict decision making) but more research is still needed to provide evidence of unique predictive validity beyond other numeracy tests. The NUMi is a more sophisticated and psychometrically sound instrument (e.g., bias-free); however, more testing is needed to determine whether the NUMi provides better, unique predictive power when compared to extant and commonly used, faster instruments like the Schwartz et al. (1997) test. A central requirement for any assessment is to demonstrate that it can predict the behavior of interest better than other tests. Absent evidence of improved predictive validity, or some other justifiable benefits (e.g., faster, more reliable, less bias), the new testing technology cannot be said to be an improvement on the former testing technology (Messick, 1995).

It is theoretically interesting that although the NUMi test provides a higher-fidelity theoretically grounded assessment of the four key numeracy components, the dimensionality analysis suggests that the NUMi assesses a unidimensional skill construct. To the extent this is true across the full range of skill (including those who are more highly risk literate that have been studied), then it is not necessary to assess all four categories of content when measuring numeracy so long as there are sufficient items from one category to provide the desired discrimination and difficulty level. This is an important theoretical point that may also clear the path to a more simplified measure. It may also help explain why the previous instruments from Lipkus et al. (2001) and Schwartz et al. (1997) have been so successful despite the fact that they primarily test people's understanding of probability and ratio concepts. Of note, however, there is some evidence of a dissociation between skills at higher levels of abilities. For example, see the chapter by Garcia-Retamero and Cokely for work showing that graph literacy and numeracy dissociate with important consequences (e.g., people with low numeracy can understand graphs but not equivalent presentations in numbers, and thus visual aids often improve risk literacy among vulnerable subpopulations like older adults or non-native speakers; Garcia-Retamero & Cokely, 2011, 2013, in press).

The Abbreviated Numeracy Scale

Another second generation test in the IRT tradition uses a one parameter Rasch approach and builds on several classical testing theory based instruments including those by Lipkus et al. (2001) and Peters et al. (2007a). Specifically, Weller and colleagues (2013) sought to address the potential redundancy of numeracy items used across various tests by combining these instruments while also refining psychometric sensitivity (e.g., creating a new composite test). Test development involved an iterative series of three studies. Study one included 1970 participants (45% women) that was reasonably representative of US residents in terms of educational attainment, and also included a wide range of adult age groups (e.g., aged 18–89; median age = 48; 3% did not complete high school; 39% had completed a college degree). Weller and colleagues had participants complete the Lipkus et al. test (including the three Schwartz et al. items) and the Peters et al. (2007a) instrument and then included the Cognitive Reflection Test (a math test often used as an assessment of cognitive impulsivity; Frederick, 2005). Confirmatory factor analysis indicated that all test items were fit equally well by either a one or two factor model, although the two factor model categorized numeracy items and cognitive reflection items as separate factors. In the interest of parsimony, a one factor model was adopted and the Rasch analysis generated a refined scale including a total of eight items. Ultimately, Weller et al. developed an abbreviated scale, which included five Lipkus items, two cognitive reflection items, and one from Peters et al. (2007a). Study 1 also provided evidence of convergent validity showing the expected correlations between education level and numeracy scores, and between numeracy score and subjective numeracy score (i.e., one's reported judgment about their own numeracy, Fagerlin et al., 2007).

In Study 2, Weller and colleagues (2013) assessed predictive validity of the new abbreviated scale as compared to two of its subcomponent scales (the cognitive reflection test and the Lipkus et al., 2001 test). Participants (N = 899) completed all numeracy instruments and made a series of judgments and decisions to assess the association between the various numeracy tests and (1) susceptibility to framing, (2) estimating bet attractiveness, and (3) a ratio bias task. All numeracy scales showed small to moderate predictive performance. Comparative analyses of the abbreviated scale with each component scale showed that the abbreviated scale was similar to component scales in most conditions, tending to demonstrate numerically if not significantly larger coefficients. However, the discriminability of the abbreviated scale was clearly superior (wider range of performance estimates). Similar results were found in Study 3 in which 165 participants' risk perceptions (e.g., risk of terrorist attacks, risk of salmon extinction) were assessed with the abbreviated scale or with either subcomponent scale (i.e., numeracy by Lipkus et al., 2001 and cognitive reflection by Frederick, 2005). Study 3 results showed a clear numeric advantage for the abbreviated test, which on average accounted for about 75% or more additional variance (i.e., ranging from about 50% to 400%).

In summary, the abbreviated scale offers a number of psychometric advantages as compared to previous numeracy tests. It provides similar or stronger predictive power when compared to the Lipkus et al. (2001) test alone, and reliability coefficients also increase. It also possesses far superior sensitivity and discriminability, particularly among higher scoring individuals, as compared to the Lipkus et al. test. The test was tuned based on samples that are relatively representative of much of the US population with respect to education, and it also included participants from a wide range of ages. These factors help explain how the abbreviated score is able to overcome the dramatic skew observed in representative sample scores on the Lipkus et al. test. Results also suggest the test is potentially well suited for use with general population and community samples. Nevertheless, as with all tests, there are also limits, bounds, and unknowns.

Although the abbreviated test is treated as if it assesses some unidimensional ability, Weller et al.'s data raise some concerns that the cognitive reflection items may be measuring a separate factor. Similarly, in studies with college educated individuals, Liberali et al. (2011) showed that the cognitive reflection test items loaded on a factor that was different from that of the Lipkus et al. (2001) test (see also Cokely et al., 2012). Theoretically, this would follow because the cognitive reflection test involves math problems that are not probabilistic in nature but rather have an intuitively appealing but inaccurate answer providing an assessment of cognitive impulsivity (Cokely et al., 2012; Cokely et al., 2009; Frederick, 2005). More research is needed to assess whether the improved distribution properties of the test reflect two different abilities rather than assessing a wider range of numeracy. There is also a need for more research to document the extent to which the abbreviated test offers improved and unique predictive power beyond other common cognitive ability measures, including general intelligence and working memory. In short, the currently available studies show at least some evidence that the abbreviated test offers modest increases in unique predictive power along with improved sensitivity among populations with wide ranges of educational attainment.

An adaptive testing approach

The Berlin Numeracy Test

Building on the work of Lipkus et al. (2001) and Schwartz et al. (1997), with support from many colleagues around the world, we have developed an adaptive numeracy test designed to predict levels of risk literacy in educated samples of adults living in industrialized countries (Cokely et al., 2012). We define risk literacy as "the ability to make good decisions based on information about risk." Our goal was not to develop a high-fidelity comprehensive test of numeracy or of its subskills. Rather, the goal was to develop a brief, valid, and easy-to-use instrument, with improved discriminability and improved predictive power. We employed a test development procedure that is similar to IRT processes but uses a decision tree algorithm (categorization tree) rather than IRT scaling procedures to identify items with optimal discriminability across the range of difficulty (with a guessing parameter of zero). Specifically, in an adaptive computerized test, questions are selected based on participants' past success in answering previous questions (see Figure 1.1 for test structure). For the Berlin Numeracy Test, the adaptive structure means that all questions have about a 50% probability of being answered correctly by moderate to highly educated participants (e.g., computer literate adults, college students, or physicians). If an answer is correct/incorrect then a harder/easier question is automatically provided. A participant's skill level can then be determined from answers to 2–3 questions in roughly half the time normally required for the Lipkus et al. (2001) numeracy test (less than 3 minutes; see Table 1.2).

The development of the Berlin Numeracy Test began with pre-testing on a pool of items including all items from both the Lipkus et al. (2001) and Schwartz et al. (1997) tests along with other items that were internally generated. Following a protocol analysis in which participants solved all numeracy problems while thinking aloud (Barton et al., 2009; see also Fox et al., 2011), we analyzed responses and retained 28 candidate questions for inclusion in the next stage of test development (i.e., 12 original items plus 16 new items). Initial testing involved 300 participants in a community sample from Berlin, Germany (57% women). Participants were primarily current or former undergraduate or graduate students from the Humboldt, Free, and Technical Universities of Berlin. Each participant completed about 6 hours of testing over the course of 2 to 3 weeks in exchange for

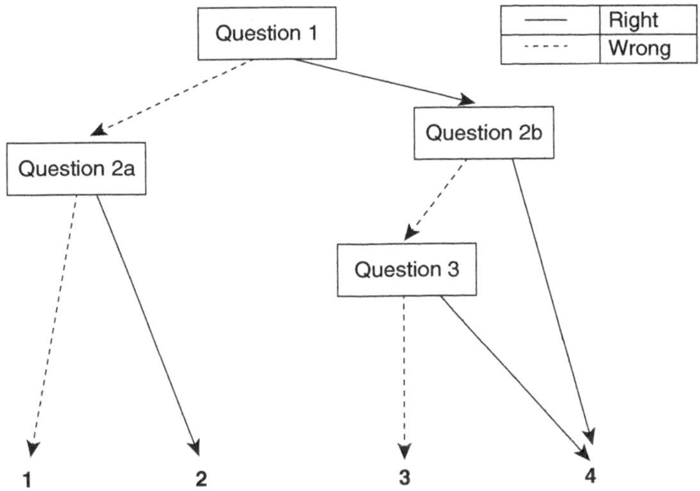

Figure 1.1. The structure of the Computer Adaptive Berlin Test. Each question has a 50% probably of being right/wrong. If a question is answered right/wrong a harder/easier question is provided that again has a 50% probability of being right/wrong.

40 euros (ca. $55). Comparative instruments and psychometrics tests used for test development are listed and described in Table 1.1.

Test construction and test items

Performance quartiles for all participants were assessed according to performance on all 28 candidate statistical numeracy questions (i.e., 12 questions from Lipkus et al., 2001 and 16 new questions). A subset of five questions with a 4-level tree structure was identified using the categorization tree application from the predictive modeling and forecasting software DTREG (Sherrod, 2003). The tree structure was constructed such that participants arriving at each branch of the tree had approximately a 50% probably of answering correctly/incorrectly. The test's tree structure was subjected to cross-validation and showed less than 10% misclassification. Subsequent analyses indicated that reducing the 4-level solution to a simpler 3-level solution (i.e., removing one problem) did not affect test classification performance or validity yet reduced test-taking time (i.e., 10% reduction), increased test format flexibility (i.e., simplified paper and pencil format scoring), and provided improved discriminability among new samples (see "cross-cultural comparisons" below). All final Berlin Numeracy Test formats are based on the four questions used for the optimal 3-level categorization tree as follows (answers provided in each blank):

Table 1.1. *Descriptions and references for tests used to establish psychometric validity.*

Measure	Description	Reference
Fluid Intelligence (RAPM)	Short form Raven's Advanced Progressive Matrices – a 12 item test of fluid intelligence.	Bors and Stokes (1998)
Cognitive Reflection (CRT)	The Cognitive Reflection Test uses three math questions to assess cognitive impulsivity.	Frederick (2005)
Crystallized Intelligence (Vocabulary)	A 37 item "spot-a-word" German vocabulary test.	Lindenberger et al. (1993)
Working Memory Capacity (Span)	A multi-item performance measure of one's ability to control attention when simultaneously solving math operations and remember words.	Turner and Engle (1989)
Understanding everyday risks	A five item battery involving interpretation of information about risks in consumer products, medical treatments, and weather forecasts.	Garcia-Retamero and Galesic (2013)
Maximizing-Satisficing	A 13 item scale measuring one's tendency to maximize vs. satisfice during decision making.	Schwartz et al. (2002)
Persistence	The Grit-S is an eight item brief measure designed to assess persistence in the face of adversity.	Duckworth and Quinn (2009)
Achievement Motivation	The AMS-R is a 10 item trait assessment of one's general achievement motivation (e.g., one's desire to achieve good grades or performance evaluations).	Lang and Fries (2006)
Self-efficacy	A10 item self-report measure of one's general sense of self efficacy.	Schwarzer and Jerusalem (1995)
Personality	A 10 item assessment of the Big Five personality traits.	Gosling et al. (2003)
Test Anxiety	The TAI-G is a 20 item assessment of test-taking anxiety.	Hodapp and Benson (1997)
Implicit theories	A four item measurement of the extent to which one believes intelligence is stable vs. changeable.	Blackwell et al. (2007)
Satisfaction with life	A five item instrument measuring self-reported levels of one's satisfaction with life.	Diener et al. (1985)

1. Out of 1000 people in a small town 500 are members of a choir. Out of these 500 members in the choir 100 are men. Out of the 500 inhabitants that are not in the choir 300 are men. What is the probability that a randomly drawn man is a member of the choir? Please indicate the probability in percent. ___25%___
2a. Imagine we are throwing a five-sided die 50 times. On average, out of these 50 throws how many times would this five-sided die show an odd number (1, 3 or 5)? __30__ out of 50 throws.
2b. Imagine we are throwing a loaded die (6 sides). The probability that the die shows a 6 is twice as high as the probability of each of the other numbers. On average, out of these 70 throws how many times would the die show the number 6? ___20___out of 70 throws
3. In a forest 20% of mushrooms are red, 50% brown and 30% white. A red mushroom is poisonous with a probability of 20%. A mushroom that is not red is poisonous with a probability of 5%. What is the probability that a poisonous mushroom in the forest is red? ___50%___

Because different research environments have different constraints such as computer-access, group-testing options, data-security requirements, etc., we designed the Berlin Numeracy Test to have multiple formats, including multiple choice, paper and pencil, median split, and computer adaptive formats. Some formats are also designed for use with the Schwartz et al. (1997) instrument, providing a wider range of skill assessment at the lower levels of numeracy. For instructions on scoring and specific recommendations about test format selection please see Cokely et al. (2012) or www.RiskLiteracy.org.

In our educated community sample, scores on the Lipkus et al. (2001) numeracy scale showed dramatic negative skew (Table 1.2). Although possible scores range from 0 to 11, the lowest observed score was 5 (45% correct). Both the mean and median were close to the measurement ceiling (i.e., 88% and 91% correct, respectively). Similar levels of skew were observed for the Schwartz et al. (1997) test. In contrast, scores on the Berlin Numeracy Test were distributed evenly across the whole range of possible scores regardless of format. Estimates of internal consistency for the Berlin Numeracy Test showed some modest improvement over other existing numeracy tests, but were not as high as either the NUMi or the abbreviated instrument, which is a consequence of having very few items. A principal axis factor analysis of the four items from the Berlin Numeracy Test indicated that all items loaded highly on a single factor explaining 45% of the observed variance. An additional study at Michigan Technological University found that when the test was taken two different times, roughly 1 week apart, it showed high levels of test–retest reliability, $r(11) = 0.91$, $p = 0.001$.

Table 1.2. *Psychometric properties of the scale: basic attributes, reliability, and discriminability.*

			Berlin Numeracy Test		
	Schwartz et al. (1997), 3 items	Lipkus et al. (2001), 11 items	Computer Adaptive Test Format, 2–4 items	Paper and Pencil Format, 4 items	Single Item Format
Basic attributes					
Range of possible scores	0–3	0–11	1–4	0–4	0–1
Range of achieved scores	0–3	5–11	1–4	0–4	0–1
Average score					
Mean	2.4	9.7	2.6	1.6	0.52
Median	3	10	3	2	1
Standard deviation	0.82	1.38	1.13	1.21	0.50
Length					
Number of items	3	11	2–3	4	1
Mean duration in minutes	1.2	4.5	2.6	4.3	1.1
Reliability					
Cronbach's alpha	0.52	0.54	–[a]	0.59	–[a]
Discriminability					
Item % correct (mean)	0.82	0.89	–[b]	0.41	0.52
Mean score of					
1st quartile	0.8	7.3	1.0	0.0	
2nd quartile	2.0	9.0	2.0	1.0	0.0
3rd quartile	3.0	10.0	3.0	2.0	
4th quartile	3.0	11.0	4.0	3.3	1.0

[a] Cronbach's alpha cannot be computed. Principal component analysis indicates that the four items used in Berlin Numeracy Test all loaded highly on a single factor explaining 45% of variance.

[b] Approximately 50%, conditional on previous responses.

Reproduced from Cokely et al., 2012.

Results of the initial study demonstrated that the Berlin Numeracy Test correlated strongly with other numeracy tests and with measures of cognitive ability (i.e., convergent validity) yet did not correlate with essentially unrelated constructs, such as motivation, personality, beliefs, or attitudes (i.e., discriminant validity) (see Table 1.3). One of the intended purposes of the Berlin Numeracy Test is predicting people's understanding of information about risk in consumer, medical, and everyday contexts – i.e., predicting risk literacy (criterion validity). To investigate the predictive validity of the Berlin Numeracy Test, we

Table 1.3. *Psychometric properties of tests: Convergent and discriminant validity (reproduced from Cokely et al., 2012).*

			Berlin Numeracy Test		
	Schwartz et al. (1997), 3 items	Lipkus et al. (2001), 11 items	Computer Adaptive Test Format	Paper and Pencil Format	Single Item Format
Convergent Validity					
Numeracy Tests					
Lipkus et al., 11 items	0.75**				
Berlin Numeracy Test Computer Adaptive	0.45**	0.49**			
Berlin Numeracy Test Paper and Pencil	0.50**	0.50**	0.91**		
Berlin Numeracy Test Single Item	0.39**	0.42**	0.90**	0.75**	
Cognitive Abilities/Styles					
Raven's Adv. Matrices	0.41**	0.37**	0.48**	0.53**	0.41**
Cognitive Reflection Test	0.40**	0.41**	0.51**	0.56**	0.41**
Vocabulary Spot-a-word	0.25**	0.21**	0.24**	0.25**	0.22**
Working Memory Span	0.14*	0.11	0.21**	0.20**	0.16**
Discriminant Validity					
Motivation Measures					
Maximizing-Satisficing	0.01	0.04	0.05	0.04	0.05
Persistence (Grit-S)	0.02	0.03	−0.05	−0.07	−0.03
Achievement Motivation	−0.08	−0.10	−0.02	0.00	−0.01
Self-efficacy	0.00	−0.01	−0.01	0.02	0.03

Table 1.3. (*cont.*)

	Schwartz et al. (1997), 3 items	Lipkus et al. (2001), 11 items	Berlin Numeracy Test: Computer Adaptive Test Format	Berlin Numeracy Test: Paper and Pencil Format	Berlin Numeracy Test: Single Item Format
Personality Traits					
Emotional Stability	–0.10	–0.05	0.01	0.05	–0.02
Conscientiousness	–0.09	–0.04	–0.09	–0.08	–0.06
Agreeableness	–0.03	–0.07	–0.14*	–0.08	–0.17**
Extraversion	–0.07	–0.06	–0.05	–0.05	–0.06
Openness to experience	–0.14*	–0.16**	–0.18**	–0.14*	–0.16**
Other measures					
Test Anxiety	–0.15*	–0.16*	–0.12	–0.16*	–0.09
Implicit Theories	–0.15*	–0.13**	–0.07	–0.10*	–0.04
Satisfaction with Life	0.14*	0.08	0.12	0.16	0.07

**p*=0.05; ***p*<0.01

administered a short battery of items dealing with information about everyday risks related to common consumer, health, and medical choices (e.g., evaluating the efficacy of toothpastes and cancer screenings), as well as information about probabilities typically used in weather forecasts (Garcia-Retamero & Galesic, 2013; see that book's appendix for examples). Table 1.4 shows correlations of available numeracy tests with the overall accuracy of interpretations of these items. All formats of the Berlin Numeracy Test were superior to the previous numeracy tests, doubling the predictive power.

We further investigated the extent to which the Berlin Numeracy Test explained additional variance in risk understanding controlling for the strongest alternative predictors of performance – i.e., fluid intelligence and cognitive reflection. As Table 1.4 shows, all formats of the Berlin Numeracy Test explained a substantial portion of additional variance after these others tests were included in a hierarchical regression model.[1] In contrast, both

[1] For comparison, risk comprehension was predicted by the Cognitive Reflection Test with a standardized beta of 0.31 and by the Raven's test with a standardized beta of 0.20. When controlling for the Berlin Numeracy Test, the cognitive reflection continued to predict unique variance 0.20, but Raven's test did not 0.05.

Table 1.4. *Psychometric properties of the tests: Predictive validity.*

			Berlin Numeracy Test		
	Schwartz et al. (1997), 3 items	Lipkus et al. (2001), 11 items	Computer Adaptive Test Format	Paper and Pencil Format	Single Item Format
Mean proportion correct answers on understanding of everyday risks, by test quartiles					
1st quartile	0.72	0.68	0.68	0.66	0.70
2nd quartile	0.74	0.66	0.70	0.70	
3rd quartile	0.78	0.78	0.74	0.78	0.78
4th quartile	0.78	0.78	0.84	0.84	
Predictive validity for correct answers on understanding of everyday risks (standardized beta coefficients)					
As a single predictor	0.20**	0.20**	0.29**	0.34**	0.25**
With Raven	0.09	0.08	0.17**	0.23**	0.14*
With CRT	0.14*	0.15*	0.24**	0.31**	0.19**

*$p<0.05$; **$p<0.01$

previous numeracy tests lose most (or all) of their predictive power when intelligence and/or cognitive reflection tests are included. Overall, results indicate that the Berlin Numeracy Test is a reliable and valid test of statistical numeracy and risk literacy, offering higher levels of discriminability and overcoming the major psychometric limitations of the Lipkus et al. (2001) test and Schwartz et al. (1997) tests.

In subsequent studies, we have found that even among very highly educated professional samples (i.e., more than 50% of the sample had a masters, professional, or advanced degree) the Berlin Numeracy Test predicted superior risky decisions, intertemporal discounting, medical judgment, and overconfidence (Ghazal et al., 2014). Results show the Berlin Numeracy Test again outperforms other instruments (e.g., Schwartz et al., 1997). In other samples of young adults, the Berlin Numeracy Test predicts differences in retirement savings, credit card re-payment decisions, understanding of economic trends, political polls, and accurate interpretation of advertisements for over-the-counter medications. More importantly for the current purposes, in a large sample of patients in the US, we found that the Berlin Numeracy Test was a unique predictor of people's health perceptions, their actual health status (i.e., Charlson Index), the number of medications they currently take, and the degree of active engagement in shared decision making. These results are independent of effects related to salary, age, education, marital status, body mass index, and race (Garcia-Retamero et al., in press).

Cross-cultural discriminability

Going beyond predicative and construct validity, we have also done extensive work on psychometric discriminability (i.e., test sensitivity). We have now assessed discriminability of the Berlin Numeracy Test in more than 30 different industrialized countries in North and South America, Europe, and Asia. These tests all involve examination of college student samples, revealing the expected high levels of discriminability and overall levels of risk literacy that accord with estimates provided by other international studies of math and science literacy (e.g., PISA; for additional details see Garcia-Retamero, Cokely, Ghazal, & Petrova, in preparation). For example, a subset of studies conducted in 14 different countries with diverse cultural backgrounds included samples from China, England, France, Germany, India, Japan, Belgium, Norway, Pakistan, Poland, Spain, Sweden, Switzerland, and the USA (N = 2685) (Cokely et al., 2012). Overall results showed the test discriminated within desirable tolerances (i.e., +/− 10%) for each benchmarked quartile (Table 1.5). Aggregating across samples, the mean test score was 51.7% correct, which closely approximated the ideal score of 50%. The observed distributions indicate that with only 2–3 statistical numeracy questions the Berlin Numeracy Test achieves good discriminability across

Table 1.5. *Proportion of participants in each quartile from 14 countries.*

Country	Language	N	1st quartile	2nd quartile	3rd quartile	Top quartile
China	English	166	0.04	0.07	0.14	0.75
Poland	Polish	205	0.14	0.20	0.22	0.44
England	English	420	0.20	0.31	0.14	0.35
Japan	Japanese	63	0.06	0.36	0.24	0.34
Sweden	Swedish	47	0.21	0.28	0.17	0.34
France	French	86	0.30	0.13	0.23	0.34
USA	English	55	0.20	0.29	0.20	0.31
Switzerland	German	503	0.26	0.23	0.23	0.28
Germany	German	173	0.29	0.21	0.22	0.28
Norway	Norwegian	156	0.25	0.24	0.25	0.26
Belgium	Dutch	50	0.30	0.30	0.16	0.24
India	English	83	0.19	0.52	0.08	0.21
Pakistan	English	114	0.29	0.41	0.19	0.11
Spain	Spanish	258	0.48	0.41	0.07	0.04
Total		2379	0.23	0.28	0.18	0.31

Quartile scores are estimated based on the computer adaptive test algorithm. Countries are ordered by their percentage of top quartile scores.

most countries even when presented in different languages or when used at elite or technological universities.

In addition to the cross-cultural data, we have also collected data on (1) medical professionals (e.g., Physician Assistants), (2) general quota samples of the general population (e.g., residents of Sweden), and (3) large samples of computer literate adults who have taken the test in paid webpanels (e.g., Mechanical Turk). See Table 1.6 for some distributional properties. Results indicate some skew in the web-panel data. To address this issue, and provide a means of assessing a wider range of skills (including less educated and less numerate individuals), we conducted a series of experiments in which we combined the Berlin Numeracy Test with the Schwartz et al. (1997) test (see Cokely et al., 2012). When scored separately, we replicated moderate negative (–0.62) and positive (0.48) skewing of scores on the two tests with the general (lower ability) samples. However, when the two scores were added together they yielded a normal distribution with no evidence of skew (–0.016). These results suggest that the combined assessment is well suited for use with Mechanical Turk and should also be appropriate for estimating the wider range of differences in numeracy that exist in samples of the general population of the USA.

Summary

The Berlin Numeracy Test has many attractive features and is among the most extensively validated tests available. Results show that the Berlin Numeracy Test provides considerable increases in predictive validity, doubling the predictive power of other cognitive ability instruments and previous numeracy tests. Indeed, it is the strongest single predictor of risk literacy and one of only three tests extensively validated for the prediction of risk literacy (i.e., the ability to make good decisions based on information about risk) (Cokely et al., 2012). Moreover, the Berlin Numeracy

Table 1.6. *Percentage of people in each quartile from three different samples estimated by the computer adaptive Berlin Numeracy Test algorithm.*

Sample	N	1st quartile	2nd quartile	3rd quartile	4th quartile
Graduating US physician assistants	51	0.16	0.39	0.29	0.16
Population sample in Sweden	213	0.20	0.36	0.24	0.20
USA web panel sample (M-Turk)	1612	0.49	0.27	0.12	0.13
Total	1876	0.28	0.34	0.22	0.16

Test provides a very fast assessment (3 minutes for the computer adaptive format; 5 minutes for the paper and pencil version), which can be completed via computer or mobile device (e.g., smart phones). The Berlin Numeracy Test is also available in multiple languages and there is an ongoing effort to develop norms across a variety of professional and community samples. Nevertheless, it is not a good tool to use alone when assessing participants who are likely to have low levels of numeracy. Although some of our results suggest that it can be used quite effectively in patient populations, we recommend including the Schwartz et al. (1997) three-item test with the Berlin Numeracy Test to increase its range of sensitivity whenever one expects a high proportion of low numeracy participants (>10%).

To facilitate access and increase awareness of risk literacy, the computer adaptive Berlin Numeracy Test is available online. The test along with other risk literacy and numeracy resources can be found at www.RiskLiteracy.org. The online forum allows the public to take the test and receive feedback on their performance relative to other college educated individuals in industrialized countries. It also provides a simple, computerized test format recommendation tool along with instructions for requesting unique links for computerized tests that can be used by researchers (e.g., embedded in ongoing experiments).

Conclusions

The research we have reviewed in this chapter details the considerable progress we have made in measuring numeracy over the last few decades. In this time, we have moved from simple, robust instruments like the Schwartz et al. (1997) and Lipkus et al. (2001) tests to sophisticated, specialized tests like the NUMi, the Abbreviated Numeracy Scale, and the Berlin Numeracy Test. These test instruments range widely in their theoretical approaches to assessment and their various other operational parameters. While some tests like the Berlin Numeracy Test are designed to be fast and valid predictors of decision making (i.e., predicting risk literacy), other numeracy tests have instead emphasized a thorough assessment of the full range of mathematical skills involved in numeracy (see Table 1.7, and Figures 1.2 and 1.3 for summary data).

In the years ahead, we envision continued progress along a number of measurement frontiers. Parallel forms of numeracy tests, or computerized adaptive tests with larger item pools, will need to be developed to allow for repeated testing and developmental studies. Greater integration with information technology should also bring computerized training programs, better estimates of population and subpopulation norms, and better decision

Table 1.7. *Properties of validated numeracy research instruments.*

Source	Test name	Theoretical approach	Test items	Test time	Components assessed	Participants
Schwartz et al. (1997)	Numeracy Assessment	Classical Test Theory	3	2 to 3 minutes	Probability ratio	Low to moderate numeracy
Lipkus et al. (2001)	Numeracy Scale	Classical Test Theory	11	5 to 10 minutes	Comparison of risk magnitudes, class inclusion	Low to moderate numeracy
Fagerlin et al. (2007)	Subjective Numeracy Scale	Classical Test Theory	8	3 to 7 minutes	Perceived ability and preferences for working with numbers	Low to moderate numeracy
Peters et al. (2007a)	Expanded Numeracy Scale	Classical Test Theory	15	6 to 15 minutes	Positive predictive value	Low to moderate numeracy
Cokely et al. (2012)	Berlin Numeracy Test	Adaptive Decision Tree	1 to 4	1 to 5 minutes	Statistical numeracy and risk literacy	Moderate-to-high numeracy
Weller et al. (2013)	Abbreviated Numeracy Scale	Rasch Model Item Response Theory	8	8 to 12 minutes	Probability, ratio, risk preference	Moderate numeracy & general population
Schapira et al. (2012)	Numeracy Understanding in Medicine Instrument (NUMi)	Two parameter Item Response Theory	20	12 to 20 minutes	Number sense, graph, probability, statistics	Low numeracy

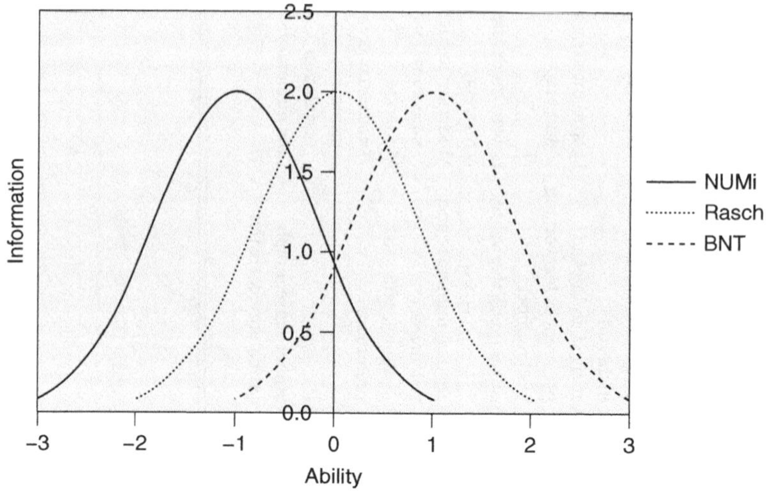

Figure 1.2. Theoretical differences in distributions of the NUMi, abbreviated numeracy test, and the Berlin Numeracy Test.

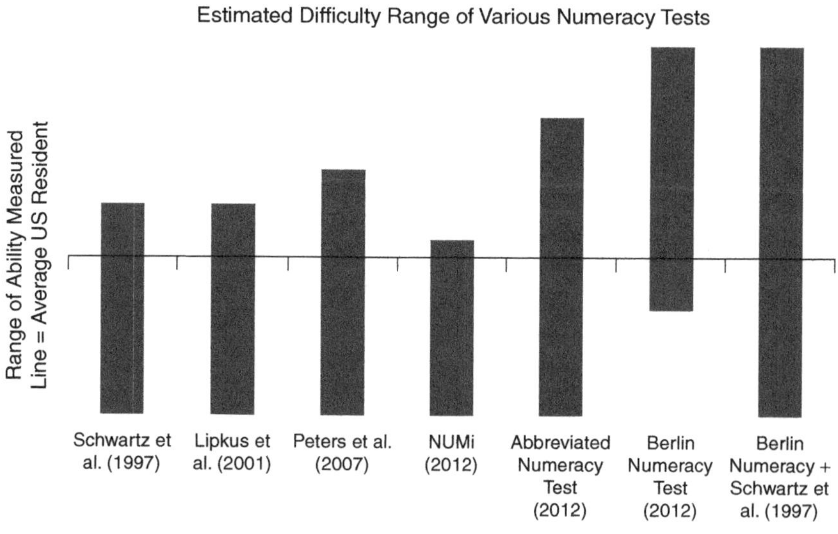

Figure 1.3. Estimated difficulty ranges for various numeracy tests. The line represents the approximated "average" US resident. Scores above the bar correspond to higher levels of numeracy whereas scores below the line correspond to lower than average numeracy levels. For example, we estimate that the NUMi has the narrowest range of skill assessment sensitivity; however, it also provides the highest fidelity assessment. Alternatively, the widest range of skill assessment comes from combining the Schwartz et al. (1997) instrument with the Berlin Numeracy Test.

support systems including custom-tailored information brochures and refined consumer protection standards (e.g., ensuring provided materials are designed at appropriate risk literacy levels). However, it is important to remember that many of these advances will come not simply because we continue to develop better tests but because we develop a better theoretical understanding of the nature of numeracy and its relationship to superior decision making (Cokely et al., 2012; Peters, 2012; Reyna et al., 2009; see also Bruine de Bruin et al., 2007; Parker & Fischhoff, 2005).

References

Barton, A., Cokely, E. T., Galesic, M., Koehler, A., & Haas, M. (2009). Comparing risk reductions: On the dynamic interplay of cognitive strategies, numeracy, complexity, and format. In: N. A. Taatgen & H. van Rijn (Eds.), *Proceedings of the 31st Annual Conference of the Cognitive Science Society*; pp. 2347–2352.

Blackwell, L., Trzesniewski, K., & Dweck, C. S. (2007). Implicit theories of intelligence predict achievement across an adolescent transition: A longitudinal study and an intervention. *Child Development*, 78, 246–263.

Bors, D. A., & Stokes, T. L. (1998). Raven's advanced progressive matrices: Norms for first-year university students and the development of a short form. *Educational and Psychological Measurement*, 58, 382–398.

Bruine de Bruin, W. B., Parker, A. M., & Fischhoff, B. (2007). Individual differences in adult decision-making competence. *Journal of Personality and Social Psychology*, 92, 938–956.

Cokely, E. T., & Kelley, C. M. (2009). Cognitive abilities and superior decision making under risk: A protocol analysis and process model evaluation. *Judgment and Decision Making*, 4, 20–33.

Cokely, E. T., Kelley, C. M., & Gilchrist, A. H. (2006). Sources of individual differences in working memory: Contributions of strategy to capacity. *Psychonomic Bulletin & Review*, 13, 991–997.

Cokely, E. T., Parpart, P., & Schooler, L. J. (2009). On the link between cognitive control and heuristic processes. In: *Proceedings of the 31st Annual Conference of the Cognitive Science Society*; pp. 2926–2931.

Cokely, E. T., Galesic, M., Schulz, E., Ghazal, S., & Garcia-Retamero, R. (2012). Measuring risk literacy: The berlin numeracy test. *Judgment and Decision Making*, 7(1), 25–47.

Del Missier, F. T., Mäntylä, T., & Bruine de Bruin, W. (2010). Executive functions in decision making: An individual differences approach. *Thinking & Reasoning*, 16, 69–97.

Del Missier, F. T., Mäntylä, T., & Bruine de Bruin, W. (2012). Decision-making competence, executive functioning, and general cognitive abilities. *Journal of Behavioral Decision Making*, 25, 331–351.

Diener, E., Emmons, R. A., Larsen, R., & Griffin, S. (1985). The satisfaction with life scale. *Journal of Personality Assessment*, 49, 71–75.

Duckworth A. L., & Quinn, P. D. (2009). Development and validation of the short grit scale (grit-s). *Journal of Personality Assessment*, 91, 166–174.

Ericsson, A., Prietula, M. J., & Cokely, E. T. (2007). The making of an expert. *Harvard Business Review*, 85, 114–121.

Fagerlin, A., Zikmund-Fisher, B. J., Ubel, P. A., Jankovic, A., Derry, H. A., & Smith, D. M. (2007). Measuring numeracy without a math test: Development of the Subjective Numeracy Scale. *Medical Decision Making*, 27, 672–680.

Fox, M. C., Roring, R., & Mitchum, A. L. (2009). Reversing the speed-IQ correlation: Intra-individual variability and attentional control in the inspection time paradigm. *Intelligence*, 37, 76–80.

Fox, M. C., Ericsson, K. A., & Best, R. (2011). Do procedures for verbal reporting of thinking have to be reactive? A meta-analysis and recommendations for best reporting methods. *Psychological Bulletin*, 137, 316–344.

Frederick, S. (2005). Cognitive reflection and decision making. *Journal of Economic Perspectives*, 19, 25–42.

Galesic, M., & Garcia-Retamero, R. (2010). Statistical numeracy for health: A cross-cultural comparison with probabilistic national samples. *Archives of Internal Medicine*, 170, 462–468.

Garcia-Retamero, R., & Cokely, E. T. (2011). Effective communication of risks to young adults: Using message framing and visual aids to increase condom use and STD screening. *Journal of Experimental Psychology: Applied*, 17, 270–287.

Garcia-Retamero, R., & Cokely, E. T. (2013). Communicating health risks with visual aids. *Current Directions in Psychological Science*, 22, 392–399.

Garcia-Retamero, R., & Cokely, E. (in press). The influence of skills, message frame, and visual aids on prevention of sexually transmitted diseases. *Journal of Behavioral Decisional Making*. http://dx.doi.org/10.1002/bdm.1797.

Garcia-Retamero, R., & Galesic, M. (2010a). How to reduce the effect of framing on messages about health. *Journal of General Internal Medicine*, 25, 1323–1329.

Garcia-Retamero, R., & Galesic, M. (2010b). Who profits from visual aids: Overcoming challenges in people's understanding of risks. *Social Science & Medicine*, 70, 1019–1025.

Garcia-Retamero, R., & Galesic, M. (2013). *Transparent Communication of Health Risks: Overcoming Cultural Differences*. New York: Springer.

Garcia-Retamero, R., & Galesic, M. (in press). Using analogies to communicate information about health risks. *Applied Cognitive Psychology*.

Garcia-Retamero, R., Wicki, B., Cokely, E. T., & Hanson, B. (in press). Factors predicting surgeon's preferred and actual roles in interactions with their patients. *Health Psychology*. doi:10.1037/hea0000061.

Ghazal, S., Cokely, E. T., & Garcia-Retamero, R. (2014). Predicting bias in very highly educated samples: Numeracy and metacognition. *Judgment and Decision Making*, 9, 15–34.

Ginsburg, L., Manly, M., & Schmitt, M. J. (2006). *The Components of Numeracy* [NCSALL Occasional Paper]. Cambridge, MA: National Center for Study of Adult Literacy and Learning.

Gosling, S. D., Rentfrow, P. J., & Swann, W. B. (2003). A very brief measure of the big-five personality domains. *Journal of Research in Personality*, 37, 504–528.

Guadagnoli, E., & Ward, P. (1998). Patient participation in decision-making. *Social Science and Medicine*, 47, 329–339.

Hanoch, Y., Miron-Shatz, T., Cole, H., Himmelstein, M., & Federman, A. D. (2010). Choice, numeracy and physicians-in-training performance: The case of Medicare part D. *Health Psychology*, 29, 454–459.

Hodapp, V., & Benson, J. (1997). The multidimensionality of test anxiety: A test of different models. *Anxiety, Stress, and Coping*, 10, 219–244.

Huff, D., & Geis, I. (1954). *How to Lie with Statistics*. New York: Norton.

Kutner, M., Greenberg, E., Jin, Y., & Paulsen, C. (2006). *The Health Literacy of America's adults: Results from the 2003 National Assessment of Adult Literacy* (NCES 2006-483). Washington, DC: National Center for Education Statistics.

Lang, J. W., & Fries, S. (2006). A revised 10-item version of the Achievement Motives Scale: Psychometric properties in German-speaking samples. *European Journal of Psychological Assessment*, 22(3), 216.

Liberali, J. M., Reyna, V. F., Furlan, S., Stein, L. M., & Pardo, S. T. (2011). Individual differences in numeracy and cognitive reflection, with implications for biases and fallacies in probability judgment. *Journal of Behavioral Decision Making*, 25(4), 361–381.

Lindenberger, U., Mayr, U., & Kliegl, R. (1993). Speed and intelligence in old age. *Psychology and Aging*, 8, 207–220.

Lipkus, I. M., Samsa, G., & Rimer, B. K. (2001). General performance on a numeracy scale among highly-educated samples. *Medical Decision Making*, 21, 37–44.

Lord, F. M. (1980). *Applications of Item Response Theory to Practical Testing Problems*. Hillsdale, NJ: Lawrence Erlbaum.

Messick, S. (1995). Validity of psychological assessment: Validation of inferences from persons responses and performances as scientific inquiry into score meaning. *American Psychologist*, 50, 741–749.

Neisser, U., Boodoo, G., Bouchard, T. J., Boykin, A. W., Brody, N., Ceci, S. J., et al. (1996). Intelligence: Knowns and unknowns. *American Psychologist*, 51, 77–101.

Novick, M. R. (1966). The axioms and principal results of classical test theory. *Journal of Mathematical Psychology*, 3, 1–18.

Okan, Y., Garcia-Retamero, R., Cokely, E. T., & Maldonado, A. (2013). Individual differences in graph literacy: Overcoming denominator neglect in risk comprehension. *Journal of Behavioral Decision Making*, 25, 390–401.

Parker, A. M., & Fischhoff, B. (2005). Decision-making competence: external validation through an individual differences approach. *Journal of Behavioral Decision Making*, 18, 1–27.

Paulos, J. A. (1988). *Innumeracy: Mathematical Illiteracy and its Consequences*. New York: Hill and Wang.

Peters, E. (2012). Beyond comprehension: The role of numeracy in judgment and decision making. *Current Directions in Psychological Science*, 21(1), 31–35.

Peters, E., & Levin, I. P. (2008). Dissecting the risky-choice framing effect: Numeracy as an individual-difference factor in weighting risky and riskless options. *Judgment and Decision Making*, 3, 435–448.

Peters, E., Västfjäll, D., Slovic, P., Mertz, C. K., Mazzocco, K., & Dickert, S. (2006). Numeracy and decision making. *Psychological Science*, 17, 407–413.

Peters, E., Dieckmann, N. F., Dixon, A., Slovic, P., Mertz, C. K., & Hibbard, J. H. (2007a). Less is more in presenting quality information to consumers. *Medical Care Research and Review*, 64, 169–190.

Peters, E., Hibbard, J. H., Slovic, P., & Dieckmann, N. F. (2007b). Numeracy skill and the communication, comprehension, and use of risk and benefit information. *Health Affairs*, 26, 741–748.

Peters, E., Slovic, P., Västfjäll, D., & Mertz, C. K. (2008). Intuitive numbers guide decisions. *Judgment and Decision Making*, 3, 619–635.

Raven, J. (2000). The Raven's Progressive Matrices: Change and stability over culture and time. *Cognitive Psychology*, 41, 1–48.

Reyna, V. F., Nelson, W. L., Han, P. K., & Dieckmann, N. F. (2009). How numeracy influences risk comprehension and medical decision making. *Psychological Bulletin*, 135, 943–973.

Schapira, M. M., Walker, C. M., & Sedivy, S. K. (2009). Evaluating existing measures of health numeracy using item response theory. *Patient Educational Counseling*, 75, 308–314.

Schapira, M. M., Walker, C. M., Cappaert, K. J., Ganschow, P. S., Fletcher, K. E., McGinley, E. L., et al. (2012). The numeracy understanding in medicine instrument: A measure of health numeracy developed using item response theory. *Medical Decision Making: An International Journal of the Society for Medical Decision Making*, 32(6), 851–865.

Schwartz, L. M. L., Woloshin, S. S., Black, W. C. W., & Welch, H. G. H. (1997). The role of numeracy in understanding the benefit of screening mammography. *Annals of Internal Medicine*, 127, 966–972.

Schwartz, B., Ward, A., Monterosso, J., Lyubomirsky, S., White, K., & Lehman, D. R. (2002). Maximizing versus satisficing: happiness is a matter of choice. *Journal of Personality and Social Psychology*, 83(5), 1178.

Schwarzer, R., & Jerusalem, M. (1995). Generalized self-efficacy scale. In: J. Weinman, S. Wright, & M. Johnston (Eds.), *Measures in Health Psychology: A User's Portfolio*. Windsor, UK: Nfer-Nelson.

Sheridan, S. L., & Pignone, M. (2002). Numeracy and the medical student's ability to interpret data. Effective clinical practice. *ECP*, 5(1), 35.

Sherrod, P. H. (2003). *DTREG: Predictive Modeling Software*. Software available at www.dtreg.com.

Steen, L. A. (1990).*On the Shoulders of Giants: New Approaches to Numeracy*. Washington, DC: National Academy Press.

Turner, M. L., & Engle, R. W. (1989). Is working memory capacity task dependent? *Journal of Memory and Language*, 28, 127–154.

Van der Linden, W. J., & Hambleton, R. K. (Eds.) (1997). *Handbook of Modern Item Response Theory*. New York, NY: Springer.

Weller, J. A., Dieckmann, N. F., Tusler, M., Mertz, C. K., Burns, W. J., & Peters, E. (2013). Development and testing of an abbreviated numeracy scale: A rasch analysis approach. *Journal of Behavioral Decision Making*, 26, 192–212.

Zikmund-Fisher, B., Smith, D. M., Ubel, P. A., & Fagerlin, A. (2007). Validation of the subjective numeracy scale: Effects of low numeracy on comprehension of risk communications and utility elicitations. *Medical Decision Making*, 27, 663–671.

2 Collective statistical illiteracy in health

Jan Multmeier, Wolfgang Gaissmaier, &
Odette Wegwarth

Introduction

National Football League athlete Tony Romo is the quarterback of the Dallas Cowboys. A few years ago, his father was diagnosed with prostate cancer. As a consequence, Romo is now supporting the non-profit organization "Prostate Conditions Education Council (PCEC)" whose goal is to increase awareness for prostate cancer prevalence and the importance of early detection, and Romo is advertising their mission in a video clip published on the PCEC's website.[1] In this video, Tony Romo and his dad are shown together, relieved that his prostate cancer was detected early so that they still had time to spend together. Tony Romo's dad advocates early detection of prostate cancer with the following statement: "But when found early, the five-year survival rate of prostate cancer is nearly 100%."

This video clip illustrates several key points that we would like to make throughout this chapter, each of which we will discuss in more detail below. The goal of this chapter is to illustrate these points rather than to provide a complete coverage of the existing literature. First, the video clip illustrates the broad phenomenon that much health information targeted at the general public does not aim to educate the public about the pros and cons of health interventions, but rather to promote and encourage health behavior change such as participation in cancer screening by means of persuasion. Second, it demonstrates that if any statistical evidence concerning the health intervention is presented, it is often incomplete in that it only presents those snippets of the data that suit the message of the sender, and it is often non-transparent in that it communicates misleading health statistics. As we will show below, although the terminology heavily suggests otherwise, 5-year survival rates are not necessarily related at all to mortality. Third, the video clip demonstrates that health campaigns not

[1] Note that the video is not available anymore on the website. However, a brochure that covers the key messages from the video can still be found at www.prostateconditions.org/images/TonyRomoTackleProstateCancer.pdf

only present health statistics in a misleading way, but often bet more strongly on what we call narrative evidence rather than statistical evidence in the first place. The term narrative evidence refers to often emotionally laden reports of single cases – here: Tony Romo's dad who believes to have been saved by early detection of prostate cancer – that are absolutely meaningless scientifically, but are known to have a strong impact on people's perception and behavior.

In sum, Tony Romo's clip is the opposite of good, balanced health information. By "good, balanced health information" we mean information that actually aims to enable people to make their own decisions rather than persuading them to do what authorities believe to be best, and this crucial distinction is what we will turn to next.

Information versus persuasion

Can the general public learn to evaluate health benefits and risks accurately, or do authorities need to steer them toward correct decisions with the presentation of persuasive information? The present research community is divided on this issue. Many specialists in the field conclude from existing research that the public will never really be capable of making the best decisions on the basis of the available scientific information, so that there is a need for a benevolent paternalism that uses methods of propaganda to persuade the public to do what is considered best for them, or by nudging them to make the "right" choices (Thaler & Sunstein, 2008). Others, in contrast, are convinced that people can be educated to improve their decision-making skills and be prepared for the complexities and uncertainties of the modern world, so that they can make informed decisions according to their values (Gigerenzer et al., 2007).

Let us illustrate the difference between those two approaches by picking up the opening example. The usual method for the early detection of prostate cancer is a blood test for the prostate-specific antigen (PSA) combined with a digital rectal examination, in the following simply referred to as PSA-screening. We have already heard that the 5-year survival rate is very high when prostate cancer is diagnosed early. But before dissecting this admittedly very difficult health statistic in detail, we would like to start out with a very simple question that one should ask about every health intervention: What evidence is available about the pros and cons for this particular health intervention?

A recent press release celebrated the results of an international randomized controlled trial on the benefits of using PSA-screening. It stated that PSA-screening would reduce the risk of dying from prostate cancer by 20% (Wilde, 2009). Just how big is 20%? It meant that out of every 1410 men who regularly participated in prostate cancer screening, one fewer died of prostate cancer than in an equally large group of men who did not participate (Schröder et al., 2009). Additionally, 48 of 1410 men were unnecessarily treated and hence subjected to risks like incontinence and impotence. What the press release omitted was that PSA-screening did not reduce overall mortality at all. That is, the one man (out of 1410) who was saved from dying from prostate cancer died from something else in the same time frame. Nor did the press release mention that there was a second large clinical trial published in the same issue of the medical journal that found no reduction in prostate cancer mortality through screening (Andriole et al., 2009). More recently, a meta-analysis summarizing the best available evidence on PSA-screening actually concluded that there is currently no indication that it is effective in reducing mortality (Djulbegovic et al., 2010). Also, a 20-year follow-up did not find a benefit of PSA-screening, while the harms such as unnecessary treatments are unquestioned (Sandblom et al., 2011).

Based on this evidence, the United States Preventive Services Task Force recently decided to recommend against routine PSA-screening for prostate cancer, yet this evidence-based recommendation was not welcome. Politicians, prostate cancer survivors, physicians, and advocacy organizations responded furiously (Arkes & Gaissmaier, 2012). It may therefore not be surprising that PSA-screening is still heavily advertised, not only by the pharmaceutical industry, but also by non-profit organizations like PCEC. To advocate PSA-screening one simply has to communicate the number that makes the effect look bigger, which is the relative risk reduction of 20% rather than communicating the more transparent but less impressive absolute risk reduction of 1 in 1410. One furthermore has to communicate the results of the most favorable study while at the same time omitting that other studies come to different conclusions, and one should probably omit the potential harms of screening such as unnecessary treatments. Many health campaigns make use of both non-transparent and incomplete information, and this does not only hold true for PSA-screening, but also for other kinds of screening such as mammography screening, and for advertising the benefits of medical treatments more generally (Gigerenzer et al., 2007).

In recent years, however, there has been a call for a paradigm shift from the traditional, paternalistic doctor–patient relationship toward educating patients to make informed medical decisions according to their own values (Barry, 1999; Gigerenzer & Gray, 2011; O'Connor et al., 2007). "An educated citizenry is the lifeblood of a modern democracy", as Gigerenzer and Gray (2011, p. 4) put it in their manifesto for a century of the patient, and they further elaborate on how such an educated citizenship may actually buy us better healthcare for less money. Moreover, patients may have very different preferences than their physicians, for instance when it comes to the acceptability of side effects (Heesen et al., 2010), and it is the patient's preference that should ultimately be most decisive.

Enabling patients to make informed medical decisions requires that patients, as well as their doctors, understand the benefits and harms of different treatment options. Unfortunately, this is often not the case (Gaissmaier & Gigerenzer, 2011). What we call statistical illiteracy in health – the inability to understand health statistics – therefore poses an existential obstacle to the ideal of informed decision making and can actually render the term "informed" obsolete. Often, precisely this lack of understanding is used to discredit the ideal of informed decision making altogether. Next, we will illustrate the collective problem of statistical illiteracy in more detail, but we will also describe ways in which clinical evidence can be communicated effectively, in order to alleviate the concerns that, as a consequence of illiteracy, one should keep patients away from important decisions.

Communicating clinical evidence

(In-)numeracy

Individual numerical competences are a key prerequisite for the understanding of clinical evidence (see Reyna et al., 2009, and Chapters 2 and 3 in this volume). In their study on numeracy and health behavior, Schwartz et al. (1997) asked the participating women three questions related to understanding uncertainty and manipulating numbers, e.g., how many heads can be expected in a number of coin flips, and converting percentages to whole numbers and vice versa. Only 16% of the participants could answer all three questions correctly, and as many as 30% could not give the right answer to at least one of the questions. Comparable results of relatively high proportions of the population who cannot answer relatively basic numerical questions have been found recently in a survey of probabilistic, representative national samples in the USA and in Germany (Galesic & Garcia-Retamero, 2010; see Table 2.1).

The ability to understand numbers has implications for understanding health information: higher numeracy is associated with more accurate judgments about the effects of prostate cancer and mammography screening (Hamm et al., 2003; Schwartz et al., 1997). Numeracy is not only important in the medical domain. In his book "Innumeracy: Mathematical Illiteracy and its Consequences," Paulos (1988) describes how behaviors such as

Table 2.1. *Basic numeracy in the USA and Germany based on nationally representative samples.*

	US adults ages 25–69	German adults ages 25–69
	% Correct answer	
In the Bingo Lottery, the chance of winning a $10 prize is 1%. What is your best guess about how many people will win a $10 prize if 1000 people each buy a single ticket for Bingo Lottery? ____ person(s) out of 1000	58%	68%
In the Daily Times Sweepstakes, the chance of winning a car is 1 in 1000. What percentage of tickets for the Daily Times Sweepstakes win a car? ____ % of tickets	24%	46%
Imagine that we flip a fair coin 1000 times. What is your best guess about how many times the coin will come up heads in 1000 flips? ____ times out of 1000	73%	73%

From Galesic & Garcia-Retamero, 2010.

belief in pseudoscience, poor risk assessment, and loss of money in gambling are related to a poor understanding of numerical concepts.

This lack of numerical understanding is indeed challenging. To tackle this issue, the literature has suggested various ways in which numbers can be presented in a comprehensible manner, and in fact the most effective remedy for the problem of statistical illiteracy in health is to use transparent representations. A few examples will be described next and can be found in Table 2.2.

Relative versus absolute risks

The press statement about PSA-screening illustrated how the same health statistic – here the reduction of prostate cancer mortality – can be presented in two different ways, either as relative risk reduction ("20%") or as absolute risk reduction ("1 in 1410"). The problem with relative risks is that they remain silent about the baseline risk, while the absolute risk makes this transparent. A 20% relative risk reduction could mean a reduction from 5 to 4 out of every 1000 men. However, it could also mean a reduction from 500 to 400 out of every 1000 men, which would clinically be a much more relevant effect. Presenting treatment benefits as relative risk reductions leads people to overestimate those benefits. This does not only hold true for patients, but also for physicians and other health professionals (Covey, 2007).

Table 2.2. *Examples of non-transparent information from a variety of sources, and simple transparent solutions.*

Source	Non-transparent information	Transparent solution
Media	Relative risk reduction "PSA screening reduces the risk of dying from prostate cancer by 20%."	Use absolute risk reduction "Out of every 1,410 men who participate in PSA screening regularly, 1 is saved from dying of prostate cancer."
Politicians	5-year survival rates "I had prostate cancer, 5, 6 years ago. My chance of surviving prostate cancer – and thank God, I was cured of it – in the United States? Eighty-two percent. My chance of surviving prostate cancer in England? Only 44 percent under socialized medicine."	Use mortality rates instead of 5-year survival rates "In 2001, about 26 of every 100,000 American men died of prostate cancer, compared to 27 out of every 100,000 in Britain."
Physicians	Single event probabilities "If you take Prozac, you have a 30 to 50% chance of experiencing a sexual problem, such as impotence or lack of interest."	Use frequency formats with a clear reference class "Out of 100 men who take Prozac, 30 to 50 will experience sexual problems."
Test results	Conditional probabilities "1% of the women in the patient's age group have breast cancer. If a woman has breast cancer, the probability that the mammography screening will detect it is 90%. If a woman does not have breast cancer, the probability that she will receive a positive test result is 9%." $p(Cancer \mid Test\,positive) = \frac{0.01 * 0.90}{0.01 * 0.90 + 0.99 * 0.09}$	Convert the information into natural frequencies "In a group of 1000 women, 10 would have breast cancer. Of the 10 women with breast cancer, 9 would receive a positive mammography. Also, 89 of the 990 women who do not have breast cancer would test positive." $p(Cancer \mid Test\,positive) = \frac{9}{9 + 89}$

Given that prostate cancer screening, as well as many other cancer screening methods, have most commonly been advocated for by communicating relative risk reductions, it is not surprising that the general public largely overestimates the benefits of cancer screening. Gigerenzer et al. (2009) surveyed about 10 000 men and women from nine European countries and asked them to estimate the benefits of PSA-screening and mammography screening, respectively. For PSA-screening, 89% of men overestimated the mortality reduction by at least one order of magnitude or answered that they did not know. This was also the case for 92% of the women with respect to mammography screening. Those who frequently consulted their physician or health pamphlets did not achieve more realistic estimates, but rather overestimated the benefits of screening even more strongly.

Why are physicians and patients systematically misinformed? How hard is it to find accurate and transparent statistical information in medical journals or patient brochures? A physician consulting a scientific medical journal is often not only misled indirectly by the use of relative risks. In some cases, the benefits and harms of treatment options are reported in different currencies: benefits are reported in relative numbers, making them look favorable, while harms are reported in absolute numbers. This technique has been termed *mismatched framing*. The *Guide to Clinical Preventive Services* of the US Preventive Services Task Force (2002), for example, states the relative risk reduction when describing the benefits of screening: "sigmoidoscopy reduced the risk of death by 59% of cancers within reach of the sigmoidoscope" (p. 93). The harms associated with sigmoidoscopy, however, are described in absolute risks: "Perforations are reported to occur in approximately 1 of 1,000 – 10,000 rigid sigmoidoscopic examinations" (p. 94). Mismatched framing is commonplace in medical journals. One in three studies which were published in the esteemed medical journals *BMJ*, *JAMA*, and *The Lancet* between 2004 and 2006 and reported both benefits and harms did so in different currencies, most often using relative risks for benefits and absolute risks for harms (Sedrakyan & Shih, 2007). A physician consulting a medical journal to generate a recommendation for his patient will thus likely be misled by the framing of benefits and harms. Are patients more likely to find unbiased information? In an analysis of Australian brochures about breast cancer screening, only 22% of the brochures included quantitative information about the benefits of screening, and always reported relative risks instead of the transparent format of absolute risks (Slaytor & Ward, 1998). Quantitative information about harms was never provided (see Gigerenzer et al., 2007 for a summary, also showing that the situation is not better in other countries).

This suggests that most information targeted at patients and physicians is misleading and persuasive rather than informative, and the next example shows that relative risk reductions are not the only misleading health statistics in this respect.

Conditional probability versus natural frequencies

Let us assume a symptom-free woman in her 50s decides to participate in mammography screening, and the mammography result is positive. Does that mean that she definitively has breast cancer? Her doctor has the following information: 1% of the women in the patient's age group have breast cancer. If a woman has breast cancer, the probability that the mammography screening will detect it is 90%. If a woman does not have breast cancer, the probability that she will receive a positive test result is 9%. What is the probability that the woman has breast cancer, given that she tested positive? Applying Bayes rule leads to the answer: about 10% (see Gigerenzer et al., 2007 for details).

Provided with this information, most women will likely fail to understand that the actual probability of having breast cancer after being tested positive is about 10%, as do most university students (Gigerenzer & Hoffrage, 1995). But turning to their doctors is also not likely to help: Gigerenzer et al. (2007) presented the same information to 160 gynecologists and asked them to estimate the probability that a woman has cancer if she received a positive test result. Only 21% picked the correct answer out of four answering options, slightly less than expected by chance. However, the situation is not hopeless. The doctors were taught to convert the information from probabilities into natural frequencies: in a group of 1000 women, 10 would have breast cancer (1%). Of the 10 women with breast cancer, 9 would receive a positive mammography (90%). Also, 89 of the 990 women who do not have breast cancer would test positive (9%). Now it is easy to see that 9 out of 98 women who receive a positive test result actually have breast cancer, which is about 10%. After learning this conversion, the confusion disappeared, and 87% could now answer the problem correctly. Figure 2.1 gives an impression of the facilitating effect of natural frequencies over conditional probabilities.

Single event probabilities versus frequencies

If the weather forecast predicts a 30% chance for rain tomorrow, what does that actually mean? Some people believe it will rain 30% of the time, other believe it will rain on 30% of the area, and yet again others believe it will rain on 30% of the days for which this forecast has been made (Gigerenzer et al., 2005). The missing reference class – time, area, or days – causes ambiguity. Clearly put, the statement meant that it will rain in 30 out of 100 days for which this forecast has been made.

Similarly, when a physician tells a patient: "If you take Prozac, you have a 30 to 50% chance of developing a sexual problem, such as impotence or lack of interest," this causes ambiguity about the reference class. Patients could interpret these numbers as meaning that every patient would have problems in about 30% to 50% of their sexual encounters, which would be quite frightening. However, the numbers actually mean that out of 100 patients 30 to 50 will experience a sexual problem – a much less

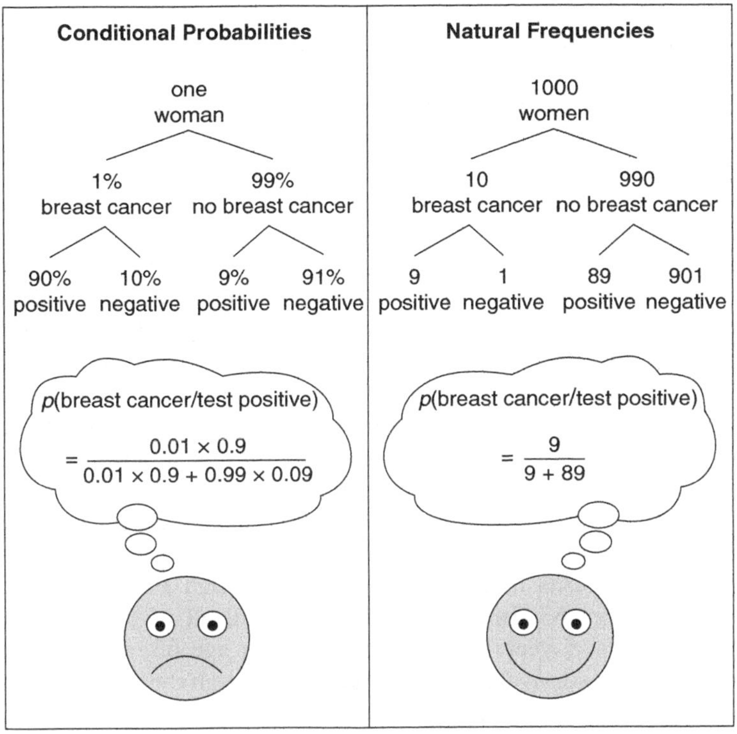

Figure 2.1. Arithmetic operations which need to be carried out with conditional probabilities (left) or natural frequencies (right) in order to determine the likelihood that a woman with a positive mammography screening result actually has breast cancer (adapted from Gigerenzer et al., 2007).

frightening statement. This example illustrates again a reference class problem: While the patients had their own sexual encounters in mind as a reference class, the doctor was referring to patients as a reference class.

Therefore, also the solution to such misunderstandings is clear: Either clearly indicate a reference class (e.g., sexual problems will occur in 30% to 50% of patients), or use a frequentist formulation (e.g., out of 100 patients, 30 to 50 will experience a sexual problem).

Survival versus mortality rates

Recall Tony Romo's dad who advocated for prostate cancer screening because the 5-year survival rate is very high when the cancer is detected early. By doing so, he is in good company: former New York City mayor

Rudi Giuliani advertised PSA-screening programs for prostate cancer in a 2007 campaign: "I had prostate cancer, 5, 6 years ago. My chance of surviving prostate cancer – and thank God, I was cured of it – in the United States? Eighty-two percent. My chance of surviving prostate cancer in England? Only 44 percent under socialized medicine" (Dobbs, 2007). Giuliani took these numbers as evidence that his chances of surviving prostate cancer were almost twice as high as in England. He was wrong. Giuliani referred to 5-year-survival rates – the proportion of patients still alive 5 years after they have been diagnosed with prostate cancer.

Two factors cause the survival rates to differ in the USA and England, and none of them has to do with prevention of deaths from prostate cancer: lead-time bias and overdiagnosis bias. Lead-time bias describes the fact that cancer is diagnosed earlier with screening, typically before any symptoms occur. Without screening, patients usually consult a physician when they are older and after certain symptoms appear. Imagine a group of prostate cancer patients who are diagnosed because of symptoms at age 67, all of whom die at age 70. Five years after their diagnosis, nobody is still alive – the 5-year-survival rate is 0%. Now imagine that the same group of patients had been diagnosed through PSA-screening 4 years earlier, at age 63. Imagine further that still all of them die at age 70. Nevertheless, 5 years after the diagnosis at age 63, all have survived so far – a 5-year-survival rate of 100%. Even though the survival rate changed dramatically, no life was saved or prolonged (see Figure 2.2).

Overdiagnosis bias refers to the detection of pseudo-disease – screening-detected abnormalities that meet the pathologic definition of cancer but will never progress to cause symptoms in the patient's lifetime. These non-progressive cancers inflate the number of diagnoses in the screening group but would have remained unnoticed if they were not detected by screenings. To illustrate this, consider 1000 men diagnosed with progressive prostate cancer. Five years later, 440 would still be alive, 560 would have died, resulting in a survival rate of 44%. Imagine that with PSA-screening, an additional 2000 non-progressive cancers would have been detected. These would be added to the 440 patients with progressive cancer who are still alive after 5 years, inflating the survival rate to 81% (2440 patients who are alive after 5 years divided by the total number of now 3000 patients diagnosed with prostate cancer, see Figure 2.3).

Differences in survival rates do not necessarily indicate differences in mortality, and in fact, changes in these two statistics over the second half of the twentieth century are not even weakly correlated with each other (Welch et al., 2000). Thus, when evaluating the success of a screening program, one should always consider mortality rates rather than survival rates: in 2001, about 26 of every 100 000 American men died of prostate cancer,

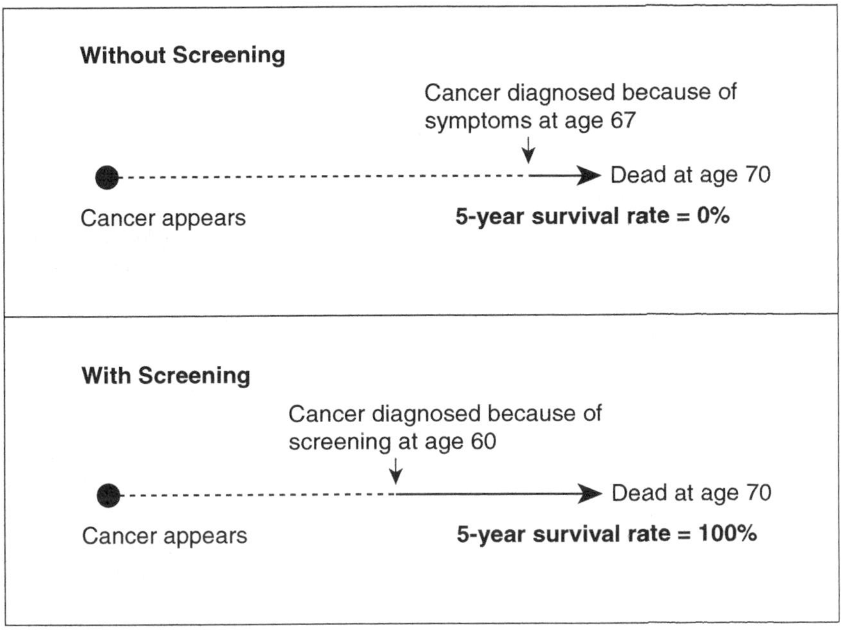

Figure 2.2. Lead-time bias (adapted from Gigerenzer et al., 2007).

compared to 27 of every 100 000 in Britain (Shibata & Whittemore, 2001). However, even most physicians are not aware of this important distinction, and they would confidently recommend a particular screening method solely based on information about survival rates although such data does not allow them to judge the method's efficacy (Wegwarth et al., 2011; Wegwarth et al., 2012).

Visual displays

Just as certain ways of presenting numbers have been found to increase transparency, a variety of graphical representations can improve the understanding of risks (Ancker et al., 2006; Kurz-Milcke et al., 2008; Zikmund-Fisher et al., 2008). Consequently, the use of visual displays is often recommended for communicating risks (e.g., Paling, 2003; Spiegelhalter et al., 2011), although research on graphical displays remains largely an atheoretical endeavor (Lipkus, 2007).

Graphical formats have been shown to be especially helpful for people with low numerical abilities (Garcia-Retamero & Galesic, 2009; Galesic et al., 2009, see Chapter 7 in this volume). They can help reduce several

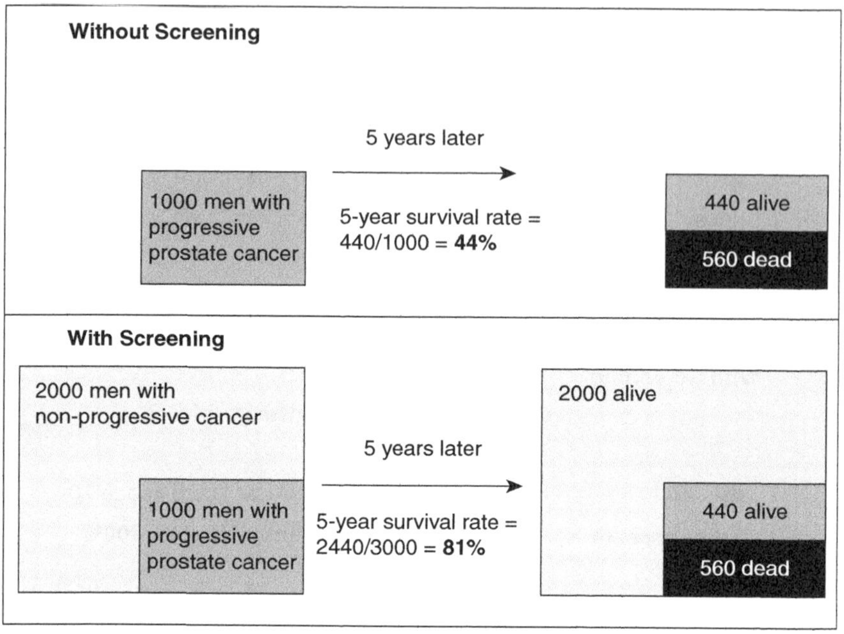

Figure 2.3. Overdiagnosis bias (adapted from Gigerenzer et al., 2007).

biases, such as denominator neglect (Garcia-Retamero, 2010), framing effects (Garcia-Retamero & Cokely, 2011; Garcia-Retamero & Galesic, 2010a), or the undue influence of narrative information (Fagerlin et al., 2005), and they can help people understand more complicated concepts such as incremental risk (Zikmund-Fisher et al., 2008). Indeed, even children in elementary school understand statistical information better when it is presented graphically than with numbers alone (Multmeier, 2013).

An important caveat is, however, that some people have problems with extracting data and meaning from visual displays. Galesic & Garcia-Retamero (2011) developed a graph literacy scale that predicts who actually profits from visual displays (Garcia-Retamero & Galesic, 2010b), and it has been shown that people who lack graph literacy could actually be better off with mere numbers (Gaissmaier et al., 2012). One solution to this could be to simplify graphs. For instance, it has been shown that graphs are more easily understandable when they do not include redundant information about mortality statistics (Zikmund-Fisher et al., 2010). At the same time, it is important to be very careful not to make graphs too flashy even though this may make them look more appealing, as too many animations can actually hinder the acquisition of knowledge about the efficacy of treatment options in comparison to static graphs (Zikmund-Fisher et al., 2012).

Overcoming low reading abilities

While research has focused mostly on low levels of numeracy and proposed presentation formats that can also be understood by people with low numerical abilities, understanding the written explanations and descriptions is just as important for making an informed decision and poses a non-trivial problem for communicating risks to non-native speakers or people with low levels of education. According to the 1992 National Adult Literacy Survey, nearly half of the adults in the United States population have limited or low literacy skills, and more than 90 million Americans lack the skills necessary for understanding health information (Kirsch et al., 1993; Paasche-Orlow et al., 2005). This means that up to 50% of the adult population in the US may not even be able to understand the written parts of the medical information properly.

One could argue that an even more basic approach is needed to address the problem of communicating clinical evidence effectively. Next, we will discuss whether presenting narrative evidence or health information in movies can help in this regard.

Statistical versus narrative evidence

As presented in the opening example of Tony Romo and his dad, a typical form of narratives is patient testimonials, and they need not represent the scientific evidence at all. What weight do those testimonials have on patients' healthcare decisions? Ubel et al. (2001) examined the impact of patient testimonials compared to statistical evidence on hypothetical treatment choices for angina. They asked participants to choose between bypass surgery and balloon angioplasty. Subjects were told that balloon angioplasty was effective in 50% of the cases, while surgery was successful in 75% of cases. In addition to the statistical information, participants also received accounts of patients who underwent surgery or angioplasty and reported their experiences. For some of the participants, the proportion of patient reports matched the statistical information: two patients were cured of angina after angioplasty and two were not, and three patients felt relief after bypass surgery, while one patient did not benefit from the treatment. Other participants received disproportionate patient testimonials where the success rates did not match the evidence for bypass surgery, making it appear less effective. Subjects who heard these disproportionate testimonials were less likely to choose bypass surgery for treatment.

From the perspective of informed decision making, the effects of testimonials on medical decisions are undesirable. Thus, it remains questionable whether testimonials could ever be part of solving problems with the communication of clinical evidence, and whether they should be used at all. Problems related to this kind of narrative evidence are probably even more pronounced for movies in which testimonials appear even more vividly. However, as the next section illustrates, this does not mean that movies need to be dismissed altogether as a means of health education even from the perspective of advocates of informed decision making.

Health information in movies

Movies displaying patient testimonials like the one about Tony Romo's dad are vehicles for transporting health messages to people, which would otherwise not be reached by written or numerical information. These movies are double-edged swords – they have the potential to mislead, but also to inform, as we will discuss next.

Movies can make it easier to understand certain health states or treatment options than verbal or written information alone, leading to a better-informed decision. El-Jawahri et al. (2010) studied how informational videos affected preferences regarding end-of-life care in patients with malignant glioma. Patients received information about life-prolonging care, basic medical care, and comfort care either in a verbal description or in a video showing patients in typical care settings in addition to the verbal description. Most patients who received only verbal information chose basic medical care, with some choosing comfort care or life-prolonging care. For those who watched the video, more than 90% favored comfort care, and none of the patients chose life-prolonging care. Patients who received the video also acquired more knowledge about the different care options and stated less uncertainty about their decision compared to patients who received the verbal information only. Volandes et al. (2010) showed a similar effect for patients when shown movies about patients with dementia, and reported that uncertainty regarding the decision decreased and knowledge about care options increased especially for patients who were less literate and had a poor understanding of medical terminology. Finally, Frosch et al. (2001) showed that sometimes being informed better and changing behavior go hand in hand. In their study, the better informed patients were about PSA testing, the less enthusiastic they were about screening. While 97.7% of men with standard written information requested a PSA test, only 50% of the men who watched an informational movie explaining the pros and cons of PSA-screening and had the opportunity to ask questions afterwards wanted to take the test.

Importantly, health information is not only acquired through educational movies. In recent years, entertainment TV shows like *Emergency Room*, *Grey's Anatomy*, *House MD*, and *Scrubs* have attracted millions of viewers with a mixture of soap opera elements and medical facts. These shows not only feature personal drama, but also convey medical information. Two studies from the Kaiser Family Foundation show how two prominent medical entertainment TV shows – *Emergency Room* and *Grey's Anatomy* – impact health knowledge in viewers. Brodie et al. (2001) interviewed regular viewers of *Emergency Room* regarding their knowledge about human papillomavirus (HPV) and emergency contraception options, which were featured in two episodes. Knowledge concerning HPV and emergency contraception increased directly after the show, compared to before the episode was aired.

In a follow-up study, Rideout (2008) worked with medical advisors of the TV series *Grey's Anatomy* to include statistical information about the transmission rate of HIV from mother to child during pregnancy in one of the episodes. Viewers learn that the chance of having a healthy baby is 98% with adequate medication and care. Before the episode was aired, only 15% of the interviewed regular viewers of *Grey's Anatomy* estimated the chance of having a healthy baby to be about as high. In the week after the episode was shown correct answers increased significantly to 61%. And knowledge was not only retained short-term: even 6 weeks afterwards, 45% of viewers still estimated the chances correctly. With an audience of about 17.5 million viewers, the additional 46% of viewers who gained knowledge about transmission rates at least short-term amount to about 8 million people who unintentionally learned about an important health topic.

In sum, health movies can change care preferences, lead to more knowledge, and help people make decisions with more certainty, especially for those who struggle to understand written information in health-related domains. Health information is not only conveyed via movies produced for that purpose, but also through entertainment media. Careful consideration of the facts stated in those shows is therefore advised.

Conclusion

Making informed health decisions requires available information on the effectiveness and risks of the options. But what patients often find is not transparently communicated data, but persuasive messages aiming at changing behavior towards the goals of the sender rather than informing the patient honestly. And even when statistical evidence is given, it is often presented in a confusing format – as survival rates, relative risks, and single event probabilities, making it unlikely that patients can derive meaningful information from these numbers. Instead, transparent numbers should be communicated – mortality rates instead of survival rates, absolute risks instead of relative ones, and natural frequencies instead of conditional probabilities (for more information see Gigerenzer et al., 2007). It would be helpful in this regard if regulators enforced the provision of complete and transparent information. For instance, to summarize the benefits and harms of drugs, Schwartz et al. (2007, 2009) developed the format of drug facts boxes – simple tabular displays of clinical evidence – and showed that they are well understood by laypeople. Educational movies, but also entertainment media, can be used as additional vehicles to provide transparent information to patients who would otherwise not be reached by written information. Only patients who understand the clinical evidence can really make informed decisions and participate in care and treatment planning.

Special attention should be devoted to information multipliers in our society – the journalists who pick up the latest developments from medical journals and make them accessible to a wide audience of doctors, patients, and the general public. Their reports can only be as good as the information on which it is based. As we have seen, neither doctors nor journalists are likely to find transparent information in medical journals or information brochures. We have also seen that a simple training can create insight in doctors. It is time that we extend the training efforts to journalists who encounter the same non-transparent representations of clinical evidence. At the same time, editors of medical journals need to enforce transparent reporting in abstracts more strictly (Gigerenzer et al., 2010), and also the issue of more high-quality press releases would help improve the situation (Schwartz et al., 2012). But even when medicine merely serves as the stage for personal drama in the entertainment media, the audience does not disregard the information presented. It will pick it up and potentially use it to make healthcare decisions for themselves or their families. This gives entertainment shows great power. But, as the movie *Spider-Man* reminds us, with great power comes great responsibility, in this case to present information *accurately* and *accessibly* for a wide range of audience to understand.

As early as the 1930s, H. G. Wells (1938/1994) predicted that for an educated citizenship in a modern democracy, statistical thinking would be as indispensable as reading and writing. At the beginning of the twenty-first century, nearly everyone in industrial societies has been taught reading and writing, but not statistical thinking. Today, statistical illiteracy is prevalent in all parts of society – patients, doctors, journalists, politicians, and students. We need programs that teach statistical thinking as early as possible to vaccinate the next generation, so that non-transparent formats can no longer mislead.

References

Ancker, J. S., Senathirajah, Y., Kukafka, R., & Starren, J. B. (2006). Design features of graphs in health risk communication: A systematic review. *Journal of the American Medical Informatics Association*, 13, 608–618.

Andriole, G. L., Crawford, E. D., Grubb, R. L., 3rd, Buys, S. S., Chia, D., Church, T. R., et al. (2009). Mortality results from a randomized prostate-cancer screening trial. *New England Journal of Medicine*, 360, 1310–1319.

Arkes, H. R., & Gaissmaier, W. (2012). Psychological research and the prostate-cancer screening controversy. *Psychological Science*, 23, 547–553.

Barry, M. D. (1999). Involving patients in medical decisions. *Journal of the American Medical Association*, 282, 2356–2357.

Brodie, M., Foehr, U., Rideout, V., Baer, N., Miller, C., Floury, R., et al. (2001). Communicating health information through the entertainment media. *Health Affairs*, 20, 192–199.

Covey, J. (2007). A meta-analysis of the effects of presenting treatment benefits in different formats. *Medical Decision Making*, 27, 638–654.

Djulbegovic, M., Beyth, R. J., Neuberger, M. M., Stoffs, T. L., Vieweg, J., Djulbegovic, B., et al. (2010). Screening for prostate cancer: systematic review and meta-analysis of randomised controlled trials. *British Medical Journal*, 341, c4543.

Dobbs, M. (2007). *Rudy was wrong on cancer survival chances*. Retrieved April 14, 2011 from: blog.washingtonpost.com/fact-checker/2007/10/rudy_miscalculates_cancer_surv.html

El-Jawahri, A., Podgurski, L. M., Eichler, A. F., Plotkin, S. R., Temel, J. S., Mitchell, S. L., et al. (2010). Use of video to facilitate end-of-life discussions with patients with cancer: a randomized controlled trial. *Journal of Clinical Oncology*, 28, 305–310.

Fagerlin, A., Wang, C., & Ubel, P. A. (2005). Reducing the influence of anecdotal reasoning on people's health care decisions: is a picture worth a thousand statistics? *Medical Decision Making*, 25, 398–405.

Frosch, D. L., Kaplan, R. M., & Felitti, V. (2001). The evaluation of two methods to facilitate shared decision making for men considering prostate-specific antigen test. *Journal of General Internal Medicine*, 16, 391–398.

Gaissmaier, W., & Gigerenzer, G. (2011). When misinformed patients try to make informed health decisions. In: G. Gigerenzer & J. A. M. Gray (Eds.), *Better Doctors, Better Patients, Better Decisions: Envisioning Healthcare 2020*. Strüngman Forum Report, Vol. 6. Cambridge, MA: MIT Press; pp. 29–42.

Gaissmaier, W., Wegwarth, O., Skopec, D., Müller, A.-S., Broschinski, S., & Politi, M. C. (2012). Numbers can be worth a thousand pictures: Individual differences in understanding graphical and numerical representations of health-related information. *Health Psychology*, 31, 286–296.

Galesic, M., Garcia-Retamero, R., & Gigerenzer, G. (2009). Using icon arrays to communicate medical risks to low-numeracy people. *Health Psychology*, 28, 210–216.

Galesic, M., & Garcia-Retamero, R. (2010). Statistical numeracy in health: A cross-cultural comparison with probabilistic national samples. *Archives of Internal Medicine*, 170, 462–468.

Galesic, M., & Garcia-Retamero, R. (2011). Graph literacy: a cross-cultural comparison. *Medical Decision Making*, 31, 444–457.

Garcia-Retamero, R., & Cokely, E. T. (2011). Effective communication of risks to young adults: Using message framing and visual aids to increase condom use and STD screening. *Journal of Experimental Psychology: Applied*, 17, 270–287.

Garcia-Retamero, R., & Galesic, M. (2009). Communicating treatment risk reduction to people with low numeracy skills: A cross-cultural comparison. *American Journal of Public Health*, 99, 2196–2202.

Garcia-Retamero, R., & Galesic, M. (2010a). How to reduce the effect of framing on messages about health. *Journal of General Internal Medicine*, 25, 1323–1329.

Garcia-Retamero, R., & Galesic, M. (2010b). Who profits from visual aids: Overcoming challenges in people's understanding of risks. *Social Science and Medicine*, 70, 1019–1025.

Garcia-Retamero, R., Galesic, M., & Gigerenzer, G. (2010). Do icon arrays help reduce denominator neglect? *Medical Decision Making*, 30, 672–684.

Gigerenzer, G., & Gray, J. A. M. (Eds.). (2011). *Better Doctors, Better Patients, Better Decisions: Envisioning Health Care 2020.* Cambridge, MA: MIT Press.

Gigerenzer, G., Gaissmaier, W., Kurz-Milcke, E., Schwartz, L. M., & Woloshin, S. (2007). Helping doctors and patients make sense of health statistics. *Psychological Science in the Public Interest*, 8, 53–96.

Gigerenzer, G., & Hoffrage, U. (1995). How to improve Bayesian reasoning without instruction: frequency formats. *Psychological Review*, 102, 684–704.

Gigerenzer, G., Hertwig, R., van den Broek, R., Fasolo, B., & Katsikopoulos, K. (2005). "A 30% chance of rain tomorrow": how does the public understand weather forecasts? *Risk Analysis*, 25, 623–629.

Gigerenzer, G., Mata, J., & Frank, R. (2009). Public knowledge of benefits of breast and prostate cancer screening in Europe. *Journal of the National Cancer Institute*, 101, 1216–1220.

Gigerenzer, G., Wegwarth, O., & Feufel, M. (2010). Misleading communication of risk. *British Medical Journal*, 341, 791–792.

Hamm, R. M., Bard, D. E., & Scheid, D. C. (2003). Influence of numeracy upon patient's prostate cancer screening probability judgments. *Annual Meeting of the Society for Judgment and Decision Making.* Vancouver, British Columbia, Canada.

Heesen, C., Kleiter, I., Nguyen, F., Schäffler, N., Kasper, J., Köpke, S., et al. (2010). Risk perceptions in natalizumab-treated multiple sclerosis patients and their neurologists. *Multiple Sclerosis*, 16, 1507–1512.

Kirsch, I., Jungblut, A., Jenkins, L., & Kolstad, A. (1993). *Adult Literacy in America: A First Look at the Results of the National Adult Literacy Survey.* Washington, DC: National Center for Educational Statistics.

Kurz-Milcke, E., Gigerenzer, G., & Martignon, L. (2008). Transparency in risk communication: Graphical and analog tools. In: W. T. Tucker, S. Ferson, A. Finkel, T. F. Long, D. Slavin, & P. Wright (Eds.), *Strategies for Risk Communication: Evolution, Evidence, Experience 1128. Annals of the New York Academy of Sciences*. New York: Blackwell; pp. 18–28.

Lipkus, I. M. (2007). Numeric, verbal, and visual formats of conveying health risks: Suggested best practices and future recommendations. *Medical Decision Making*, 27, 696–713.

Multmeier, J. (2013). Representations facilitate Bayesian reasoning: Computational facilitation and ecological design revisited. PhD thesis, Free University, Berlin.

O'Connor, A. M., Wennberg, J. E., Legare, F., Llewellyn-Thomas, H. A., Moulton, B. W., Sepucha, K. R., et al. (2007). Towards the 'tipping point': decision aids and informed patient choice. *Health Affairs*, 26, 716–725.

Paasche-Orlow, M. K., Parker, R. M., Gazmararian, J. A., Nielsen-Bohlman, L. T., & Rudd, R. R. (2005). The prevalence of limited health literacy. *Journal of General Internal Medicine*, 20, 175–184.

Paling, J. (2003). Strategies to help patients understand risks. *British Medical Journal*, 327, 745–748.

Paulos, J. A. (1988). *Innumeracy: Mathematical Illiteracy and its Consequences*. New York: Hill and Wang.

Reyna, V. F., Nelson, W. L., Han, P. K., & Dieckmann, N. F. (2009). How numeracy influences risk comprehension and medical decision making. *Psychological Bulletin*, 135, 943–973.

Rideout, V. (2008). *Television as a Health Educator: A Case Study of Grey's Anatomy*. The Henry J. Kaiser Family Foundation.

Sandblom, G., Varenhorst, E., Rosell, J., Löfman, O., & Carlsson, P. (2011). Randomised prostate cancer screening trial: 20 year follow-up. *British Medical Journal*, 342, d1539.

Schröder, F. H., Hugosson, J., Roobol, M. J., Tammela, T. L., Ciatto, S., Nelen, V., et al. (2009). Screening and prostate-cancer mortality in a randomized European study. *New England Journal of Medicine*, 360, 1320–1328.

Schwartz, L. M., Woloshin, S., Black, W. C., & Welch, H. G. (1997). The role of numeracy in understanding the benefit of screening mammography. *Annals of Internal Medicine*, 127, 966–972.

Schwartz, L. M., Woloshin, S., & Welch, H. G. (2007). The drug facts box: Providing consumers with simple tabular data on drug benefit and harm. *Medical Decision Making*, 27, 655–662.

Schwartz, L. M., Woloshin, S., & Welch, H. G. (2009). Using a drug facts box to communicate drug benefits and harms. *Annals of Internal Medicine*, 150, 516–527.

Schwartz, L. M., Woloshin, S., Andrews, A., & Stukel, T. A. (2012). Influence of medical journal press releases on the quality of associated newspaper coverage: retrospective cohort study. *British Medical Journal*, 344, d8164.

Sedrakyan, A., & Shih, C. (2007). Improving depiction of benefits and harms: analyses of studies of well-known therapeutics and review of high-impact medical journals. *Medical Care*, 45(10 Suppl 2), S23–28.

Shibata, A., & Whittemore, A. S. (2001). Re: prostate cancer incidence and mortality in the United States and the United Kingdom. *Journal of the National Cancer Institute*, 93, 1109–1110.

Slaytor, E. K., & Ward, J. E. (1998). How risks of breast cancer and benefits of screening are communicated to women: analysis of 58 pamphlets. *British Medical Journal (Clinical research ed.)*, 317(7153), 263–264.

Spiegelhalter, D., Pearson, M., & Short, I. (2011). Visualizing uncertainty about the future. *Science*, 333, 1393–1400.

Thaler, R. H., & Sunstein, C. R. (2008). *Nudge: Improving Decisions About Health, Wealth, and Happiness*. New Haven, CT: Yale University Press.

Ubel, P., Jepson, C., & Baron, J. (2001). The inclusion of patient testimonials in decision aids: effects on treatment choices. *Medical Decision Making*, 21, 60–68.

US Preventive Services Task Force. (2002). *Guide to Clinical Preventive Services: Report of the US Preventive Services Task Force* (3rd edn.). Baltimore, MD: Williams & Wilkins.

Volandes, A. E., Barry, M. J., Chang, Y., & Paasche-Orlow, M. K. (2010). Improving decision making at the end of life with video images. *Medical Decision Making*, 30, 29–34.

Wegwarth, O., Gaissmaier, W., & Gigerenzer, G. (2011). Deceiving numbers: Survival rates and their impact on doctors' risk communication. *Medical Decision Making*, 31, 386–394.

Wegwarth, O., Schwartz, L. M., Woloshin, S., Gaissmaier, W., & Gigerenzer, G. (2012). Do physicians understand cancer screening statistics? A national survey of primary care physicians in the U.S. *Annals of Internal Medicine*, 156, 340–349.

Welch, H. G., Schwartz, L. M., & Woloshin, S. (2000). Are increasing 5-year survival rates evidence for success against cancer? *Journal of the American Medical Association*, 283, 2975–2978.

Wells, H. G. (1994). *World Brain*. London: Cambridge University Press. (Original work published in 1938.)

Wilde, J. (2009). *PSA screening cuts deaths by 20%, says world's largest prostate cancer study*. Retrieved April 14, 2011 from: www.erspc-media.org/release090318.php

Zikmund-Fisher, B. J., Ubel, P. A., Smith, D. M., Derry, H. A., McClure, J. B., Stark, A. T., et al. (2008). Communicating side effect risks in a tamoxifen prophylaxis decision aid: The debiasing influence of pictographs. *Patient Education and Counseling*, 73, 209–214.

Zikmund-Fisher, B. J., Fagerlin, A., & Ubel, P. A. (2010). A demonstration of "less can be more" in risk graphics. *Medical Decision Making*, 30, 661–671.

Zikmund-Fisher, B. J., Witteman, H. O., Fuhrel-Forbis, A., Exe, N. L., Kahn, V. C., & Dickson, M. (2012). Animated graphics for comparing two risks: a cautionary tale. *Journal of Medical Internet Research*, 14, e106.

3 Physicians' understanding and use of numeric information

Britta L. Anderson & Jay Schulkin

Introduction

Whether they are reading test results, discussing risks with their patients, or evaluating the evidence used to develop guidelines, physicians are constantly working with numbers. Their role as medical providers requires that they be able to not only read and understand numeric information and statistics, but also communicate this information to their patients. Throughout this chapter we use the term "numeracy" to refer to the basic ability to convert numbers between formats and answer questions about basic probability and we use the term "statistical literacy" to refer to the ability to use, understand, and apply statistics and biostatistics information. Though these terms are used interchangeably in the literature, we distinguish between the two for this chapter because in physician samples, statistical literacy tests have assessed knowledge about statistical concepts or the application of statistics, whereas numeracy tests have assessed basic math abilities and computations.

The beginning of this chapter reviews research on physician numeracy. Studies with the general population have examined the association between numeracy and medical decision making (see Chapter 4 by Zikmund-Fisher and colleagues). However, only a few studies have examined numeracy and medical decision making in physicians. We will review this literature and compare it to research with the general population. The majority of this chapter will focus on statistical literacy. Many studies have assessed physicians' understanding of statistical concepts and their ability to complete statistical tasks. We provide examples of studies on physicians' statistical literacy and then examine the evolving role of statistics in clinical medicine, physicians' statistical literacy training, finally, we conclude by making suggestions for future research.

Physician numeracy

As reviewed by Zikmund-Fisher and colleagues in Chapter 4 of this volume, the numeracy skills (i.e., the basic ability to convert numbers between formats and answer questions about basic probability) of patients are associated with their health decisions, reasoning about health risks, and health outcomes. Corresponding research on physicians is sparse. This is due in part to the belief that physicians have advanced training and should have no difficulties with basic number problems. However, results from initial studies suggest that this is not the case for all physicians.

Objective numeracy: As discussed in Chapter 1 by Cokely and colleagues, the initial objective numeracy measures (the measures that have typically been used with physicians) assess the ability to complete questions about basic probability and to convert between frequencies and percentages (Schwartz et al., 1997; Lipkus et al., 2001). Examples of the questions include "If Person A's risk of getting a disease is 1% in ten years, and Person B's risk is double that of A's, what is B's risk?," or "If the chance of getting a disease is 20 out of 100, this would be the same as having a ____% chance of getting the disease."

Though these measures include only basic numeracy questions that all physicians should be able to answer, only 53–75% of physician samples answered all the questions correctly over four studies (Estrada et al., 1999; Hanoch et al., 2010; Anderson et al., 2011; Anderson & Schulkin, 2011). The samples in these studies varied: some were convenience samples at grand rounds and others were volunteer survey participants. The question items and length of the questionnaires differed as well (ranging from 3 to 11 questions). A recent study directly compared the numeracy skills of physicians with those of their patients and found that physicians had significantly higher scores on the numeracy test than patients: of the twelve possible points, physicians' mean score was 10.6 (SD = 1.3) and the patients' mean score was 8.9 (SD = 1.8) (Garcia-Retamero & Hoffrage, 2013).

Two studies have assessed how objective numeracy was associated with physicians' judgments and decision making. One study assessed whether physicians' numeracy scores were associated with their recommendations about the most beneficial Medicare Part D plan. Physicians were provided with information about a hypothetical patient as well as information about either 3, 10, or 20 Medicare Part D plans. They were then asked to choose which plan would be best for that patient. Both the number of plans that they reviewed and the physicians' numeracy scores were significant predictors of whether or not physicians recommend the more optimal plan. Physicians who received information about fewer plans and physicians with higher numeracy were more likely to recommend the more optimal plan (Hanoch et al., 2010). These results were in line with similar studies with the general population, where patients also make more optimal decisions when they are provided with only the most important information rather than all the information (Peters et al., 2007; Wood et al., 2011).

Another study examined whether patient and physician numeracy scores were associated with the ability to make diagnostic inferences about the results of a screening test and whether visual aids facilitated understanding (Garcia-Retamero & Hoffrage, 2013). A Bayesian reasoning task was used where participants were provided with the relevant statistical information (prevalence, sensitivity, and false-positive rate) and asked to estimate the chances that the patient had the condition if they received a positive screening test result. Some of the doctors also received visual aids. Not only did more numerate patients and physicians have more accurate responses, but visual aids helped both patients and physicians. These results, along with the results of Hanoch et al. (2010), suggest that the differences in reasoning and decision making between high and low numerate physicians are similar to the differences in reasoning and decision making between high and low numerate patients, though more research needs to be done with physicians to examine this further.

Subjective numeracy: When objective numeracy measures are intimidating or too time consuming for study participants, subjective measures can be used. Subjective numeracy scales gather information about individuals' self-reported abilities with numbers. The Subjective Numeracy Scale is a validated eight question measure (Fagerlin et al., 2007; Zikmund-Fisher et al., 2007) that asks participants to rate their own numeracy ability and preference for using number information. For example, one question asks, "How good are you at working with fractions?," to which respondents answer on a 6-point scale from 1 (not at all good) to 6 (extremely good). When administered to a physician sample, the mean subjective numeracy scale score was 4.9 (SD = 0.7) out of a possible of 6 (Anderson et al., 2011). Along with measuring performance on the subjective numeracy scale, this study also examined whether higher subjective numeracy was associated with a preference to communicate using numeric information (as opposed to qualitative information). Indeed, the higher ob-gyns rated their numeracy skills, the more likely they were to indicate that they use quantitative information.

In sum, the findings of the limited number of studies on physician numeracy thus far show that, although physicians perform better than the general population, not all physicians have mastered basic numeracy skills. Findings also show that physicians' objective numeracy is associated with reasoning and decision making, and that subjective numeracy is associated with physicians' reported communication. However, given that physicians in different specialties and practice locations perform considerably different tasks in their day-to-day practices, associations between number skills and decision making or communication may differ across specialties and practice locations.

Physicians' statistical literacy

Physicians recognize the relevance of statistics to their practice (Windish et al., 2007; Swift et al., 2009). For example, in one study, around 90% of physicians indicated that an understanding of probabilities and statistics would help them with such clinical tasks as explaining the levels of risks to patients, interpreting results of screening tests, and accessing clinical guidelines (Swift et al., 2009). Yet, physicians also report that they do not have the necessary statistical skills and that they would like to improve their abilities (Windish et al., 2007; Swift et al., 2009). Ninety-five percent of residents in one sample indicated that it was important to understand all of the statistics that they encounter in journal articles, but 75% indicated that they could not currently do so (Windish et al., 2007). Indeed, many studies have found that not all physicians have mastered the statistical skills that are relevant to their practice (Lancet, 1937; Weiss & Samet, 1980; Friedman & Phillips, 1981; Wulf et al., 1987; Estrada et al., 1999; Young et al., 2002; Halvorsen et al., 2003; Ghosh et al., 2004; Bramwell et al., 2006; Gigerenzer et al., 2007; Anderson et al., 2011; Wegwarth et al., 2011, 2012; Obrecht et al. 2012).

The sections below review our research with obstetricians and gynecologists and similar studies from other physician samples in order to provide examples of recent research on physicians' statistical literacy. These studies measured physicians' range of statistical literacy abilities as well as their understanding of screening statistics and Bayesian Reasoning. We also discuss a study on physicians' communication of statistical information.

Range of statistical literacy abilities: Research studies assessing statistical knowledge and abilities have shown that only a minority of physicians have broad statistical skills. One recent study surveyed a national sample of obstetrician gynecologists to evaluate their statistical literacy skills using a 14 item multiple-choice questionnaire. The items were either statistical facts (e.g., the number of women in the USA who have HIV), statistical concepts (e.g., identifying whether a statistic is the prevalence or incidence), or number relationships (e.g., converting between frequencies and percentages), and were tailored to clinical topics that were relevant to the specialty.

Performance on the statistical facts questions was quite variable. Many physicians over- or underestimated the number of women in the USA living with HIV/AIDS and the number of women diagnosed with cancer each year by twofold or more (Anderson et al., 2012). Physicians were better able to answer questions in which they were asked to convert and compute numbers (relationship questions) than those in which they were asked to identify the correct statistical terms (concept questions). Where 21% answered all the concept questions correctly, 36% of respondents answered all of the relationship questions correctly. Though few ob-gyns answered all of the concept questions correctly, each item was answered correctly by the majority of the sample. For example, two questions asked participants to indicate whether the numeric information was the incidence rate (the number of new cases of a disease within a specified time interval (e.g., over 1 year)) or the prevalence (the total number of cases of a disease at a certain point in time (e.g., the day that the sample was tested)). When the statement had an incidence rate, 74% identified it correctly, and when the statement had a prevalence rate, 68% identified it correctly. The question that was the most difficult for participants to answer was one that asked them to calculate the number needed to treat (often abbreviated NNT), which is the number of people who need to receive an intervention in order to save one person from an adverse outcome. Though it has been shown to be a difficult concept to grasp (e.g., Halvorsen et al., 2003), number needed to treat (and similar terms like number needed to invite to screen (NNI)) continues to be used in guidelines and other health literature.

In another study, which surveyed internal medicine residents (Windish et al., 2007), a questionnaire was developed that assessed statistical terminology, knowledge of study design, and interpretation of study results. For example, one question asked participants to recognize a continuous variable, another asked them to indicate which statistical method should be used to test the hypothesis that there were mean differences across groups, and another asked them to choose which of four options best described the purpose of a double-blind study. The mean score on this test was 41% correct. When asked to interpret the meaning of a *p*-value, only 59% of respondents were able to do so. The authors of this study also identified characteristics that were associated with better performance on the questionnaire. Those who had an advanced medical degree, had completed medical school more recently, belonged to a university-based program, had biostatistics training, and were male tended to perform better on the questionnaire.

Screening statistics: In addition to assessing the breadth of physicians' statistical skills, recent studies have also investigated abilities and understanding of specific concepts like screening statistics. For example, Wegwarth and colleagues (2012) assessed whether a national sample of US physicians knew which statistics they should use to determine if a screening test is beneficial. Although the 5-year survival rate is commonly used to report progress in treating cancer, it can be a misleading statistic when comparing groups who participate in screening to groups who do not. As described previously (see Chapter 2), the lead-time bias and overdiagnosis bias are two ways in which screening statistics can exaggerate the benefits of screening when comparing those that screen and those that do not. To conduct this study Wegwarth and colleagues developed two hypothetical screening tests about prostate cancer and paired them with 5-year survival statistics and mortality statistics. They then assessed what impact the statistics had on the physicians' recommendation of the screening test to a hypothetical patient. The type of cancer and the kind of screening test were purposely not mentioned in the study to prevent physicians' from basing their recommendations on prior knowledge or opinions about the type of cancer or screening test.

When the hypothetical screening tests were paired with a 5-year survival rate, the tests were more likely to be recommended than when the tests were paired with the cancer mortality statistic. In fact, physicians were three times more likely to recommend the test when the impact of the test was described in terms of a 5-year survival rate than when it was presented as a change in mortality rate (Wegwarth et al., 2012).

In a similar study with a sample of 65 German physicians, Wegwarth and colleagues (2011) found similar trends. Screening tests that were described in terms of an increased 5-year survival were recommended to hypothetical patients more often (66%) than tests that were described in terms of reduced mortality (8%). This study also found that only 2 of the 54 responders provided the correct definition for "lead-time bias" (i.e., that screening may impact the amount of time until diagnosis without increasing the time to death) and none of the responders provided the correct definition for "length-time bias" (i.e., detecting a slow progressing cancer that would never become clinically significant; also referred to as overdiagnosis bias).

Bayesian Reasoning: Physicians also need to understand the likelihood that a patient has the disease when they get a positive screening test result, or the positive predictive value, which can be derived using Bayes Theorem (see Ashby, 2006; Fischhoff and Beyth-Marom, 1983; Baron 2000 for application of Bayes Theorem to decision making).

Figure 3.1 provides an example of a Bayesian problem written in two different formats and an explanation of how to calculate the correct answer (taken from Bramwell et al., 2006).

Two recent studies have manipulated elements of Bayesian problems to assess their impact on clinically relevant contexts (Bramwell et al., 2006; Obrecht et al., 2012). Bramwell and colleagues (2006) compared performance when the problem provided numeric information in natural frequency format with performance when the same information was presented in the percentage format. The natural frequency format is thought to improve performance on Bayesian problems because it provides information about the reference class, while the other formats such as percentages have been

Version 1: Percentages

The serum test screens pregnant women for babies with Down syndrome. The test is a very good one, but not perfect. Roughly 1% of babies have Down syndrome. If the baby has Down syndrome, there is a 90% chance that the result will be positive. If the baby is unaffected, there is still a 1% chance that the result will be positive. A pregnant woman has been tested and the result is positive. What is the chance that her baby actually has Down syndrome?

_____%

Version 2: Frequencies

The serum test screens pregnant women for babies with Down syndrome. The test is a very good one, but not perfect. Roughly 100 babies out of 10 000 have Down syndrome. Of these 100 babies with Down syndrome, 90 will have a positive test result. Of the remaining 9900 unaffected babies, 99 will still have a positive test result. How many pregnant women who have a positive result to the test actually have a baby with Down syndrome?

___ out of ____

An explanation of how to derive the correct answer

* If 10 000 pregnant women were tested, we would expect 100 (1% of 10 000) to have babies with Down syndrome.
* Of these 100 babies with Down syndrome, the test result would be positive for 90 (90% of 100) and negative for 10
* Of the 9900 unaffected babies, 99 (1% of 9900) will also test positive, and 9801 will have a negative test result
* So, out of the 10 000 pregnant women tested, we would expect to see 189 (90+99) positive test results. Only 90 of these actually have babies with Down syndrome, which is 47.6%
* Therefore, 47.6% of pregnant women who have a positive result to test would actually have a baby with Down syndrome

Figure 3.1. Example of a Bayesian problem and an explanation of how to calculate the correct answer. (Reproduced with permission from Bramwell et al., 2006.)

normalized. Physicians in this study performed much better when information was provided in the frequency format: 65% answered correctly with frequency format while only 5% were able to do so with percentage format (this is similar to what was found by Hoffrage and Gigerenzer, 1998. See also Gigerenzer & Hoffrage, 1995). Interestingly, the study also assessed how confident physicians were in their response and found that confidence did not correlate with performance. On a scale from 1 (not at all confident) to 6 (very confident), almost half (49%) of those who answered the Bayesian question incorrectly rated their confidence as 5 or 6.

In another study (Obrecht et al., 2012), researchers assessed whether physicians had more accurate Bayesian estimates when thinking about past events than when making predictions about future events. Ob-gyns were asked to estimate the posterior probability that a patient has a fetus with Down syndrome given a positive test result. They were then asked to estimate the prevalence of Down syndrome in their practice, the sensitivity of the test (i.e., if the fetus has Down syndrome, what are the chances that the test will be positive?), and the false-positive rate of the test (i.e., if the fetus does not have Down syndrome, what are the chances that the test will be positive?). These three estimates were used to calculate a posterior probability, which was then compared to the physicians' estimated posterior probability as a measure of consistency. Physicians were asked to make these estimates under one of these three conditions: (1) by thinking about patients in general (single event probability), (2) by thinking about patients they had seen in the past year (retrospective natural frequency, which provides a reference class), and (3) by thinking about patients they will see in the next year (prospective natural frequency, which also provides a reference class). See Table 3.1.

As shown in Figure 3.2, physicians who made estimates by thinking about their past experiences (retrospective condition) tended to be the most consistent in their estimates. These results suggest that, not only does the format of numeric information impact Bayesian reasoning, but the way in which physicians draw information to think about various situations can also impact their Bayesian reasoning.

Table 3.1. *Instructions for the three conditions in a study assessing physicians' Bayesian estimates.*

	Retrospective natural frequency	Prospective natural frequency	Single event probability
Question format	In the past year some of your pregnant patients received positive results. . .about how many of them	In the next year some of your pregnant patients will receive positive results. . .about how many of them	One of your pregnant patients received a positive result. . .how likely
Response	____ cases of Down out of____positive second trimester test results	____ cases of Down out of ____ positive second trimester test results	____ % chance

Obrecht et al., 2012.

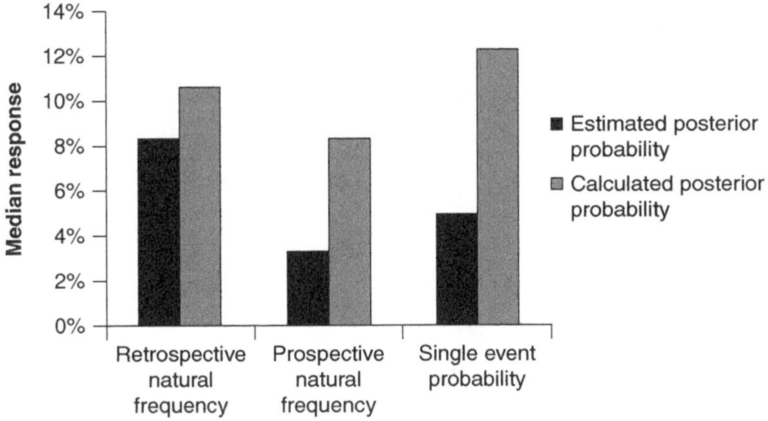

Figure 3.2. The way physicians draw information about their patient population (by thinking about future patients or past experiences) will impact their reasoning and their accuracy in their Bayesian inferences. There were smaller differences in the estimated and calculated probabilities among those who were asked to answer the questions by thinking about patients they had seen in the past year (retrospective natural frequency) than the two other conditions. (Created using median scores from Obrecht et al., 2012.)

Communication of statistical information: Along with using and understanding numeric information, the communication of numeric information is also an important role of a clinician. In order to determine which numeric information physicians would choose to communicate to patients when a variety of statistics were available to them, we examined ob-gyns' communication to hypothetical patients about the benefits and side effects of antidepressants (Gaissmaier et al., 2014).

Participants received statistical information from a clinical trial about the benefit of taking an antidepressant as well as the possible side effects (dry mouth and sexual problems). Physicians received the event rates (rate of depression or the side effect under treatment and placebo), the relative risk reduction/increase, and the absolute risk reduction/increase of the drug and each of the two side effects.

They were asked to imagine a hypothetical patient for whom the drug would be safe and then asked which pieces of information they would point out to their patients. Next, the participants were asked to imagine another patient, for whom the drug was *not* safe, and asked whether they would provide the same information to this second patient or whether they would provide different information. If they indicated that they would provide different information, they were asked to specifiy what

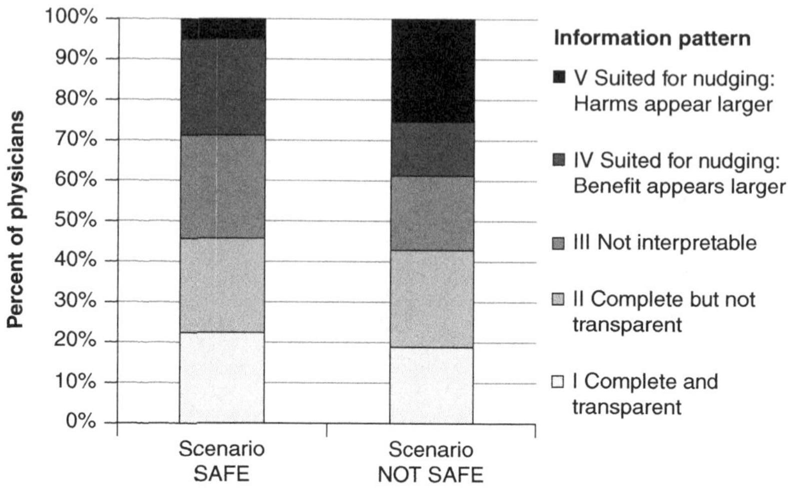

Figure 3.3. Patterns of numeric benefit and risk information in two scenarios. Physicians were asked to indicate which information they would show to a patient for whom the antidepressant was safe and a patient for whom the antidepressant was not safe (N = 142) (created from data presented in Gaissmaier et al., 2014).

information they would provide. We examined the responses to determine whether the information that they provided was complete (communicating both benefit and side effects), transparent (clearly indicating which proportion of people is actually affected by the antidepressant), or persuasive (nudging patients toward a particular option).

Of physicians who provided the same information for both patient scenarios (87 of the total sample of 142), only 24% (or 21 respondents) supplied information that was both complete and transparent (meaning that their choice of information included both benefit and side effect information and that their choice of information made clear which proportion of people was affected by the antidepressant). Physicians who provided the same information across scenarios supplied complete information more often and persuasive information less often than those who provided information differently across scenarios. See Figure 3.3 for patterns of numeric benefit and risk information.

The findings reviewed here are examples of the larger body of literature assessing that physicians' knowledge and communication of statistical terminology and concepts could be improved. It should be noted that none of the studies on physician statistical literacy or numeracy discussed in this chapter, or published elsewhere to our knowledge, measure physicians' actual performance in real patient interactions or how their statistical literacy impacts the quality of care they provide patients or their actual patient outcomes.

Physicians' use of statistics in the evolving medical context

To provide a context for the results of the studies on physicians' statistical literacy, we now consider some of the ways in which the use of statistics has changed in the evolving medical context.

Evidence-based medicine: Evidence-based medicine has become an important part of clinical practice (e.g., Elstein, 2004; Schulkin, 2000; 2008). It can be defined as "the conscientious, explicit, and judicious use of current best evidence in making decisions about the care of individual patients. The practice of evidence-based medicine means integrating individual clinical expertise with the best available external clinical evidence from systematic research" (Sackett et al., 1996). Statistical abilities are essential for many of the tasks that are required for practicing evidence-based medicine, including critically appraising the evidence, gaining a full understanding of the results, and integrating evidence into patient care (Guyatt & Rennie, 2002; Rao & Kanter, 2010). The Cochrane Reviews provide the widest collection of systematic reviews of medical evidence. Each systematic review states a clear problem/goal (e.g., to evaluate the effectiveness of decision aids for people facing treatment and screening decisions) and reports a summary of results. Reviews are carried out after structured searches are conducted to obtain the most current literature, and the evidence has been critically appraised.

The use of statistics in medical research publications has evolved over the past few decades. Hellems and colleagues reviewed 171 articles in the journal *Pediatrics* and found that the percentage of articles using inferential statistical procedures in selected volumes of *Pediatrics* was growing substantially in the past decades, increasing from 13% in 1952 to 89% in 2005 (see Figure 3.4) (Hayden, 1983; Hellems et al., 2007). Put another way, in 1952 over 60% had only basic descriptive statistics, compared to less than 5% of articles in 2005.

Not only have the proportion of articles using advanced statistics grown in this time period, but there is also greater diversity in the types of statistics being used. Few of the articles used the same statistical methods. In fact, according to the review of *Pediatrics* articles, a physician who understands the 20 most commonly used statistics may recognize, and therefore evaluate, the statistics in only 70% of the articles she encounters (Hellems et al., 2007). A review of the *New England Journal of Medicine* found similar trends in the difficulty of the statistics in that journal. In

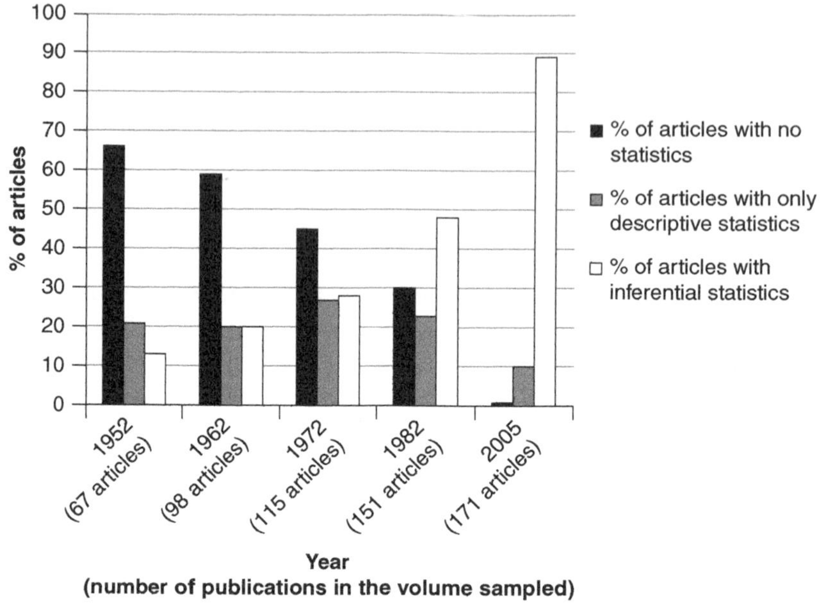

Figure 3.4. Characteristics of statistics in selected volumes of *Pediatrics*, 1952–2005. (Adapted from Hayden, 1983 and Hellems et al., 2007.)

2005, authors noted that over half of the articles in the *New England Journal of Medicine* used sophisticated statistics that would not be covered in standard statistics courses (Horton & Switzer, 2005).

Obtaining statistical information from sources other than evidence-based reviews and journals, such as pharmaceutical companies and health campaigns, poses a distinct set of challenges. "Mismatched framing" is an example of a communication strategy that is often used to mislead individuals about the benefits and harms of a drug or a treatment. When mismatched framing is employed, statistical information for benefits and risks is provided in different number formats in order to make the disadvantages look small and benefits look large. Consider this hypothetical example. A patient brochure might say that the treatment can reduce the risk of breast cancer by 50% but increase the risk of colon cancer by seven in a thousand. This is mismatched framing because the 50% value is a relative risk reduction but the seven in a thousand is an absolute risk increase. This makes the benefit (50%) look large, but, if the clinical trial found that 8 in 1000 patients in the control group got breast cancer and that 4 in 1000 patients in a treatment group got cancer, the absolute risk reduction of the treatment would actually be 4 in 1000 (8–4 = 4).

Using the mismatched framing makes the benefit of the treatment look significantly greater than the risk (50% sounds bigger than seven in a thousand), when it is actually not.

A review of high-impact journals found that while a majority of articles present benefit and harm data in the same metric, one-third present benefit and harm information in different formats, most often presenting harms using absolute risks and benefits using relative risk reductions (Sedrakyan & Shih, 2007). A meta-analysis of 31 experiments found that physicians are just as likely to be influenced by the format of numeric information as medical students, other medical professionals, and the general public (Covey, 2007).

Statistics and Medical Decision Making: Another way in which the medical context has evolved is that medical decision making has become a cooperative and collaborative endeavor between the patient and physician. Scientific evidence and the patient's preferences are evaluated by the patient and the physician together, and then decisions are made either by the patient or by agreement between the patient and physician (Rayburn & Schulkin, 2011). This cooperative medicine (which can also be referred to as shared decision making or patient-centered care) is in stark contrast with the paternalistic patient–physician relationship common a few decades earlier, in which a physician would make decisions that he/she thought would be best for the patient. Making decisions with patients, rather than for patients, requires physicians to take on the important role of communicating information to their patients so that patients understand the evidence and can apply it to their situation.

Counseling patients about genetic screening is one context in which physicians are responsible for being educators and communicators of statistical information to help their patients make decisions (Wilkins-Haug et al., 2000; Driscoll et al., 2009). Physicians need to understand the statistical information about genetic tests in order to explain results to their patients and give valid clinical advice. This can be challenging because: (1) genetic risks may be presented in confusing numeric formats, and (2) understanding genetic risks requires some knowledge about the genetic tests themselves (e.g., specificity and sensitivity of the test). As discussed by Dukhovny and Wilkins-Haug in Chapter 6 in this volume, opportunities to test for genetic predispositions have grown substantially in recent years. This growth not only increases the need for counseling services, it also makes genetic counseling more challenging; physicians have indicated that keeping up with rapid changes in genetic testing is the greatest obstacle to providing genetic information to patients (Wilkins-Haug et al., 1999).

Though medical decision making and evidence-based medicine both strive to improve quality of care, they do so in different ways (Elstein,

2004). While evidence-based medicine focuses on the knowledge and practices of providers, medical decision making examines how providers and patients apply that knowledge and integrate it with patient values or preferences. While medical decision making uses utility assessment, cost-effectiveness analysis, and decision psychology, these are largely ignored by evidence-based knowledge. Though we discuss the relevance of statistics to reading publications, evidence-based medicine, and medical decision making, physicians' statistical literacy and numeracy are relevant to any aspect of medical care where numeric information and/or risk or uncertainty information is involved. With no shortage of such contexts, statistical skills are essential for physicians.

Statistical literacy education

A formal review of statistical literacy training of physicians during undergraduate education, medical school, residency, and postgraduate training is beyond the scope of this chapter. Instead, in the paragraphs below, we provide some brief information about the current statistical literacy training at each level of education (from pre-medicine through continuing medical education).

Calculus is the traditional mathematics prerequisite for medical school. However, in 1998 none of the 100 surveyed US medical schools required biostatistics or statistics for admission (Looney et al., 1998), even though statistics and numeracy are arguably more relevant to medical practice than traditional calculus courses (Nusbaum, 2006). An informal review of the current medical admission requirements found that several schools now accept statistics in place of the calculus requirement; some schools even require statistics prior to starting medical school.

Out of the 100 medical school progams included in the 1998 data, 74 programs reported that they required a biostatistics course as part of their curriculum (Looney, 1998). More recent information from the American Association of Medical Colleges (AAMC) Curriculum Management and Information Tool (CurrMIT), which collects information about medical school curricula, suggests that the majority of schools include statistics or biostatistics in their curricula: of the 106 medical schools participating in the 2012 graduation year (which is 56% of the total number of medical schools), 85 (80%) required "statistics" (note this does not include research methods or evidence-based medicine training, or epidemiology). Most of the reported courses were in the first two years of the curriculum.

When surveyed about statistical literacy training during residency, resident directors as well as residents report that formal training is limited (Morreale et al., 2012; Anderson et al., 2013). A convenience sample of

10 psychiatry resident directors was surveyed about the statistical literacy training in their programs. Seven of the 10 programs incorporated statistical literacy training for their non-research-track residents, with journal clubs being the most common method. Only one program offered a semester-long formal course on statistical literacy, though four offered short courses on the topic. Eight of the 10 directors indicated that competing priorities are important barriers to statistical literacy education, but all of the directors indicated that it is at least minimally important to teach statistical literacy to their psychiatry residents (Morreale et al., 2012).

In another study, the entire US cohort of ob-gyn residents was surveyed about their statistical literacy training during residency (Anderson et al., 2013). When asked how they received statistical literacy training, about half (50.7%) indicated having training through a journal club, 29% had informal training, 15% had training as part of a course, and 11% had no training. About 66% rated the quality of their training as adequate, while 23.7% rated it as inadequate. Females were more likely to rate their statistical literacy training poorly, with 25.1% of the females indicating that their training was inadequate compared to only 17.9% of the males. There were no significant differences between males and females on any questions assessing their statistical literacy performance.

Because statistical literacy facilitates the understanding of evidence-based medicine recommendations, evidence-based medicine training is one setting where statistical literacy could be taught. Reviews of evidence-based medicine curricula show that they do not currently integrate much statistical literacy training. Instead, critical appraisal is most often the primary focus, receiving the most attention of all the evidence-based medicine skills (Green, 1999, 2000; Rao & Kanter, 2010). Rao and Kanter (2010) reviewed evidence-based medical school curricula and found that only 9 of the 28 curricula incorporated training on statistical skills.

One group has designed an evidence-based medicine curriculum focused on physicians' abilities with numbers (Rao & Kanter, 2010; Rao, 2007, 2008). The 32 hour curriculum uses a combination of tailored lectures and small group sessions for instruction on biostatistics and diagnostic reasoning such as applications of Bayes Theorem. For more information on the curriculum, see Rao and Kanter, 2010. The impact of statistical literacy training, through evidence-based medicine or via other means, should continue to be assessed and developed.

Continued training is needed for physicians in practice in order to help them to stay up-to-date. Continuing medical education opportunities support physicians in the lifelong learning that is essential to the practice of medicine (Abrahamson et al., 1999). Because medical decision making and the use of statistics evolve with new innovations, continuing medical education lies at the heart of maintaining state-of-the-art medical decision making and statistical literacy among physicians.

Continuing medical education opportunities can be offered in a variety of formats. "Enduring Materials" are printed, electronic, or video instructional materials designed for physicians that are reviewed and kept up-to-date on a regular basis. "Journal continuing medical education" requires physicians to read a journal article and then answer a set of questions about the material. A third type of continuing medical education is the "Regularly Scheduled Series (RSS)," which are multiple ongoing sessions such as grand rounds or morbidity and mortality conferences. Continuing medical education is provided in these and a variety of other formats (e.g., online "webinars").

To foster statistical literacy throughout a physician's career, opportunities for continuing medical education on statistical literacy need to be readily available. We searched the websites of some of the major health-care organizations and continuing medical education providers to identify continuing medical education offerings on statistical literacy. Though we did not find many offerings focused specifically on statistical literacy, we did find opportunities for journal continuing medical education about statistics and research (e.g., jama.com).

Because statistics are presented in formats such as mismatched framing in journal articles and the media, it will be a useful educational goal for physicians to be trained on how to recognize and interpret these misleading messages. Doing so will not only improve the quality of the information that physicians provide to their patients, but it will also reduce the collective statistical illiteracy (as discussed by Multmeier and colleagues in Chapter 2 of this volume).

Statistical literacy education has evolved as the field of medicine continues to change. However, we still do not know what level of statistical literacy skills physicians need. Does every physician need to be able to understand the advanced statistics in each journal article they read? Is it possible that physicians can provide high quality care with only basic statistical knowledge? These are questions that need to be addressed before determining to what extent statistical literacy training is inadequate.

Directions for future research

A useful next step to addressing physician statistical literacy is to conduct studies that connect physicians' statistical skills with quality of care in actual practice as well as actual patient outcomes. This research is important for at least two reasons: (1) To develop evidence-based standards for statistical literacy training. By defining how much and/or which knowledge leads to improved patient outcomes, education standards can be clearly established to ensure that all physicians are adequately trained. (2) To better define the magnitude of the problem. Should a large impact be seen, this research should bolster the calls for improved statistical literacy education. Given the many competing topics on which medical students and doctors need to be educated, empirical data showing the impact of specific statistical literacy skills on the quality of care and patient outcomes could motivate educators to make statistical literacy a higher priority throughout medical training.

Linking specific statistical literacy skills to actual patient care and patient outcomes would require gathering a range of data in real clinical contexts. For example, information would need to be gathered on physicians' abilities as well as patients' decision making, outcomes, and their perceptions of the quality of care. The typical healthcare setting may find it difficult to incorporate the collection of this type of data. However, healthcare systems such as the Geisinger system (discussed in Chapter 9), which is already collecting detailed data on physicians and patients and using that data to inform quality improvement efforts, may find it easy to do so.

Once statistical skills most essential to physicians are identified, a well validated statistical literacy assessment for physicians can be developed. Though some measures have included a few advanced statistical tasks, there is no validated measure that assesses physicians' abilities on a wide range of advanced statistics or biostatistics tasks. If a standard statistical literacy scale is established, it would allow researchers to compare results across studies as well as over time.

Improving physicians' comfort and confidence with communicating numerical information will likely enhance their interactions with their patients. Only 36% of physicians in one study indicated that they could communicate risk effectively in the numerical format (Gramling et al., 2004). One way to improve confidence could be to teach physicians specific strategies for communicating numeric information (Sedgwick & Hall, 2003; Apter et al., 2008). A recent review of communication training programs found that role-play, feedback, and small group discussions were the most effective teaching strategies (Berkhof et al., 2011). Programs are beginning to incorporate "integrated training" in which skills are acquired in clinical contexts rather than in the classroom (Coomarasamy & Kahn, 2004; Hatala et al., 2006). In a systematic review, integrated evidence-based medicine was found to positively impact knowledge, skills, attitudes, and behavior, whereas standalone courses on evidence-based medicine only impacted knowledge (Coomarasamy & Kahn, 2004).

References

Abrahamson, S., Baron, J., Elstein, A. S., Hammond, W. P., Holzman, G. B., Marlow, B., et al. (1999). Continuing medical education for life: eight principles. *Academic Medicine*, 74(12), 1288–1294.

Anderson, B. L., & Schulkin, J. (2011). Physicians' perceptions of patients' knowledge and opinions regarding breast cancer: Associations with patient education and physician numeracy. *Breast Care*, 6(4), 285–288.

Anderson, B. L., Obrecht, N. A., Chapman, G., Driscoll, D. A., & Schulkin, J. (2011). Physicians' communication of Down syndrome screening test results: The influence of physician numeracy. *Genetics in Medicine*, 13(8), 744–749.

Anderson, B. L., Gigerenzer, G., Parker, S., & Schulkin, J. (2014). Statistical literacy in obstetrics and gynecology. *Journal for Healthcare Quality*, 36(1), 5–17.

Anderson, B. L., Williams, S., & Schulkin, J. (2013). Statistical Literacy of Obstetrics-Gynecology Residents. *Journal of Graduate Medical Education*, 5(2), 272–275.

Apter, A. J., Paasche-Orlow, M. K., Bennett, I. M., Ben-Joseph, E. P., Batista, R. M., & James Hyde, S. M. (2008). Numeracy and communication with patients: They are counting on us. *Journal of General Internal Medicine*, 23(12), 2117–2124.

Ashby, D. (2006). Bayesian statistics in medicine: A 25 year review. *Statistics in Medicine*, 25(21), 3589–3631.

Baron, J. (2000). *Thinking and Deciding* (3rd edn.). Cambridge: Cambridge University Press.

Berkhof, M., van Rijssen, H. J., Schellart, A. J. M., Anema, J. R., & van der Beek, A. J. (2011). Effective training strategies for teaching communication skills to physicians: An overview of systematic reviews. *Patient Education and Counseling*, 84, 152–162.

Bramwell, R., West, H., & Salmon, P. (2006). Health professionals' and service users' interpretation of screening test results: Experimental study. *British Medical Journal*, 333(7562), 284.

Coomarasamy, A., & Kahn, K. S. (2004). What is the evidence that postgraduate teaching in evidence based medicine changes anything? A systematic review. *British Medical Journal*, 329(7473), 1017.

Covey, J. (2007). A meta-analysis of the effects of presenting treatment benefits in different formats. *Medical Decision Making*, 27, 638–654.

Driscoll, D. A., Morgan, M. A., & Schulkin, J. (2009). Screening for Down syndrome: changing practice of obstetricians. *American Journal of Obstetrics and Gynecology*, 200(4), 459.e1–459.e9.

Elstein, A. S. (2004). On the origins and development of evidence-based medicine and medical decision making. *Inflammation Research*, 53(2), S184–S189.

Estrada, C., Barnes, V., Collins, C., & Byrd, J. C. (1999). Health literacy and numeracy. *JAMA*, 282(6), 527.

Fagerlin, A., Zikmund-Fisher, B. J., Ubel, P. A., Jankovic, A., Derry, H. A., & Smith, D. M. (2007). Measuring numeracy without a math test: development of the Subjective Numeracy Scale. *Medical Decision Making*, 27(5), 672–680.

Fischhoff, B., & Beyth-Marom, R. (1983). Hypothesis evaluation from a Bayesian perspective. *Psychological Review*, 90(3), 239–260.

Friedman, S. B., & Phillips, S. (1981). What's the difference? Pediatric residents and their inaccurate concepts regarding statistics. *Pediatrics*, 68(5), 644–646.

Gaissmaier, W., Anderson, B. L., & Schulkin, J. (2014). How do physicians provide statistical information about antidepressants to hypothetical patients? *Medical Decision Making*, 34(2), 206–215.

Garcia-Retamero, R., & Hoffrage, U. (2013). Visual representation of statistical information improves diagnostic inferences in doctors and their patients. *Social Science & Medicine*, 83, 27–33.

Ghosh, A. K., Ghosh, K., & Erwin, P. J. (2004). Do medical students and physicians understand probability? *QJM*, 97(1), 53–55.

Gigerenzer, G., & Hoffrage, U. (1995). How to improve Bayesian reasoning without instruction: Frequency formats. *Psychological Review*, 102(4), 684–704.

Gigerenzer, G., Gaissmaier, W., Kurz-Mielke, E., Schwartz, L. M., & Woloshin, S. (2007). Helping doctors and patients make sense of health statistics. *Psychological Science in the Public Interest* 8(2), 53–96.

Gramling, R., Irvin, J. E., Nash, J., Sciamanna, C., & Culpepper, L. (2004). Numeracy and medicine: Key family physician attitudes about communicating probability with patients. *The Journal of the American Board of Family Practice*, 17(6), 473–473.

Green, M. L. (1999). Graduate medical education training in clinical epidemiology, critical appraisal, and evidence-based medicine: A critical review of curricula. *Academic Medicine*, 74(6), 686–694.

Green, M. L. (2000). Evidence-based medicine training in graduate medical education: past, present and future. *Journal of Evaluation in Clinical Practice*, 6(2), 121–138.

Guyatt, G., & Rennie, D. (Eds). (2002). *Users' Guides to the Medical Literature: A Manual for Evidence-Based Practice*. Chicago, IL: AMA Press.

Halvorsen, P. A., Kristiansen, I. S., Aasland, O. G., & Førde, O. H. (2003). Medical doctors' perception of the "number needed to treat" (NNT). *Scandinavian Journal of Primary Health Care*, 21(3), 162–166.

Hanoch, Y., Miron-Shatz, T., Coles, H., Himmelstein, M., & Federman, A. D. (2010). Choice, numeracy, and physicians-in-training performance: The case of Medicare Part D. *Health Psychology*, 29(4), 454–459.

Hatala, R., Keitz, S. A., Wilson, M. C., & Guyatt, G. (2006). Beyond journal clubs. *Journal of General Internal Medicine*, 21(5), 538–541.

Hayden, G. F. (1983). Biostatistical trends in Pediatrics: Implications for the future. *Pediatrics*, 72, 84–87.

Hellems, M. A., Gurka, M. J., & Hayden, G. F. (2007). Statistical literacy for readers of Pediatrics: A moving target. *Pediatrics*, 119(6), 1083–1088.

Hoffrage, U., & Gigerenzer, G. (1998). Using natural frequencies to improve diagnostic inferences. *Academic Medicine*, 73(5), 538–540.

Horton, N. J., & Switzer, S. S. (2005). Statistical methods in the journal. *NEJM*, 353(18), 1977–1979.

Lancet. (1937). Mathematics and medicine. *The Lancet*, 229(5914), 31.

Lipkus, I. M., Samsa, G., & Rimer, B. K. (2001). General performance on a numeracy scale among highly educated samples. *Medical Decision Making*, 21(1), 37–44.

Looney, S. W., Grady, C. S., & Steiner, R. P. (1998). An update on biostatistics requirements in US medical schools. *Academic Medicine*, 73(1), 92–94.

Morreale, M. K., Balon, R., & Arfken, C. L. (2012). Teaching statistical literacy to psychiatry residents: A pilot study of training directors. *Academic Psychiatry*, 36(2), 152–153.

Nusbaum, N. J. (2006). Mathematics preparation for medical school: Do all premedical students need calculus? *Teaching and Learning in Medicine*, 18(2), 165–168.

Obrecht, N. A., Anderson, B., Schulkin, J., & Chapman, G. B. (2012). Retrospective frequency formats promote consistent experience-based bayesian judgments. *Applied Cognitive Psychology*, 26(3), 436–440.

Peters E., Dieckmann, N., Dixon A., & Hibbard J. H. (2007). Less is more in presenting quality information to consumers. *Medical Care Research Review*, 64(2), 169–190.

Rao, G. (2007). *Rational Medical Decision Making: A Case-Based Approach*: New York, NY: McGraw-Hill.

Rao, G. (2008). Physician numeracy: Essential skills for practicing evidence-based medicine. *Family Medicine*, 40(5), 354–358.

Rao, G., & Kanter, S. L. (2010). Physician numeracy as the basis for evidence-based medicine curriculum. *Academic Medicine*, 85(11), 1794–1799.

Rayburn, W. F., & Schulkin, J. (Eds.). (2011). *Changing Landscape of Academic Women's Health Care in the United States*. Netherlands: Springer Science+ Business Media.

Sackett, D. L., Rosenberg, W. M., Muri Gray, J. A., Haynes, R. B., & Richardson, W. S. (1996). Evidence based medicine: What it is and what it isn't. *British Medical Journal*, 312, 71–72.

Schulkin, J. (2000). Decision sciences and evidence-based medicine – two intellectual movements to support clinical decision making. *Academic Medicine*, 75(8), 816–818.

Schulkin, J. (2008). *Medical Decisions, Estrogen, and Aging*. New York: Springer.

Schwartz, L. M., Woloshin, S., Black, W. C., & Welch, H. G. (1997). The role of numeracy in understanding the benefit of screening mammography. *Annals of Internal Medicine*, 127(11), 966–972.

Sedgwick, P., & Hall, A. (2003). Teaching medical students and doctors how to communicate risk. *British Medical Journal*, 327(7417), 694–695.

Sedrakyan, A., & Shih, C. (2007). Improving depiction of benefits and harms: Analyses of studies of well-known therapeutics and review of high-impact medical journals. *Medical Care*, 45(10), S23–S28.

Swift, L., Miles, S., Price, G. M., Shepstone, L., & Leinster, S. J. (2009). Do doctors need statistics? Doctors' use of and attitudes to probability and statistics. *Statistics in Medicine*, 28(15), 1969–1981.

Wegwarth O., Gaissmaier, W., & Gigerenzer, G. (2011). Deceiving numbers: Survival rates and their impact on doctors' risk communication. *Medical Decision Making*, 31, 386–394.

Wegwarth, O., Schwartz, L., Woloshin, S., Gaissmaier, W., & Gigerenzer, G. (2012). Do physicians understand cancer screening statistics? A national survey of primary care physicians in the United States. *Annals of Internal Medicine*, 156, 340–349.

Weiss, S. T., & Samet, J. M. (1980). An assessment of physician knowledge of epidemiology and biostatistics. *Journal of Medical Education*, 55(8), 692.

Wilkins-Haug, L., Hill, L., Schmidt, L., Holzman, G. B., & Schulkin, J. (1999). Genetics in Obstetricians' Offices: A Survey Study. *Obstetrics and Gynecology*, 93, 642–647.

Wilkins-Haug, L., Erickson, K., Hill, L., Power, M., Holzman, G. B., & Schulkin, J. (2000). Obstetrician-gynecologists' opinions and attitudes on the role of genetics in women's health. *Journal of Women's Health & Gender-Based Medicine*, 9(8), 873–879.

Windish, D. M., Huot, S. J., & Green M. L. (2007). Medicine residents' understanding of biostatistics and results in the medical literature. *JAMA*, 298(9), 1010–1022.

Wood, S., Hanoch, Y., Barnes, A., Liu, P., Cummings, J., Bhattacharya, C., & Rice, T. (2011). Numeracy and Medicare Part D: Decision making for Medicare's prescription drug program. *Psychology and Aging*, 26(2), 295–307.

Wulf, H. R., Andersen, B., Brandenhoff, P., & Guttler, F. (1987). What do doctors know about statistics? *StatMed*, 6(1), 3–10.

Young, J. M., Glasziou, P., & Ward, J. E. (2002). General practitioners' self-rating of skills in evidence based medicine: a validation study. *British Medical Journal*, 324, 950.

Zikmund-Fisher, B. J., Smith, D. M., Ubel, P. A., & Fagerlin, A. (2007). Validation of the subjective numeracy scale (SNS): Effects of low numeracy on comprehension of risk communications and utility elicitations. *Medical Decision Making*, 27(5), 663–671.

4 Patient numeracy: what do patients need to recognize, think, or do with health numbers?

Brian J. Zikmund-Fisher, Gillian Mayman, & Angela Fagerlin

In modern medicine, it is clear that being an effective clinician requires significant numeracy skills. In a single clinic shift, a primary care clinician might, for example, be required to adjust one patient's medication dose based on his blood counts, to interpret another patient's serum hormone levels as part of diagnosing her condition, and to estimate a third patient's future cancer risks. These types of quantitative data are the heart of patient medical records and the core of the practice of evidence-based medicine. In order to be effective clinicians, doctors, nurses, and other medical personnel must have sufficient knowledge, training, and numeracy skills to make sense of the data they receive.

Yet, it is worth asking the important question: what do *patients* need to recognize, think, or do with health numbers? One might argue that clinicians are the interpreters of health data and tell patients what to do based on that data. Do patients need to think about health numbers?

We argue that *patient numeracy*, the ability of patients to understand and use quantitative health data, is as important to patient health as clinician numeracy is. Patients must understand how their actions can prevent disease and help them live healthier lives. Once diagnosed with disease, patients need to understand how and when their own actions can help them heal or prevent complications. Often, they also need to make medical treatment decisions that depend on their preferences and values. Each of these needs can be met, in part, through effective use of medical and health data. Thus, the most fundamental role of patient numeracy is to enable patients to understand how, when, and why numerical information is relevant to their health and through that

Dr. Zikmund-Fisher was supported by Mentored Research Scholar Grant MRSG-06–130–01-CPPB from the American Cancer Society.

Table 4.1. *Key functions of patient numeracy and examples of how these functions enable patients to act on health data.*

Functions of patient numeracy	Examples of what patients need to recognize, think, or do with health numbers
Understand the uncertainty yet predictability of health	• Understand the concept of a disease risk factor • Understand the difference between population rates and individual risk propensity • Understand that clinical trials may not provide benefit to individual participants
Understand risk information	• Translate between risk formats • Interpret visual displays of risk • Interpret medical data such as body mass index
Be able to make better health decisions	• Recognize the relevance of health data to individual medical decisions • Identify personally relevant data out of larger sets • Evaluate the meaning of health data by comparing it with reference standards • Vary risk perceptions as risk estimates change • Adjust decisions based on magnitude of risk or treatment benefit
Complete tasks that require number skills	• Accurately interpret medication dosing schedules • Calculate appropriate medication doses based on body weight or age • Interpret nutrition labels • Record and use self-monitoring data such as blood pressure or blood glucose readings • Use a risk calculator • Complete health utility elicitations

understanding to encourage their use of such data in health management and decision making.

Several excellent recent papers have examined the conceptual elements of numeracy and identified functions that numeracy serves in decision making (Ancker & Kaufman, 2007; Peters et al., 2007a; Apter et al., 2008; Schapira et al., 2008; Lipkus & Peters, 2009; Reyna et al., 2009). In this chapter, we will touch upon these perspectives but take a more practical focus. We present evidence that numeracy is related to specific types of understanding (e.g., of the predictability of health) and specific skills (such as interpreting risk information or medical test results) that are more relevant to health behaviors and health decision making than scoring highly on a math test is (Table 4.1). In so doing, we hope to trace the dots from measures of numeracy in individuals to health abilities, on to health actions, and then ultimately to health outcomes.

Numeracy should help patients understand the uncertainty yet predictability of health

In 2006, Nick Kurzon, a young filmmaker living in New York City, wrote a short piece in *Newsweek* that describes how he came to terms with the risks associated with his diagnosis of lymphoma by playing poker (Kurzon, 2004). He compares being told that he has a 90% chance of surviving 10 years to playing a hand where he knows that he has a 90% chance of winning and a 10% chance of his opponent drawing one of the only four cards that could beat him. In fact, Kurzon tells the story of getting just such a poker hand, betting big, yet nonetheless losing. The experience helped Kurzon to understand the difference between having good odds and experiencing good outcomes. In other words, he came to understand how risk data can accurately describe the chances of a population of patients like him yet be unable to tell him whether he will live or die. Such data helped Kurzon to understand "how predictable it is to be as lucky as I am"(Kurzon, 2004).

Kurzon's story is an example of how a relatively numerate person can grasp the concept of randomness as it applies to understanding his own health. Patients like Kurzon need to understand randomness in order to grasp the concept of a risk factor, i.e., to understand that different people are more or less likely to have things happen to them *and* that medical data can clarify whether an individual patient is in a higher or lower risk group. Without such understanding, patients are likely to be more susceptible to believing that outcomes are predetermined, and such fatalism undermines the meaningfulness of all types of health information. After all, why should a patient care about the abstract concept of her "risk," or even the more concrete measures of her cholesterol level or her calorie intake, if she doesn't see how changing those numbers might change her health outcomes? We should be clear, however, that it is not understanding randomness in the sense of a coin flip or lottery that is important for patients. Patients need to understand the multiple types of uncertainty in health: health outcomes (good or bad) are (a) *possible*, yet not assured, (b) *predictable* in the sense that certain characteristics or actions make them more or less likely to occur, and (c) potentially *modifiable* by their own or their healthcare providers' actions.

Logically, patient numeracy should be closely related to patients' abilities to understand the uncertainty, yet predictability, of health. In other words, numeracy should help patients to make the connection between data about what happened to other patients and what might happen to them, thereby providing the seeds of motivation to change behavior, seek medical attention, and adhere to treatment or prevention regimens.

Unfortunately, there appears to be a dearth of research examining the relationship between numeracy and beliefs that health is predictable and modifiable. Identifying such relationships should be a priority for future research.

What is known is that numeracy appears related to understanding uncertainty as it relates to medical research trials. Clinical trials have uncertain outcomes: By definition, they are attempting to assess interventions for which benefit is *not* known and/or assured. Yet some patients appear to believe that clinical trials can be expected to provide individual benefit to participants (Weinfurt et al., 2008), and numeracy appears related to such beliefs: Weinfurt and colleagues found that a single numeracy question included in a study of cancer patients significantly predicted belief in assumptions of benefit from Phase I clinical trials, with less numerate patients being more likely to assume individual benefit from trial participation (Weinfurt et al., 2003).

Numeracy helps people understand risk information

Much of the research examining patient numeracy has focused on its effect on patients' ability to accurately comprehend or recall risk and benefit information. Some of these studies have focused on identifying the mechanisms that impede risk communication to less numerate patients. For example, multiple studies have shown that people with lower numeracy skills are particularly prone to variations in the way risk information is presented, e.g., gain versus loss frames or percentages versus frequencies (Peters et al., 2006). In particular, they are more susceptible to variations in the denominator used to represent a risk frequency and may, for example, view a 40 out of 800 risk as larger than 10 out of 100 (Garcia-Retamero & Galesic, 2009). People with low statistical confidence (a marker of subjective numeracy) also prefer risk information to be presented in words rather than numerical formats (Smith et al., 2010).

Numeracy also directly impacts patients' ability to identify and interpret key statistics from visual displays such as line graphs or other risk graphics. The evidence base on this issue is both substantial and growing. People with higher numeracy skills are more likely to accurately interpret or recall data in survival curves (Zikmund-Fisher et al., 2007), risk ladders (Hess et al., 2011a), bar charts, and icon arrays ("pictographs") (Zikmund-Fisher et al., 2007; Wright et al., 2009). However, less numerate people appear better able to interpret icon arrays than other types of risk graphics (Hawley et al., 2008; Galesic et al., 2009b; McCaffery et al., 2012) and thus numeracy differences tend to be reduced when they are used (Galesic et al., 2009b).

Of note, more numerate people appear to process risk graphics in a different way to less numerate people. In one line of work using eye-tracking methods, highly numerate people presented with a risk ladder (showing risks associated with radon exposure) had higher visual efficiency, spending proportionately more time looking at relevant frequency, textual, and comparative risk information than less numerate people did (Hess et al., 2011a; Keller, 2011). Another paper by the same research group showed that highly numerate people presented with icon array graphics were more likely to count the icons than less numerate people (Hess et al., 2011b). More numerate people also relied on a counting-based process to derive their risk perceptions, whereas less numerate people were actually distracted by instructions to count the icons.

Another important note is that Galesic and Garcia-Retamero have recently argued that patients can have graphical literacy skills (the ability to read and interpret visual representations) independent of numeracy skills, although the two are correlated with each other (r = 0.51) (Galesic & Garcia-Retamero, 2011a). Research using their graphical literacy scale suggests that visual displays like icon arrays or bar graphs can be particularly helpful to the less numerate if and only if they have the graphical literacy abilities to use them (Garcia-Retamero & Galesic 2010; Gaissmaier et al., 2012). Conversely, patient difficulties comprehending medical graphics may be caused not only by numeracy deficits but also by limited graphical literacy skills as well.

Numeracy skills are directly related to people's ability to make sense of data regarding cancer risks. When considering screening tests, more numerate patients are better able to comprehend risk reduction information (Schwartz et al., 1997) and other types of online cancer risk information (Donelle et al., 2008). In one study, numeracy was significantly associated with accurate interpretation of graphical representation of breast cancer risk among a cohort of women with personal or family history of breast cancer (Brown et al., 2011). Of particular note, after adjusting for numeracy in multivariate linear regression, education added little to the prediction of graph interpretation accuracy. People with better numeracy skills are also better able to translate data about the sensitivity and specificity of different screening tests into an accurate calculation of positive predictive value (Galesic et al., 2009a).

Numeracy skills also affect patients' abilities to interpret many other types of medical data. For example, less numerate patients make larger errors when interpreting medication side effect risk information (Gardner et al., 2011). Oettinger et al. found that less numerate parents (as measured with the WRAT-3) had greater difficulty in interpreting charts that mapped body mass index (BMI) to children's age to determine if a particular BMI represented a healthy versus overweight child (Oettinger et al., 2009). Another study found that parents of children scheduled for elective surgery who rated themselves higher on the Subjective Numeracy Scale were able to retain higher gist knowledge and verbatim (specific) knowledge when presented with data about the risks and benefits of different hypothetical pediatric anesthesia agents (Tait et al., 2010a). And these are only some of the research studies that have linked numeracy to comprehension of health risk.

In principle, numeracy should also have other effects related to risk information. For example, because more numerate people better understand probability and randomness in general, they should also be more tolerant of ambiguity (uncertainty about what the true level of risk is). Yet, the research evidence for such an effect is not yet present. Nonetheless, what is clear is that current numeracy measures are effective at distinguishing those people who are likely to understand health risk information presented to them from those who may find risk data to be confusing and perhaps unintelligible. For further detail on numeracy-related barriers to health communication, please see the chapter by Peters in this volume.

Numeracy enables patients to make better health decisions

Patients use quantitative data to address specific needs, which include identifying dominant options (e.g., equally effective treatments with lower side effect rates), providing motivation to act (e.g., if a risk calculator shows a need for intervention), and making magnitude-dependent trade-off choices (e.g., whether the incremental risk reduction of a cancer prevention intervention is worth its associated side effects) (Zikmund-Fisher, 2013). Improved health outcomes do not occur simply because patients have greater awareness of their health status but because such awareness is translated into improved health decisions and health management. While the evidence that such translation occurs is unfortunately limited, some studies have started to elaborate the linkages between numeracy and decision making.

To start, less numerate patients appear to be less willing to engage in the very process of medical decision making. In national samples of both US and German patients, a significant minority of low numeracy patients preferred more passive roles in medical decision making, while high numeracy patients were more satisfied with their current role (Galesic & Garcia-Retamero, 2011b). This could be because less numerate patients feel uncomfortable with health data and ill prepared to use it effectively in decision making.

Research has also documented that less numerate patients have more difficulty identifying personally relevant information out of larger sets or tables. For example, when presented with tables of data regarding various attributes of different hospitals, less numerate people had significantly greater difficulty identifying the objectively best hospitals from the set when the tables included non-essential information in addition to decision-critical data (Peters et al., 2007b). This may help to explain the observed fact that less numerate older patients appear less able to accurately answer questions after being given information about multiple Medicare Part D Prescription drug plans (Wood et al., 2011), less likely to choose to enroll in such programs (Szrek & Bundorf, 2011), and more willing to pay extra simply to preserve choice options in the future (Szrek & Bundorf, 2011).

It is quite common to present patients with tabular health data as part of "helping" them to make better health decisions. For example, patients are commonly presented with tables to "help" them calculate their BMI, determine medication dosages, choose health insurance plans, compare the side effects of different medications or treatment options, etc. Yet a BMI table is only useful if you can figure out which height row applies to you, use your weight to find the current BMI value, and assess within that row how changes in weight might result in changes in BMI. Similarly, a chart of medication side effects observed in clinical trials is only useful for decision making if you can recognize that the incremental effect of treatment is the difference between the risks experienced by the intervention and control groups, are able to calculate those differences, and understand the distinction between relative and absolute risk differences. All of these steps require numeracy skills to complete.

Furthermore, numeracy should improve the "evaluability" of quantitative health information, thereby enabling patients to become more sensitive to variations and better able to use such information in decision making. Research on information evaluability has shown that merely having access to relevant data does not mean that patients will be able to use that information to inform their decisions (Hsee et al., 1999). Data can be hard to evaluate (i.e., difficult to determine whether the number or attribute should be seen as good or bad and to what degree) when people lack relevant expertise, context, and/or reference standards. When people are presented with both hard-to-evaluate and easy-to-evaluate data, they tend to rely only on the data that are easier to interpret in making their decisions. Such information evaluability effects have been shown in healthcare decisions in addition to consumer choices (Hsee, 1996; Zikmund-Fisher et al., 2004).

A key element of evaluability is recognizing when higher numbers represent better versus worse outcomes. Unfortunately, less numerate people are more likely to be confused in this regard, leading to worse decision performance when attempting to choose a hospital from tables of quality and cost data (Peters et al., 2007b). The previously mentioned susceptibility of less numerate people to changes in risk denominators is related to this effect (Garcia-Retamero & Galesic, 2009, 2011). For example, a question in the Lipkus et al. numeracy measure asks respondents to identify the largest risk from the following set: 1 in 100, 1 in 10, 1 in 1000 (Lipkus et al., 2001). While the correct answer is, of course, 1 in 10, less numerate people are less likely to understand that a larger denominator implies a smaller risk and see 1 in 1000 as the largest risk.

Numeracy also changes how people perceive the same data. Multiple studies have shown that more numerate people tend to see risks (e.g., chances of side effects) as less concerning than less numerate patients do (Zikmund-Fisher et al., 2008; Tait et al., 2010b; Peters et al., 2011). This is possibly because more numerate patients recognize that the risk is possible *but unlikely* whereas a less numerate person only knows that something bad "might happen."

Perhaps more importantly, several recent research studies have shown that, when presented with a range of risk statistics, more numerate patients *vary* their risk perceptions to a greater degree than less numerate patients do. For example, Lipkus et al. recently did an analysis of two pilot studies of 105 women with early stage breast cancer who received information about survival chances and potential treatment effectiveness from the online decision aid Adjuvant Online (Lipkus et al., 2010). The authors found that not only did more numerate patients provide estimates of cancer-free survival that more closely matched those provided by Adjuvant Online, but also the correlations of both survival estimates and perceived treatment benefit to the objective data were significantly higher among the more numerate patients.

The ability of more numerate patients to be aware of variations in risk can also translate into greater use of risk information in making medical treatment choices. In a large Internet-administered study, women age 40–75 were asked to imagine that they had just had breast cancer surgery and were then presented with the same type of survival and treatment benefit data available from Adjuvant Online regarding adjuvant therapies (Zikmund-Fisher et al., 2011). These women were then asked to choose among four treatment options: no adjuvant therapy, hormonal therapy only, chemotherapy only, and combined hormonal and chemotherapies. As shown in Figure 4.1, when all four options were presented at once, women with lower numeracy skills were equally likely to choose

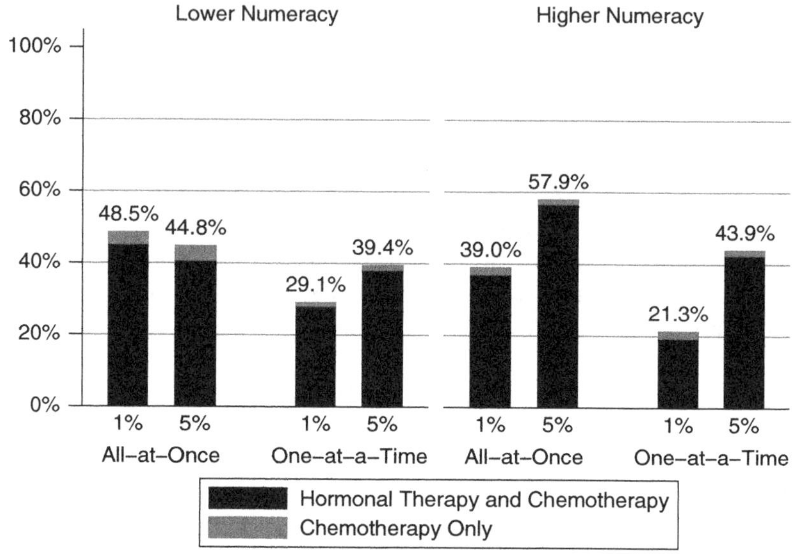

Figure 4.1. Percentage of women choosing chemotherapy in a hypothetical scenario regarding choice of adjuvant therapies following breast cancer surgery, by incremental benefit of chemotherapy (1% vs. 5%), by whether options were presented all-at-once versus sequentially, and by numeracy level. (Reprinted from *Breast Cancer Research and Treatment*, 129(1), Jan 1, 2011, "The benefits of discussing adjuvant therapies one at a time instead of all at once" by Brian J. Zikmund-Fisher, with kind permission from Springer Science and Business Media.)

chemotherapy when there was a 1% benefit as when there was a 5% benefit. In other words, risk data had no impact on their treatment decisions. By contrast, women with higher numeracy skills were significantly more likely to choose chemotherapy when the benefit was, in fact, larger.

However, the treatment decisions of less numerate women can be made more sensitive to variations in benefit by simplifying how data are presented. While some study participants saw data about four treatment options simultaneously, others learned about them one at a time (i.e., statistics and decisions about hormonal therapy first, followed by data about the incremental benefit of chemotherapy). Less numerate women who learned about treatment options one at a time were more likely to choose chemotherapy when it offered a larger benefit, although they were not as sensitive to the variation in effectiveness as more numerate women were.

Numeracy helps patients to complete tasks that require number skills

Numeracy is also fundamental to patients' ability to complete tasks that require basic computational skills. Two everyday examples of this issue are management of medications and use of nutrition information to guide dietary choices. More generally, we would expect numeracy to be related to patients' ability to perform a variety of self-monitoring tasks. In the research context, we would also expect numeracy to be related to patients' ability to make value judgments about different health states, a process often described as utility elicitations.

To start, it is important to acknowledge that being able to translate frequency of dosing instructions requires numeracy skills. The phrases "2 times a day," "every 12 hours," and "in the morning and evening" may be equivalent in meaning to a highly numerate person, but such cannot be assumed for a less numerate patient. Patients taking multiple medications, especially those with different dosing schedules, face even more difficult tasks. Low literacy patients have been shown to be easily confused by different ways of stating equivalent dosing frequencies (Wolf et al., 2007, 2011a, 2011b). Although numeracy was not measured specifically in these studies, it seems likely that at least part of this effect is related to low numeracy skills.

Both reading a thermometer and calculating appropriate medication doses for children are even more directly related to numeracy. Because infant and child doses are a function of the child's weight (often proxied for by age), less numerate parents run a significant risk of over- or under-dosing their children if they cannot follow the provided formulas to determine the appropriate amounts to give (Yin et al., 2010). Kumar et al. measured the ability to perform such tasks in the Parental Health Literacy Activities Test (PHLAT) and found that numeracy (as measured with the Wide Range Achievement Test (WRAT-3)) was highly correlated ($r = 0.55$) with the PHLAT (Kumar et al., 2010). Furthermore, the correlation with numeracy was much higher than with either education or health literacy.

In addition, while research in this area is limited, two early studies show clear relationships between performance on numeracy measures and ability to interpret nutrition labels to make healthy dietary choices. A study of primary care patients found that numeracy (measured with the WRAT-3) was highly related to ability to answer questions about nutrition labels (Rothman et al., 2006). Common errors involved misapplication of serving size and incorrect calculations, both tasks that require arithmetic operations. As was true in the medication study cited above,

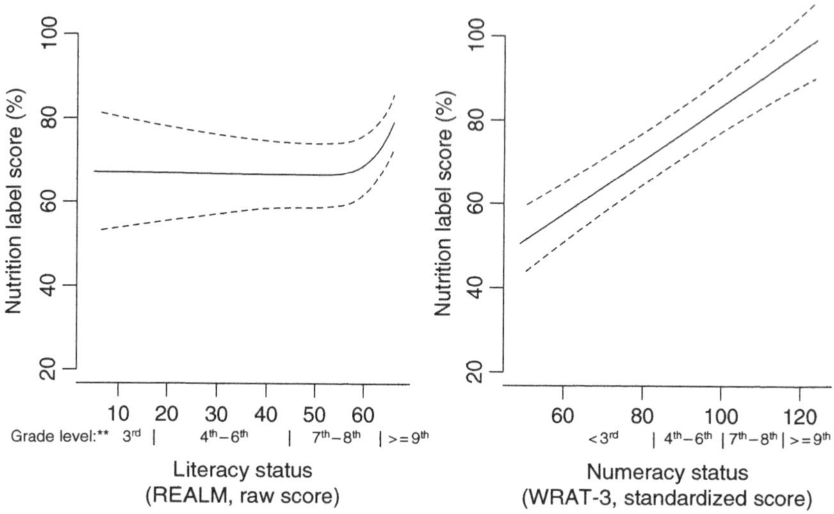

Figure 4.2. Predicted ability to interpret nutrition labels by literacy or numeracy status. Models were adjusted for age, gender, race/ethnicity, income, insurance status, presence of chronic disease, education level, literacy or numeracy, status of being on a specific diet, and label reading frequency. Dashed lines represent 95% confidence intervals. **Grade levels are approximations based on the REALM and WRAT-3 scores. REALM, Rapid Estimate of Adult Literacy in Medicine; WRAT-3, Wide Range Achievement Test, edition 3. (Reprinted from *American Journal of Preventive Medicine*, 31(5), November 2006, "Patient understanding of food labels: the role of literacy and numeracy" by Russell L. Rothman et al., with permission from Elsevier.)

the numeracy correlation (rho = 0.67, shown in Figure 4.2) was substantially higher than the correlations of comprehension score with income, education, or health literacy. In another study, less numerate Swiss consumers (as determined by ratings on the Subjective Numeracy Scale) presented with nutrition labels appeared less able to differentiate reduced-fat products from regular-fat products than more numerate consumers (Visschers & Siegrist, 2010). Both studies suggest that numeracy helps people both to find relevant nutrition information and to make use of such data in assessing the healthfulness of their dietary options.

More generally, numeracy skills affect patients' interest in and ability to accurately gather relevant health data. Analyses of Health Information National Trends Survey (HINTS) data show that numeracy is related to how easy or hard patients find searching for online health information (Manganello & Clayman, 2011) and familiarity with direct-to-consumer genetic testing (Langford et al., 2012) suggesting that less numerate people may avoid seeking out health information because they lack confidence in their ability to interpret their meaning. Because numeracy includes a preference component (some people like numbers more than others) in addition to an ability component (Fagerlin et al., 2007), highly numerate people are likely to find regular health measurements (such as dietary intake logs, growth charts, blood pressure readings, or blood glucose test result records) to be intuitively meaningful. While we are unaware of specific evidence to support this, we therefore expect that numeracy would be correlated with the amount and quality of health data collected by patients when participating in self-monitoring plans. More research is clearly needed to examine whether and how patient numeracy might impact health data gathering by patients and patients' abilities to use such data in self-management decisions.

For similar reasons, we also expect that numeracy will be related to interest in, and use of, health risk calculators. Such calculators require patients to either remember or find a variety of input data, and less numerate patients are likely to be less able and less interested in gathering such inputs if the result is just another (meaningless-to-them) number. In addition, in one study of people's responses to hypothetical risk calculators, less numerate people perceived the risk estimates they received to be both less believable and larger in magnitude than more numerate people did (Witteman et al., 2011). While some research has attempted to identify optimal formats for presenting risk calculator outputs (e.g., Witteman et al., 2011; Waters et al., 2007), further research is clearly needed to determine how the design of calculators might need to be adjusted to make them useful even for less numerate patients. Such research may also help to explain recent findings that a pre-diabetes risk calculator, while popular with users, did not appear to improve the accuracy of risk perceptions among patients receiving higher-than-expected estimates or influence immediate health behaviors (Harle et al., 2012).

Multiple studies have also shown that numeracy is related to patients' ability to provide quantitative ratings of different health states, a task often referred to as a "utility elicitation." For example, patients might be asked to assess how much worse it is to live with a colostomy than with perfect health (Smith et al., 2006). Such utility values are key inputs into many types of medical decision analyses. Unfortunately, less numerate patients are less likely to complete such tasks (resulting in potential biases to the results) (Zikmund-Fisher et al., 2007) and provide less reliable answers (e.g., by having the correlation between ratings and health states in the wrong direction) (Woloshin et al., 2001; Schwartz et al., 2004).

Table 4.2. *Examples of patient health outcomes related to patient numeracy.*

- Hemoglobin A1c values among type 1 or type 2 diabetic patients
- Degree of anticoagulation control among patients on anticoagulation therapy
- Frequency of hospitalization or emergency department visits among patients with asthma
- Receiving a kidney transplant or being on the transplant waitlist among patients with chronic kidney disease
- Ability to manage HIV medication regimens among HIV-positive patients
- Smoking cessation rates among smokers

Numeracy is related to improved patient health outcomes

Ultimately, our interest in patient numeracy depends on identifying its relationship to improved health outcomes. While research demonstrating such associations is limited, evidence is building that numeracy can be directly related to outcomes in a variety of health domains (Table 4.2).

Diabetes

As Cavanaugh discusses in more detail in her chapter of this volume, effective diabetes self-management requires patients to engage in a range of quantitative tasks, particularly in the areas of controlling glucose levels and taking insulin. To maintain appropriate blood glucose levels, patients with diabetes must monitor their food intake by calculating grams of carbohydrates and tracking calories, interpret the results of blood glucose tests, and manage multiple medications. Patients requiring insulin need to understand their insulin-to-carbohydrate ratio and adjust their individual dose based on changing blood glucose levels.

In recognition of the likely relationship between diabetes and numeracy, Huizinga et al. developed the Diabetes Numeracy Test (DNT) as a reliable and valid instrument to test numeracy skills specifically related to diabetes self-management (Huizinga et al., 2008). The 43 items on the scale were designed to simulate typical daily tasks encountered by patients with diabetes and assess the five major areas of diabetes self-management, including nutrition, exercise, glucose monitoring, oral medication, and insulin skills. Examples include counting carbohydrates (e.g., "What is the total amount of carbohydrate eaten if 1 cup of pasta and 1 cup of carrots are eaten together?"), adjusting insulin (e.g., "The doctor tells you to take 2 units of insulin for every 1 serving of carbohydrate you eat. How many units of insulin do you take for 6 servings of carbohydrate?"), and calculating supplies needed (e.g., "You test your blood sugar four times a day. How many strips do you need to take with you on a 2-week vacation?").

While Cavanaugh's chapter reviews the research evidence more broadly, we note here an illustrative study that highlights the potential impact of numeracy on diabetes outcomes. In a study of 398 adults aged 18 to 85 with type 1 or type 2 diabetes, scores on the DNT were found to be weakly associated with hemoglobin A1c levels, even after controlling for age, sex, race, income, diabetes type, years of diabetes diagnosis, and clinic site (Cavanaugh et al., 2008). Among patients with the lowest numeracy scores, the median HbA1c level was 7.7%, while median HbA1c was 6.3% among patients with the highest numeracy scores. For patients who use insulin, higher diabetes-related numeracy was found to be associated with adjustment of insulin dose for blood glucose level or carbohydrate intake. Higher perceived self-efficacy of self-management skills was associated with higher diabetes-related numeracy in patients. However, DNT score was not found to be significantly associated with diet, physical activity, or medication behaviors.

More recently, in a smaller study, Marden et al. studied glycemic control in 112 patients with type 1 diabetes living in the UK (Marden et al., 2012). Using the Literacy and Numeracy Initial Assessments from the UK Skills for Life Programme, they found that low numeracy scores were significantly associated with higher HbA1c levels. Furthermore, the relationship between numeracy and HbA1c was found to be independent of socioeconomic factors.

Anticoagulation control

Patients using warfarin for anticoagulation control are required to follow a changing dosing regimen set by their physicians with frequent monitoring and adjustment of doses. A key measure that patients need to understand is the international normalized ratio (INR), which is a measurement of the time blood takes to clot in comparison to an average. The INR is used to monitor the impact of anticoagulation medications. If the INR is too high, there is a risk of uncontrolled bleeding. An INR that is too low indicates that the medication may not be having a strong enough effect. Patients are given a range for their INR that they try to stay within. Staying within this set range is an indication that the patient's illness is well controlled.

Thus, patients taking anticoagulant medications need to (a) understand the meaning of the INR, (b) understand the importance of maintaining an INR within a range, (c) identify when their INR is out of range, (d) understand what medication changes are needed to adjust the INR in the appropriate direction, and (e) follow and implement changing medication doses.

All of these tasks require significant patient numeracy, and thus we can expect that more numerate patients would achieve better outcomes than less numerate patients.

As evidence of the importance of numeracy to these tasks, Estrada et al. measured numeracy among 143 patients enlisted in anticoagulation management units and taking warfarin for at least 1 month (Estrada et al., 2004). General numeracy was measured using the three-item numeracy scale developed by Schwartz et al. (1997), and three questions specific to anticoagulation therapy were added. These questions measured task-specific multiplication and addition skills (e.g., "If you have 5 mg pills of Coumadin and you take 7.5 mg a day, how many of those pills should you take every day?") and assessment of INR values relative to target (e.g., "Your normal INR should be 2 to 3. If your INR today is 3.5, would your INR be [Low/Normal/High]?").

Estrada et al. measured patients' INR an average of 5.8 times during a 3-month follow-up period and found that patients with low levels of numeracy spent more time above their INR range and less time within their range (Figure 4.3) (Estrada et al., 2004). Patients with the lowest scores had a 46% higher INR variability than patients with the highest scores. INR variability continued to be higher for patients with low numeracy after adjusting for age although the time in range was similar among patients at varying levels of numeracy.

Asthma

Similar to other chronic diseases, patients with moderate or severe asthma must engage in multiple self-management tasks. Many of these tasks are quantitatively based, including understanding percentages to interpret peak flow meter results, applying algorithms to determine when to take oral steroids, and understanding correct doses of medications on an asthma action plan. In fact, Apter et al. developed the Asthma Numeracy Questionnaire (ANQ) to measure such abilities. The ANQ asks questions about determining the amount of a medication to be taken (e.g., "Your doctor asks you to take 30 mg of prednisone every day for a week. The pharmacist gives you a bottle of 5 mg tablets. How many pills should you take each day?"), understanding risk, and reading a peak flow meter ("You have a peak flow meter. Your Danger or Red Zone is 50% of your best reading. Your best reading is 400 L/min. What is your Danger Zone?") (Apter et al., 2006).

A couple of recent studies have documented the relationship between numeracy and management of asthma symptoms. In a study of 73 adult asthma patients, low ANQ scores were found to be significantly associated

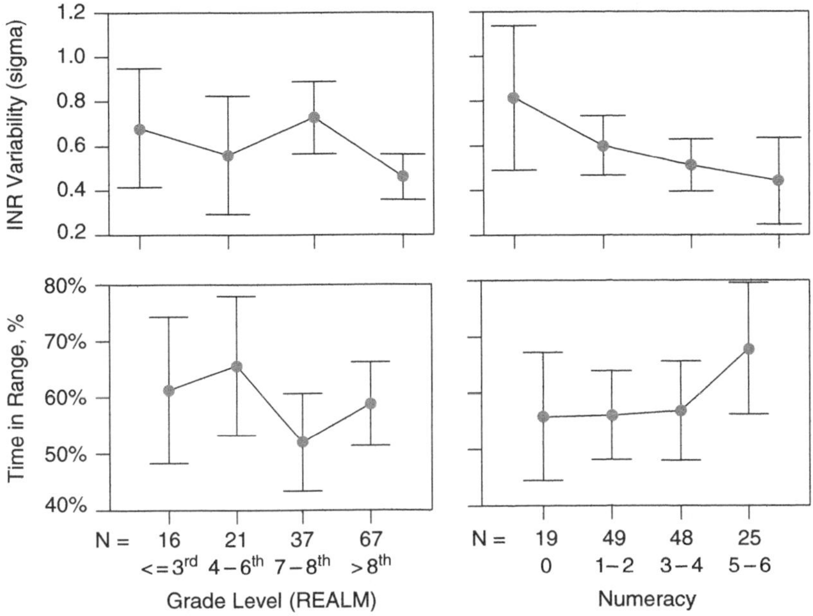

Figure 4.3. Anticoagulation control according to literacy grade level and numeracy level. Error bars represent 95% confidence intervals. INR, international normalized ratio; REALM, Rapid Estimate of Adult Literacy in Medicine. (Reprinted from *The American Journal of the Medical Sciences*, 328(2), Jan 1, 2004, "Literacy and numeracy skills and anticoagulation control" by Carlos Estrada et al., with permission from Wolters Kluwer Health.)

with a history of hospitalizations and ED visits even when controlling for age, sex, educational attainment, and household income (Apter et al., 2006). Furthermore, a study of 28 emergency departments across 17 states found a higher prevalence of limited numeracy among patients presenting with acute asthma symptoms than the general outpatient population (Ginde et al., 2008).

Chronic kidney disease

Patients with chronic kidney disease (CKD) or end stage renal disease (ESRD) are faced with difficult decisions regarding their treatment options, including the possibility of kidney transplantation. Abdel-Kader et al. studied 187 patients with stage 4 or 5 CKD or ESRD and found that high numeracy was associated with receipt of a kidney transplant or being listed as active status on the transplant waitlist, even after adjusting for age, sex, race, and duration of follow-up (Abdel-Kader et al., 2010). These results suggest that low numeracy may be a barrier to patient interest in kidney transplantation, perhaps by affecting patients' ability to understand the risks and benefits of transplantation. Alternately, clinicians may see less numerate patients as less viable candidates for transplantation.

HIV

Given that patients with HIV must often manage particularly complex multi-drug medication regimens in order to effectively treat their condition, we would expect that numeracy skills would be important for HIV management. In fact, numeracy abilities have been shown to mediate observed disparities among female and African-American HIV patients and their ability to answer questions about a mock HIV medication regimen (Waldrop-Valverde et al., 2009a, 2009b). Furthermore, the cognitive dysfunction that can be associated with HIV infection has the potential to interfere with patients' ability to accurately manage their disease. Waldrop-Valverde et al. tested 191 HIV-positive patients for neurocognitive functioning, health literacy, and numeracy to assess effects on a simulated HIV medication regimen. The results showed that measures relating to "Executive Skill," which include numeracy scores from the Applied Problems subtest of the Woodcock Johnson-III Tests of Achievement, were significantly associated with patients' scores on the medication management task (Waldrop-Valverde et al., 2010).

Cancer screening

Given the previously discussed findings of relationships between numeracy and comprehension of the risks of cancer and the benefits of cancer screening, it is certainly plausible that patients with higher numerical abilities will also have higher rates of compliance with cancer screening guidelines. However, the results of three studies show conflicting results. Using cross-sectional data from the 2007 Health Information National Trends Survey (HINTS), Ciampa et al. found that adults 50 years or older with low numeracy skills also had significantly lower odds of self-reported up-to-date CRC screening in comparison to those with higher numeracy abilities (Ciampa et al., 2010). Yet, when Shapira et al. measured health numeracy using the Lipkus scale (Lipkus et al., 2001), they found no association between health numeracy and breast, cervical, or colorectal cancer screening in a sample of 359 individuals aged 40 years or older (Schapira et al., 2011). Another study examined an urban population of 264 women aged 40 years or older and also found no association between either breast or colorectal cancer screening and numeracy (Aggarwal et al., 2007).

Smoking

Although numeracy is not associated with becoming a regular smoker, poor numeracy has been found to be significantly associated with smoking cessation. In one study, among people who had ever been regular smokers, the odds of participants quitting smoking increased by about 24% (OR = 1.24) for every point increase in an 8-item numeracy score (Martin et al., 2012).

Conclusion: patient numeracy matters

The measurement and study of numeracy has historically been most associated with efforts to communicate health risk data (such as cancer or side effect risks) to patients and to enable patients to complete complex number-based tasks such as utility elicitations. The reasons are obvious: Both tasks require patients to receive quantitative data, process it in certain ways, and then often return answers in quantitative forms. The abilities and preferences that are components of patient numeracy enable people to do those tasks in meaningful, and hence medically useful, ways. Measures of numeracy consistently perform better than broader measures of education in predicting such abilities.

The focus on numeracy in medical risk communication and decision making situations, however, has left many people unclear about the relevance of numeracy to real-world health outcomes. *We need to convince clinicians, patients and health policy makers alike that more numerate patients are not just better able to make value-concordant health decisions (e.g., by better comprehending the risk trade-offs in pregnancy or cancer treatment) but more importantly are better able to live healthier lives (e.g., by better managing their chronic diseases and better understanding which health risks are more significant and modifiable).*

Numbers are a fundamental part of an enormous number of patient healthcare tasks and patient health maintenance activities, and hence numeracy is an important determinant of patient health outcomes. If we wish to improve these outcomes, we must identify numeracy-related barriers and take active steps to overcome them. Such steps might include greater use of visual aids to help transform numbers into more meaningful pictures. They might include using evaluative labels to help patients interpret the meaning of health data. In many situations, using simpler messages instead of more detailed numerical data communications might help less numerate patients to grasp the "gist" of what they need to know for health management. In addition, numeracy screening tests could be used to identify patients needing assistance with health data, thereby preventing numeracy-related health disparities.

Because numbers are a fundamental part of healthcare, numeracy research must be a fundamental part of health services research. Demonstrating that numeracy is related to patient abilities is a good initial step, but the value of such research is multiplied when the mediational pathway from numeracy to ability to outcome is fully described and documented. To this end, we urge systematic measurement and analysis of patient numeracy in all types of patient medical research, not just those focused on medical risk communication. In particular, the effectiveness of interventions related to chronic disease management (including cancer survivorship) appears particularly likely to be influenced by patient numeracy. Researchers in this area need to measure patient numeracy consistently and to consider whether it is a potential moderating factor that may explain variations in certain types of patient outcomes perhaps even better than standard demographics (e.g., race, gender, ethnicity) do.

More importantly, we need to acknowledge the impact of numeracy on the design of health informatics systems. Simply providing patients (and, for that matter, clinicians) with accurate health data reports is not enough. We need to provide health data in easy-to-understand and easy-to-evaluate formats and to work with patients to build their general and context-specific numeracy skills if we expect them to use that information in self-management and medical decision making. As a result, we sorely need research that systematically identifies when and why patients need quantitative health data and when they don't (e.g., Zikmund-Fisher, 2013). Such findings could then be used to develop templates for health data communications in electronic medical record systems that specifically meet the needs of less numerate patients.

Both patient access to health data (e.g., through patient portals to their electronic health records) and requirements that patients use health data for self-monitoring (e.g., risk calculators, blood glucose meters) are increasing dramatically (Bonander & Gates, 2010; Ahern et al., 2011; CLIA Program, 2011). As a result, less numerate patients are at an ever-greater disadvantage as they try to navigate through the healthcare system and manage their own care. Only once all partners in the healthcare system recognize the central role of numeracy in health behaviors will there be willingness to change established practices to make many different types of health data more intuitively meaningful for *all* patients, not just those with higher numeracy. By such actions, a broader understanding of the impact of numeracy on patient actions and outcomes holds the potential to improve not just specific types of medical care but to help to address many of our most pressing public health objectives.

References

Abdel-Kader, K., Dew, M. A., Bhatnagar, M., Argyropoulos, C., Karpov, I., Switzer, G., et al. (2010). Numeracy skills in CKD: correlates and outcomes. *Clinical Journal of the American Society of Nephrology*, 5(9), 1566–1573.

Aggarwal, A., Speckman, J. L., Paasche-Orlow, M. K., Roloff, K. S., & Battaglia, T. A. (2007). The role of numeracy on cancer screening among urban women. *American Journal of Health Behavior*, 31(Suppl 1), s57–s68.

Ahern, D. K., Woods, S. S., Lightowler, M. C., Finley, S. W., & Houston, T. K., (2011). Promise of and potential for patient-facing technologies to enable meaningful use. *American Journal of Preventive Medicine*, 40(5), S162–S172.

Ancker, J. S., & Kaufman, D. (2007). Rethinking health numeracy: a multidisciplinary literature review. *Journal of the American Medical Informatics Association*, 14(6), 713–721.

Apter, A. J., Cheng, J., Small, D., Bennett, I. M., Albert, C., Fein, D. G., et al. (2006). Asthma numeracy skill and health literacy. *Journal of Asthma*, 43(9), 705–710.

Apter, A. J., Paasche-Orlow, M. K., Remillard, J. T., Bennett, I. M., Ben-Joseph, E. P., Batista, R. M., et al. (2008). Numeracy and communication with patients: they are counting on us. *Journal of General Internal Medicine*, 23(12), 2117–2124.

Bonander, J., & Gates, S. (2010). Public health in an era of personal health records: opportunities for innovation and new partnerships. *Journal of Medical Internet Research*, 12(3), e33.

Brown, S. M., Culver, J. O., Osann, K. E., MacDonald, D. J., Sand, S., Thornton, A. A., et al. (2011). Health literacy, numeracy, and interpretation of graphical breast cancer risk estimates. *Patient Education and Counseling*, 83(1), 92–98.

Cavanaugh, K., Huizinga, M. M., Wallston, K. A., Gebretsadik, T., Shintani, A., Davis, D., et al. (2008). Association of numeracy and diabetes control. *Annals of Internal Medicine*, 148(10), 737–746.

Ciampa, P. J., Osborn, C. Y., Peterson, N. B., & Rothman, R. L. (2010). Patient numeracy, perceptions of provider communication, and colorectal cancer screening utilization. *Journal of Health Communication*, 15 (Suppl 3), 157–168.

CLIA Program and HIPAA Privacy Rule: Patients' access to test reports. (2011). *Federal Register*, 76(178), 56712–56724.

Donelle, L., Arocha, J. F., & Hoffman-Goetz, L. (2008). Health literacy and numeracy: key factors in cancer risk comprehension. *Chronic Diseases in Canada*, 29(1), 1–8.

Estrada, C. A., Martin-Hryniewicz, M., Peek, B. T., Collins, C., & Byrd, J. C., (2004). Literacy and numeracy skills and anticoagulation control. *American Journal of Medical Science*, 328(2), 88–93.

Fagerlin, A., Zikmund-Fisher, B. J., Ubel, P. A., Jankovic, A., Derry, H., & Smith, D. M. (2007). Measuring numeracy without a math test: Development of the subjective numeracy scale (SNS). *Medical Decision Making*, 27(5), 672–680.

Gaissmaier, W., Wegwarth, O., Skopec, D., Müller, A.-S., Broschinski, S., & Politi, M. C. (2012). Numbers can be worth a thousand pictures: Individual differences in understanding graphical and numerical representations of health-related information. *Health Psychology*, 31(3), 286–296.

Galesic, M., & Garcia-Retamero, R. (2011a). Graph literacy: A cross-cultural comparison. *Medical Decision Making*, 31(3), 444–457.

Galesic, M., & Garcia-Retamero, R. (2011b). Do low-numeracy people avoid shared decision making? *Health Psychology*, 30(3), 336–341.

Galesic, M., Gigerenzer, G., & Straubinger, N. (2009a). Natural frequencies help older adults and people with low numeracy to evaluate medical screening tests. *Medical Decision Making*, 29(3), 368–371.

Galesic, M., Garcia-Retamero, R., & Gigerenzer, G. (2009b). Using icon arrays to communicate medical risks: overcoming low numeracy. *Health Psychology*, 28(2), 210–216.

Garcia-Retamero, R., & Galesic, M. (2009). Communicating treatment risk reduction to people with low numeracy skills: a cross-cultural comparison. *American Journal of Public Health*, 99(12), 2196–2202.

Garcia-Retamero, R., & Galesic, M. (2010). Who profits from visual aids: Overcoming challenges in people's understanding of risks. *Social Science and Medicine*, 70(7), 1019–1025.

Garcia-Retamero, R., & Galesic, M. (2011). Using plausible group sizes to communicate information about medical risks. *Patient Education and Counseling*, 84(2), 245–250.

Gardner, P. H., McMillan, B., Raynor, D. K., Woolf, E., & Knapp, P. (2011). The effect of numeracy on the comprehension of information about medicines in users of a patient information website. *Patient Education and Counseling*, 83(3), 398–403.

Ginde, A. A., Clark, S., Goldstein, J. N., & Camargo, Jr., C. A. (2008). Demographic disparities in numeracy among emergency department patients: Evidence from two multicenter studies. *Patient Education and Counseling*, 72(2), 350–356.

Harle, C. A., Downs, J. S., & Padman, R. (2012). Effectiveness of personalized and interactive health risk calculators: a randomized trial. *Medical Decision Making*, 32(4), 594–605.

Hawley, S. T., Zikmund-Fisher, B. J., Ubel, P. A., Jankovic, A., Lucas, T., & Fagerlin, A. (2008). The impact of the format of graphical presentation on health-related knowledge and treatment choices. *Patient Education and Counseling*, 73(3), 448–455.

Hess, R., Visschers, V. H. M., Siegrist, M., & Keller, C. (2011a). How do people perceive graphical risk communication? The role of subjective numeracy. *Journal of Risk Research*, 14(1), 47–61.

Hess, R., Visschers, V. H. M., Siegrist, M. (2011b). Risk communication with pictographs: The role of numeracy and graph processing. *Judgment and Decision Making*, 6(3), 263–74.

Hsee, C. K. (1996). The evaluability hypothesis: An explanation for preference reversals between joint and separate evaluations of alternatives. *Organizational Behavior and Human Decision Processes*, 67(3), 247–257.

Hsee, C. K., Blount, S., Loewenstein, G. F., & Bazerman, M. H. (1999). Preference reversals between joint and separate evaluations of options: A review and theoretical analysis. *Psychological Bulletin*, 125(5), 576–590.

Huizinga, M. M., Elasy, T. A., Wallston, K. A., Cavanaugh, K., Davis, D., Gregory, R. P., et al. (2008). Development and validation of the Diabetes Numeracy Test (DNT). *BMC Health Services Research*, 8, 96.

Keller, C. (2011). Using a familiar risk comparison within a risk ladder to improve risk understanding by low numerates: A study of visual attention. *Risk Analysis*, 31(7), 1043–1054.

Kumar, D., Sanders, L., Perrin, E. M., Lokker, N., Patterson, B., Gunn, V., et al. (2010). Parental understanding of infant health information: Health literacy, numeracy, and the Parental Health Literacy Activities Test (PHLAT). *Academic Pediatrics*, 10(5), 309–316.

Kurzon, N. (2004). A poker player's guide to beating cancer. *Newsweek*, 19, 12.

Langford, A. T., Resnicow, K., Roberts, J. S., & Zikmund-Fisher, B. J. (2012). Racial and ethnic differences in direct-to-consumer genetic tests awareness in HINTS 2007: Sociodemographic and numeracy correlates. *Journal of Genetic Counseling*, 21(3), 440–447.

Lipkus, I. M., & Peters, E. (2009). Understanding the role of numeracy in health: Proposed theoretical framework and practical insights. *Health Education and Behavior*, 36(6), 1065–1081.

Lipkus, I. M., Samsa, G., & Rimer, B. K. (2001). General performance on a numeracy scale among highly educated samples. *Medical Decision Making*, 21(1), 37–44.

Lipkus, I. M., Peters, E., Kimmick, G., Liotcheva, V., & Marcom, P. (2010). Breast cancer patients' treatment expectations after exposure to the decision aid program adjuvant online: The influence of numeracy. *Medical Decision Making*, 30, 464–473.

Manganello, J. A., & Clayman, M. L. (2011). The association of understanding of medical statistics with health information seeking and health provider interaction in a national sample of young adults. *Journal of Health Communication*, 16(Suppl 3), 163–176.

Marden, S., Thomas, P. W., Sheppard, Z. A., Knott, J., Lueddeke, J., & Kerr, D. (2012). Poor numeracy skills are associated with glycaemic control in Type 1 diabetes. *Diabetic Medicine*, 29(5), 662–669.

Martin, L. T., Haas, A., Schonlau, M., Derose, K. P., Rosenfeld, L., Rudd, R., et al. (2012). Which literacy skills are associated with smoking? *Journal of Epidemiology and Community Health*, 66(2), 189–192.

McCaffery, K. J., Dixon, A., Hayen, A., Jansen, J., Smith, S., & Simpson, J. M. (2012). The influence of graphic display format on the interpretations of quantitative risk information among adults with lower education and literacy: A randomized experimental study. *Medical Decision Making*, 32(4), 532–544.

Oettinger, M. D., Finkle, J. P., Esserman, D., Whitehead, L., Spain, T. K., Pattishall, S. R., et al. (2009). Color-coding improves parental understanding of body mass index charting. *Academic Pediatrics*, 9(5), 330–338.

Peters, E., Västfjäll, D., Slovic, P., Mertz, C. K., Mazzocco, K., & Dickert, S. (2006). Numeracy and decision making. *Psychological Science*, 17(5), 407–413.

Peters, E., Hibbard, J., Slovic, P., Dieckmann, N. (2007a). Numeracy skill and the communication, comprehension, and use of risk-benefit information. *Health Affairs*, 26(3), 741–748.

Peters, E., Dieckmann, N., Dixon, A., Hibbard, J. H., & Mertz, C. K. (2007b). Less is more in presenting quality information to consumers. *Medical Care Research and Review*, 64(2), 169–190.

Peters, E., Hart, P. S., & Fraenkel, L. (2011). Informing patients: The influence of numeracy, framing, and format of side effect information on risk perceptions. *Medical Decision Making*, 31(3), 432–436.

Reyna, V. F., Nelson, W. L., Han, P. K., & Dieckmann, N. F. (2009). How numeracy influences risk comprehension and medical decision making. *Psychological Bulletin*, 135(6), 943–973.

Rothman, R. L., Housam, R., Weiss, H., Davis, D., Gregory, R., Gebretsadik, T., et al. (2006). Patient understanding of food labels. The role of literacy and numeracy. *American Journal of Preventive Medicine*, 31(5), 391–398.

Schapira, M. M., Fletcher, K. E., Gilligan, M. A., King, T. K., Laud, P. W., Matthews, B. A., et al. (2008). A framework for health numeracy: How patients use quantitative skills in health care. *Journal of Health Communication*, 13(5), 501–517.

Schapira, M. M., Neuner, J., Fletcher, K. E., Gilligan, M. A., Hayes, E., & Laud, P. (2011). The relationship of health numeracy to cancer screening. *Journal of Cancer Education*, 26(1), 103–110.

Schwartz, L. M., Woloshin, S., Black, W. C., & Welch, H. G. (1997). The role of numeracy in understanding the benefit of screening mammography. *Annals of Internal Medicine*, 127(11), 966–972.

Schwartz, S. R., McDowell, J., & Yueh, B. (2004). Numeracy and the shortcomings of utility assessment in head and neck cancer patients. *Head and Neck*, 26(5), 401–407.

Smith, D. M., Sherriff, R. L., Damschroder, L., Loewenstein, G., & Ubel, P. A. (2006). Misremembering colostomies? Former patients give lower utility ratings than do current patients. *Health Psychology*, 25(6), 688–695.

Smith, S. G., Wolf, M. S., & Wagner, C. V. (2010). Socioeconomic status, statistical confidence, and patient-provider communication: An analysis of the Health Information National Trends Survey (HINTS 2007). *Journal of Health Communication*, 15(Suppl 3), 169–185.

Szrek, H., & Bundorf, M. K. (2011). Age and the purchase of prescription drug insurance by older adults. *Psychology and Aging*, 26(2), 308–320.

Tait, A. R., Voepel-Lewis, T., Zikmund-Fisher, B. J., & Fagerlin, A. (2010a). Presenting research risks and benefits to parents: Does format matter? *Anesthesia and Analgesia*, 111(3), 718–723.

Tait, A. R., Zikmund-Fisher, B. J., Fagerlin, A., & Voepel-Lewis, T. (2010b). Effect of various risk/benefit trade-offs on parents' understanding of a pediatric research study. *Pediatrics*, 125(6), e1475–e1482.

Visschers, V. H. M., & Siegrist, M. (2010). When reduced fat increases preference. How fat reduction in nutrition tables and numeracy skills affect food choices. *Appetite*, 55(3), 730–733.

Waldrop-Valverde, D., Jones, D. L., Jayaweera, D., Gonzalez, P., Romero, J., & Ownby, R. L. (2009a). Gender differences in medication management capacity in HIV infection: The role of health literacy and numeracy. *AIDS Behavior*, 13(1), 46–52.

Waldrop-Valverde, D., Osborn, C. Y., Rodriguez, A., Rothman, R. L., Kumar, M., & Jones, D. L. (2009b). Numeracy skills explain racial differences in HIV medication management. *AIDS and Behavior*, 14(4), 799–806.

Waldrop-Valverde, D., Jones, D. L., Gould, F., Kumar, M., & Ownby, R. L. (2010). Neurocognition, health-related reading literacy, and numeracy in medication management for HIV infection. *AIDS Patient Care and STDs*, 24(8), 477–484.

Waters, E. A., Weinstein, N. D., Colditz, G. A., & Emmons, K. M. (2007). Reducing aversion to side effects in preventive medical treatment decisions. *Journal of Experimental Psychology: Applied*, 13(1), 11–21.

Weinfurt, K. P., Castel, L. D., Li, Y., Sulmasy, D. P., Balshem, A. M., Benson, A. B. 3rd, et al. (2003). The correlation between patient characteristics and expectations of benefit from Phase I clinical trials. *Cancer*, 98(1), 166–175.

Weinfurt, K. P., Seils, D. M., Tzeng, J. P., Compton, K. L., Sulmasy, D. P., Astrow, A. B., et al. (2008). Expectations of benefit in early-phase clinical trials: implications for assessing the adequacy of informed consent. *Medical Decision Making*, 28(4), 575–581.

Witteman, H. O., Zikmund-Fisher, B. J., Waters, E. A., Gavaruzzi, T., & Fagerlin, A. (2011). Risk estimates from an online risk calculator are more believable and recalled better when expressed as integers. *Journal of Medical Internet Research*, 13(3), e54.

Wolf, M. S., Davis, T. C., Shrank, W., Rapp, D. N., Bass, P. F., Connor, U. M., et al. (2007). To err is human: Patient misinterpretations of prescription drug label instructions. *Patient Education and Counseling*, 67(3), 293–300.

Wolf, M. S., Curtis, L. M., Waite, K., Bailey, S. C., Hedlund, L. A., Davis, T. C., et al. (2011a). Helping patients simplify and safely use complex prescription regimens. *Archives of Internal Medicine*, 171(4), 300–305.

Wolf, M. S., Davis, T. C., Curtis, L. M., Webb, J. A., Bailey, S. C., Shrank, W. H., et al. (2011b). Effect of standardized, patient-centered label instructions to improve comprehension of prescription drug use. *Medical Care*, 49(1), 96–100.

Woloshin, S., Schwartz, L. M., Moncur, M., Gabriel, S., & Tosteson, A. N. A. (2001). Assessing values for health: numeracy matters. *Medical Decision Making*, 21(5), 382–390.

Wood, S., Hanoch, Y., Barnes, A., Liu, P.-J., Cummings, J., Bhattacharya, C., et al. (2011). Numeracy and Medicare Part D: The importance of choice and literacy for numbers in optimizing decision making for Medicare's prescription drug program. *Psychology and Aging*, 26(2), 295–307.

Wright, A. J., Whitwell, S. C. L., Takeichi, C., Hankins, M., & Marteau, T. M. (2009). The impact of numeracy on reactions to different graphic risk presentation formats: An experimental analogue study. *British Journal of Health Psychology*, 14(Pt 1), 107–125.

Yin, H. S., Wolf, M. S., Dreyer, B. P., Sanders, L. M., & Parker, R. M. (2010). Evaluation of consistency in dosing directions and measuring devices for pediatric nonprescription liquid medications. *JAMA*, 304(23), 2595–2602.

Zikmund-Fisher, B. J., Fagerlin, A., & Ubel, P. A. (2004). "Is 28% good or bad?" Evaluability and preference reversals in health care decisions. *Medical Decision Making*, 24(2), 142–148.

Zikmund-Fisher, B. J., Smith, D. M., Ubel, P. A., & Fagerlin, A. (2007). Validation of the subjective numeracy scale (SNS): Effects of low numeracy on comprehension of risk communications and utility elicitations. *Medical Decision Making*, 27(5), 663–671.

Zikmund-Fisher, B. J., Fagerlin, A., Roberts, T. R., Derry, H. A., & Ubel, P. A. (2008). Alternate methods of framing information about medication side effects: Incremental risk versus total risk occurence. *Journal of Health Communication*, 13(2), 107–124.

Zikmund-Fisher, B. J., Angott, A. M., & Ubel, P. A. (2011). The benefits of discussing adjuvant therapies one at a time instead of all at once. *Breast Cancer Research and Treatment*, 129(1), 79–87.

Zikmund-Fisher, B. J. (2013). The right tool is what they need, not what we have: a taxonomy of appropriate levels of precision in patient risk communication. *Medical Care Research and Review*, 70(1 Suppl), 37S–49S.

5 Application of numeracy in diabetes mellitus chronic disease care

Jillian Berkman & Kerri L. Cavanaugh

The epidemic of diabetes mellitus is recognized worldwide, is estimated to affect 366 million adults, and this burden is projected to increase to more than 550 million people by 2030 (Whiting et al., 2011). While strategies to prevent the development of diabetes will be a necessary priority, successful management of diabetes and its related conditions will be fundamental to optimizing overall health. Employment of available therapies to treat diabetes mellitus is often substandard (Saaddine et al., 2006), and in part contributes to the persistence of poor health outcomes in diabetes. Self-care is a fundamental component of the plan to treat diabetes, including tasks related to adherence and manipulation of medication schedules, diet choices, engagement in physical activity, preventive care, and health coping (Funnell et al., 2012). Patients and multidisciplinary providers including physicians or other clinical primary providers, dietitians, nurses, and social workers must collaborate to effectively approach the dynamic, and often complex, management of diabetes. Understanding the factors that promote a productive connection between patients, providers, and the overall health system is important to developing resources to engage patients with diabetes in successful care.

Literacy is more than just the ability to read, but rather includes a variety of skills related to processing information that is printed, verbally communicated, and also that which is quantitative. In the USA, it is estimated that more than 90 million people have basic or below basic literacy skills, and more than 110 million people specifically have limited mathematical skills (Kutner et al., 2006). Health literacy is one concept that characterizes the interactions between patients and the health system, and has been defined as, "the degree to which individuals can obtain, process, understand and communicate about health-related information needed to make informed health decisions" (Berkman et al., 2010). Vulnerable patient populations where diabetes is particularly prevalent are at risk for lower health literacy, where basic or below basic skills were reported in 59% of those greater than 65 years old, 66% of Hispanics, and

Table 5.1. *Diabetes tasks and related numeracy domains.*

Diabetes task	Diabetes care domain	Numeracy skill(s)
Dietary choices, carbohydrate counting, calculation of total calories	Nutrition	Numeration/Counting/Hierarchy Operations Fractions/decimals Multistep mathematics
Engagement in physical activity, monitoring of level of activity and its effect on diabetes, associated medication and dietary modifications	Exercise	Numeration/Counting/Hierarchy Operations Fractions/decimals Time/rates Multistep mathematics
Assessment of current diabetes status, interpretation of value and application for adjusting diet or medications if needed	Blood glucose monitoring	Numeration/Counting/Hierarchy Operations Time Multistep mathematics
Adhering to or adjustment of medications	Oral medication or insulin use	Numeration/Counting/Hierarchy Operations Time Multistep mathematics

58% of Black participants (Kutner et al., 2006). Perhaps more concerning is that even in the setting of adequate health literacy, mathematical skills may be poor (Rothman et al., 2006). Delivery of information about a person's health status, relative risks of therapeutic choices, executing medication schedules, and navigating the physical environment as well as processing of documents requires facility with mathematical skills and concepts, especially in diabetes (Table 5.1). The interpretation of the commonly used marker for glycemic control, glycated hemoglobin (A1C), requires basic math skills. People with lower numeracy skills may be more at risk for poor health outcomes, and require unique resources to support their care.

Identification of patients with poor health literacy in clinical practice is challenging. While the efficiency of assessments has been improved by the introduction of brief subjective screening tools (Chew et al., 2008), this and other health literacy assessments do not primarily aim to characterize the broad range of a person's numeracy skills needed in diabetes management. This chapter reviews specifically the available tools to measure numeracy in diabetes, the prevalence and associations of lower numeracy skills, and tested resources and strategies to overcome related barriers to diabetes care.

Measuring numeracy in patients with diabetes

There are several tools to measure numeracy skills in patients with diabetes mellitus. These include objective measures that assess actual numeracy skills of patients, including generally non-disease-specific and also diabetes-specific assessments, as well as subjective surveys characterizing the confidence patients have with processing quantitative information. The experience with these measures specifically in patients with diabetes is described here, where we first describe the performance of the measures and characteristics associated with numeracy and follow this with a comprehensive review of the relationship between each of the measures and health-related outcomes. To enhance the context of these results, a full review of numeracy measures is available in detail in Chapter 1.

General objective numeracy measures

Although the Test of Functional Health Literacy in Adults (TOFHLA) includes numeracy items in both its full version and its shortened version (Davis et al., 1991, 1993), these are often omitted as they contribute little to the variance of the overall score (Kandula et al., 2009) and have not been reported separately related specifically to diabetes outcomes. There is one report where the four items of the short-TOFHLA were administered to 518 older patients with diabetes and scored separately from the reading portions of the instrument (Kirk et al., 2011). Each of the four items was valued at 7 points for a total possible score of 28. Significantly lower average scores were observed among those with less education (19.9 ± 8.1) and lower income (21.0 ± 7.5) compared to participants with either more education or higher reported annual income (Kirk et al., 2011). Another consideration includes the Newest Vital Sign (NVS), a valid six-item measure of health literacy based upon interpretation of a nutrition food label that includes items directed at a numeracy component of health literacy. However, it does not offer the opportunity to evaluate the performance of these quantitative items independently (Osborn et al., 2007). A review of the performance of these general measures of health literacy in diabetes is reported elsewhere (Al Sayah et al., 2013).

Assessment of computational mathematical skills, including numeration, hierarchy, basic operations, fractions, and more advanced multistep calculations may be evaluated with the math component of the Wide Range Achievement Test (WRAT) standardized test (Wilkinson & Robertson, 2006). This 15-minute traditional exam with 40 items was not specifically developed to evaluate health literacy or health-specific numeracy skills, nor is it feasible to administer in routine clinical practice. Two research studies have examined general numeracy scores using this measure in patients with diabetes. In one sample of 398 patients, 69% had quantitative skills less than 9th grade level (Cavanaugh et al., 2008). In the second sample of 144 self-identified Latino patients with spoken Spanish fluency, 94% demonstrated a WRAT score equivalent to 7th grade or lower skills. No evaluation of associations with diabetes health outcomes was reported in either study. While the WRAT may have limitations as a general numeracy measure, it is a standardized objective assessment that can be administered across a range of ages and other patient characteristics. In addition, it has two forms permitting re-testing within study designs if desired. There are no studies comparing specifically the performance of the WRAT among the general population and patients with diabetes, although at least in the USA this is an age standardized test to then estimate grade-level performance. Objective assessments of general health numeracy are limited. A recent contribution, the *Numeracy Understanding in Medicine Instrument* (NUMi), is a 20-item applied quantitative skills assessment developed using item response theory methodology and validated in a sample of 1000 participants (Schapira et al., 2012). This test was not specifically designed for the context of diabetes care and the proportion of respondents with diabetes was not included, but 3 of the 20 items are centered on issues in diabetes management. Future studies may consider this instrument when assessing general numeracy.

Internationally the attention on the impact of numeracy in chronic disease is growing. In the UK, one study described the assessment of general numeracy skill among 112 patients with type 1 diabetes mellitus (Marden et al., 2012). Similar to the use of the WRAT, this study assessed functional numeracy with a component of the UK Skills for Life Programme (The Excellence Gateway, 2006), which included 25 items that were formatted as culturally appropriate word problems. A limitation of this assessment is its requirement to be administered by a trained professional. The psychometric properties of this assessment in this sample, including any associations between numeracy, patient demographic characteristics, and health literacy, were not reported.

Objective measures that evaluate predominantly skills with interpretation of risk or probabilities have demonstrated associations with health (Lipkus et al., 2001; Schwartz et al., 1997), but have received limited attention related to diabetes management or outcomes. One study created a numeracy measure by combining two items from the Lipkus numeracy measure assessing risk and percentages(Lipkus et al., 2001), and also two items from the TOFHLA evaluating understanding of medication timing and interpretation of blood glucose results (Brega et al., 2012). Internal reliability of this numeracy measure was not reported; however, low item-total correlations among the four items suggested lower magnitude of association among the items. Associations between lower numeracy and higher age ($p \leq 0.001$), less education ($p \leq 0.001$), and lower income ($p \leq 0.0001$) were observed and consistent with previous reports (Brega et al., 2012). Perhaps the overall applied quantitative nature of clinical care has driven the interest in a more functional assessment of health numeracy in diabetes.

Diabetes-specific objective numeracy measures

Previous research reports the development and use of disease-specific numeracy assessments in other chronic conditions. The Asthma Numeracy Questionnaire is a four-item survey developed to assess asthma-specific numeracy skills (Apter et al., 2006). Another example is the administration and management of warfarin therapy where a modified version of the brief Schwartz numeracy scale, adding three items specific to anticoagulation therapy, was administered and its association with successful treatment was examined (Estrada et al., 2004). In the effort to understand the underlying factors that drive the processing of information and its application in daily diabetes care, the Diabetes Numeracy Test (DNT) was developed to assess diabetes-specific numeracy (Huizinga et al., 2008). Prior to the DNT, there were no other scales that were designed to assess diabetes-related numeracy.

The DNT was created through a step-wise systematic process of development, starting with item generation by a group of experts. Specifically, this group consisted of diabetologists, certified diabetes educators, primary care providers, registered dietitians, behavioral researchers in diabetes, and literacy and numeracy experts. As with most projects, an inspired project leader is essential to spark and coordinate the development of a new measure. Assembly of diverse, but invested experts covering clinical, health communication, and survey development is essential. Initially for the DNT, 70 items were created that addressed five diabetes self-management behaviors (nutrition, exercise, glucose monitoring, oral medication, and insulin use). After piloting the items to assess understandability and cognitive interviewing with patients, the survey was reduced to its final full form consisting of 43 items (Huizinga et al., 2008). Inclusion of representatives from the target population is also essential. Participants may even be a consideration at the developmental stage if appropriate. Examples of the functional numeracy tasks within the DNT are nine nutrition items that require patients to interpret food labels and count carbohydrates, four questions addressing blood glucose

1. If you ate the entire bag of chips, how many total grams of carbohydrates would you eat?

Nutrition Facts	
Serving size 1 oz (28 g/About 10 chips)	
Servings Per Container 3.5	
Amount Per Serving	
Calories 140	Calories from Fat 60
	% Daily Value
Total Fat 6 g	10%
Saturated Fat 0.5 g	4%
Cholesterol 0 mg	0%
Sodium 150 mg	7%
Total Carbohydrate 18 g	6%

Answer: 63 grams

2. Your target blood sugar is between 60 and 120. Please circle the values below that are in the target range (circle all that apply):

55 145 118

Answer: 1 18 only

3. You have a prescription for Metformin 500-mg tablets. The label says, "Take 1 tablet with supper each night for the first week. Then, increase by 1 tablet each week for a total of 4 tablets daily with supper." How many tablets should you take with supper each night the second week?

Answer: 2 tablets

4. You check your blood sugar just before eating. You take 1 unit of insulin for every 10 grams of carbohydrates you eat. You are also given the sliding scale shown below. The sliding scale indicates the amount of insulin you should add to your usual dose on the basis of your blood sugar levels:

- If your blood sugar is greater than 120 points at breakfast, lunch, or supper, add 2 units of insulin.
- If your blood sugar is greater than 150 points at breakfast, lunch, or supper, add 4 units of insulin.
- If your blood sugar is greater than 180 points at breakfast, lunch, or supper, add 6 units of insulin.

1 unit of insulin per 10 grams of carbohydrates

If your blood sugar is:	Breakfast	Lunch	Dinner
>120 >150 >180	+2 +4 +6	+2 +4 +6	+2 +4 +6

Your blood sugar is 140 and you will eat 50 grams of carbohydrates at lunch. How much total insulin do you need to take?

Answer: 7 units

Figure 5.1. Examples of items from the Diabetes Numeracy Test.

monitoring including number hierarchy and calculations, five items assessing oral medication use, refill patterns and dates, and oral titration schemes (Figure 5.1). Numeracy domains include the use of addition, subtraction, multiplication, division, fractions/decimals, multistep mathematics, time, and numeration/counting/hierarchy. To model actual practice, the use of calculators is permitted when administering this assessment.

In 398 patients with diabetes, DNT scores were examined for associations with an a priori construct validity model that included education, income, diabetes knowledge, general numeracy, and health literacy (Figure 5.2). Analyses demonstrated significant correlations between the DNT and education ($\rho = 0.52$), income ($\rho = 0.51$), health literacy ($\rho = 0.54$), diabetes knowledge ($\rho = 0.71$), and general numeracy as measured by the WRAT ($\rho = 0.62$), with all p-values < 0.0001. Furthermore, DNT scores were associated with diabetes care behaviors that require quantitative skills including the frequency of blood sugar testing ($\rho = 0.15$, $p = 0.003$), performing adjustments of insulin for carbohydrate intake ($\rho = 0.51$, $p < 0.0001$) or blood glucose ($\rho = 0.28$, $p < 0.0001$) (Huizinga et al., 2008). In addition, internal consistency was excellent with a Kuder-Richardson-20 score of 0.95. Factor

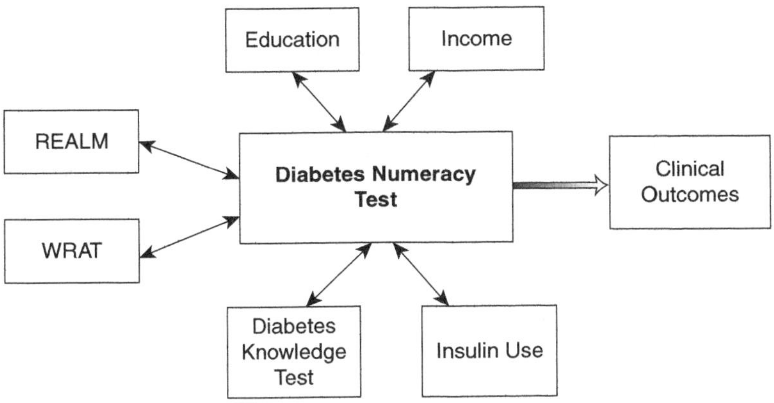

Figure 5.2. Construct validity model for the Diabetes Numeracy Test.

analyses supported one primary underlying latent construct explaining 65% of total score variance.

A significant limitation of the initial DNT instrument was its length and administration burden. The survey itself often required more than 60 minutes to complete, and often longer in those with more limited skills. Thus, the DNT scale was shortened from 43 to 15 items (DNT-15). The validity of the DNT-15 was established through random split sample analysis in which the overall initial sample data were randomly equally divided into two smaller sub-samples. Sub-sample 1 was used to develop the shortened scale and sub-sample 2 was used for confirmation of results. Principal component factor analysis using sub-sample 1 determined which items to retain in the shortened scale. Items with greater than 0.6 loading on the primary component were included, and additionally items with more than 80% mean correct score were discarded. The DNT-15 retained representation of all five diabetes care domains. Ultimately, the DNT-15 also showed good reliability (KR-20 = 0.89) and construct validity, and discriminated among patients with varying diabetes-related numeracy skills. Although the timing of administration of this shortened assessment was approximately 15–20 minutes, this may still limit its practical use in clinical settings. A further reduced version with only five items has subsequently been developed, and research evaluating its use and impact is currently ongoing.

In order to reach the growing vulnerable population of Latino patients with diabetes, the Diabetes Numeracy Test has been adapted and validated for use in Spanish-speaking individuals (White et al., 2011). The DNT-15 Latino was developed initially as an iterative translation and back-translations for each of the DNT-15 items. In a sample of 144 self-identified Latino patients with diabetes, correlations with education ($\rho = 0.35$, $p < 0.0001$), income ($\rho = 0.27$, $p = 0.001$), health literacy ($\rho = 0.29$, $p < 0.001$), and general numeracy ($\rho = 0.50$, $p < 0.001$) supported construct validity of the DNT-15 Latino. Internal reliability was also strong (KR-20 = 0.78), and average administration time was 20–25 minutes (White et al., 2011). The DNT-15 Latino and the other versions of the DNT are available for use (available at: www.mc.vanderbilt.edu/root/vumc.php?site=CDTR&doc=37816).

Subjective numeracy

The Subjective Numeracy Scale (SNS) is the only available assessment of subjective numeracy at this time (Fagerlin et al., 2007; Zikmund-Fisher et al., 2007). This eight-item assessment indirectly measures numeracy skill by querying subjects about how good they are at working with more complicated quantitative concepts, and demonstrates good correlations with objective numeracy measures. Its brevity and ease of administration are favorable characteristics for its use in diverse research and healthcare settings. The SNS is a general assessment that is not specific to diabetes, or to health or healthcare. Only one study specific to diabetes has reported use of the SNS, assessing it as a covariate related to computer use (Mayberry et al., 2011). In the 61 participants sampled with type 2 diabetes mellitus, numeracy scores ranged from 2.4 to 6.0 with a mean of 4.7 (SD = 0.9). No association in this small study was found between SNS and subjective health literacy (Mayberry et al., 2011). There is limited information about the performance of the SNS even in the general public, and there are no current studies available that directly compare patients with diabetes and those with other health conditions or varying health status. The validation study of the SNS, which enrolled mostly White (91%) patients from two hospital waiting rooms, reported a mean score 4.03 (SD 1.04), similar to the findings described above (Fagerlin et al., 2007). Additional research is needed to determine the strength of the SNS as an assessment of numeracy, and its relationship with outcomes in diabetes care.

Summary

There is a reasonable experience with measuring numeracy in a variety of studies in patients with diabetes, and includes both objective and subjective general measures, as well as diabetes-specific objective measures. However, the total number of participants evaluated remains small and there is not a dominant measure that has been adopted and applied for measuring numeracy in patients with diabetes. Burden related to the length, format, or administration requirements have limited consideration of integration of these measures into both clinical and perhaps even research settings. Information regarding the use and performance of the shortened DNT to only five items may be of significant value to advance beyond this hurdle and further our understanding of the impact of numeracy in the care of patients with diabetes.

Associations between diabetes-related numeracy and outcomes

Diabetes-related numeracy performance

Numeracy scores on nearly all measures generally are lower among patients with diabetes when compared to measures of literacy. However, the granularity of the translation of those scores to risk related to successful self-care or health outcomes remains in development. A summary of the available results describing available numeracy scores among patients with diabetes is shown in Table 5.2. The WRAT general numeracy assessment at least provides a national standard with associated US school grade equivalents for a measure of comparison. As reported previously, the two studies in patients with diabetes reporting WRAT scores found substantial deficits in quantitative skills with 69% having less than 9th grade skills in one sample, and 94% less than 7th grade skills in the other (Cavanaugh et al., 2008; White et al., 2011). In older adults with diabetes administered the four numeracy items of the S-TOFHLA the mean score was 22.2 ± 6.8 (Kirk et al., 2011). The four-item objective numeracy assessment combining two S-TOFHLA items and two risk-related items was administered in 3033 American Indians or Alaskan Natives with diabetes and found 69.8% of the participants answered the numeracy items correctly. Individual item results showed that most were able to identify the correct time to self-administer a second tablet (88.3%), convert a proportion to a percent (70.2%), and identify a normal blood sugar (69.8%), and fewer were able to identify the lowest risk value (52.2%) (Brega et al., 2012). Differences by literacy level were not reported, which might further our understanding of the compounding barrier of limited literacy in conjunction with numeracy deficiencies. For example, a previous study of 3260 Medicare patients reported that 63.4% correctly answered the item identifying normal blood sugar (Gazmararian et al., 1999). But when further examined by health literacy, among those with inadequate health literacy only 32.3% correctly responded to this question. Vulnerable populations may be even more at risk for a high prevalence of poor numeracy skills.

Table 5.2. *Summary of numeracy assessments in patients with diabetes.*

Patient characteristics	Numeracy assessment	Score	Reference
N = 398 51% Female 63% White 86% T2DM 43% ≤HS education	WRAT DNT	69% < 9th grade Median score 65% (IQR 42–81%)	Cavanaugh et al. 2008
N = 144 62% Female 100% Latino 87% T2DM 91% HS or less	WRAT DNT-15 Latino	94% <7th grade Mean (SD) 26% (19%)	White et al. 2011
N = 112 53% Female 100% T1DM UK	UK Skills for Life Programme Numeracy component	47% < Level 2 (equivalent to <14 years of schooling)	Marden et al. 2012
N = 3033 66% Female 100% American Indian or Alaska Natives 44% HS or less	4-item Numeracy Assessment 2 TOFHLA items 2 Lipkus Risk items	70% correct	Brega et al. 2012
N = 61 68% Female 65% White	Subjective Numeracy Scale	Mean (SD) 4.7 (0.9)	Mayberry et al. 2011
N = 198 64% Female 57% White 49% ≤ HS education	DNT	Median score 59% (IQR 26–86%)	Cavanaugh et al. 2009
N = 95 51% Female 50% White 96% T2DM	DNT-15	Mean (SD) 57% (30%)	Green et al. 2012

Diabetes-related numeracy has been evaluated in three studies. In the initial validation study, the median score was 65% (IQR (interquartile range) 42% to 81%) with a possible range of 0–100%. Further evaluations were performed by DNT score quartile where ranges for scores were 0–42% for 1st quartile, 43–65% for the 2nd quartile, 66–81% for the 3rd quartile, and 82–100% for the highest quartile. Areas of poor performance in individual item domains were found for calculation of total grams of carbohydrates in one food item based on information in a nutrition label (44% correct), calculation of insulin dosing accounting for blood glucose levels and carbohydrate intake (41% correct), and deficiencies were even observed for tasks often considered to be basic such as marking specific units on a diagram of a syringe (66% correct) (Cavanaugh et al., 2008). Participants with literacy and general numeracy skills less than 9th grade equivalent had lower median DNT scores (40 (IQR 23–58) and 51 (35–70), respectively).

The DNT and its shorter version, the DNT-15, were administered as a component of a clinical trial (Cavanaugh et al., 2009). In this study, the two groups administered the full version of the DNT had median (IQR) scores of 83 (65–90; N = 53) and 69 (44–84; N = 52). The other site, where the participants varied in respect to their socioeconomic and educational characteristics, were administered the DNT-15 and found no difference in scores by group (median 33 (13–70); N = 93 total). In a small study of 95 participants with diabetes derived from a primary care setting, the DNT-15 demonstrated a similar mean (SD) score of 57% (30%) (Green et al., 2011). One study of nine participants used a five-item version of the DNT and found that the majority of participants scored 20% correct, with a range from 0 to 100% (Gerber et al., 2010). In the sample of 144 subjects completing the DNT-15 Latino, the mean score was 26.4% (SD 18.9%) correct, substantially less than that observed in the other English-speaking administrations of the assessment.

Associations between DNT and outcomes

Glycemic control

The majority of the self-care activities for patients with diabetes are ultimately performed with the primary goal of glycemic control, including both dietary and medication management. Because of the common underlying reliance on numeracy skills to successfully execute many of these applied tasks, it is further hypothesized that numeracy may be associated with glycemic control. The primary validation study of the DNT examined its association with glycated hemoglobin (A1C), and found a modest significant association (Cavanaugh et al., 2008). In unadjusted analyses, the lowest quartile of DNT score had a median (IQR) A1C of 7.6% (6.5–9.0%), and the highest quartile of DNT score A1C was 7.1% (6.3–8.1%). In addition, those with lower DNT scores who also had fewer years of education, fewer years of diabetes, or used insulin had higher A1C levels. Among those with lower health literacy (<9th grade reading level), A1C in those scoring in the lowest DNT quartile was significantly higher than those in the highest quartile (Q1: 7.7% (6.7–9.3%) vs. Q4: 6.3% (5.5–8.1%); $p = 0.014$) (Cavanaugh et al., 2008). Finally, in analyses adjusted for age, sex, race, income, diabetes type, years of diabetes diagnosis, and clinic site, DNT score was modestly associated with A1C where a 10%-point decrease in DNT score predicted an increase in A1C level of 0.09% (95% CI: 0.01–0.16%, $p = 0.027$). The DNT-15 Latino did not demonstrate an association with A1C, but may have been limited by a smaller sample size (White et al., 2011).

General numeracy measures have been examined related to glycemic control in two studies. The UK Skills for Life Initial Assessments showed that numeracy skills at level 2 or higher were associated with statistically significantly lower A1C levels ($p = 0.027$) (Marden et al., 2012). However, when examining the relationship between the WRAT categorized as either <9th grade or ≥9th grade levels, no differences were observed in glycemic control (7.7% ± 1.7% vs. 7.5% ± 1.6%, $p = 0.28$). Path models adjusting for age, race, years of diabetes, and insulin use further demonstrated that no direct association between numeracy and glycemic control was observed, but rather an indirect association through diabetes self-efficacy (Osborn et al., 2010a). Higher numeracy skills were associated with greater self-efficacy of diabetes self-management skills, which was in turn significantly related to lower A1C. In addition, when health literacy is included in the evaluation, only numeracy remains associated with self-efficacy and with glycemic control (Osborn et al., 2010a). These findings reinforce the consideration that self-efficacy may be a target to improve glycemic control especially among people with low numeracy skills. The lack of a direct association between A1C and general numeracy is in contrast to that observed for diabetes-related numeracy. One explanation may be that the numeracy assessment of the DNT more closely replicates real-world applications and activities of patients with diabetes, thus deficiencies of this scale may more strongly correlate with clinical status. This may be an advantage when considering its use to identify patients most at risk for suboptimal diabetes control.

Diabetes knowledge, self-efficacy, and self-care behaviors

Health literacy is commonly positively associated with knowledge of general health as well as disease-specific information. Similarly, both general numeracy as well as diabetes-specific numeracy are significantly related to higher scores on diabetes knowledge tests (Brega et al., 2012; Cavanaugh et al., 2008). For example, those in the lowest quartile of DNT score had a median diabetes knowledge test score of 52% (IQR 43–81%) and those in the highest quartile of DNT score had a median knowledge score of 86% (IQR 78–93%). The format of the DNT consists of word problems and indeed contains common applications of diabetes quantitative issues. Therefore, its positive association with knowledge was expected and contributed to the construct validity of the assessment itself. If future novel disease-specific scales are developed, it is recommended to include a disease-specific knowledge measure if available.

As discussed previously, DNT score is also significantly associated with factors that contribute to diabetes control, including self-efficacy and self-care behaviors. Additional evaluation in larger patient groups is needed to confirm these observations. Among the patients assessed by the DNT-15 Latino, no associations were found with self-efficacy or self-care behaviors. However, diabetes numeracy in this cohort was associated with acculturation ($\rho = 0.28$, $p = 0.001$). Acculturation represents the varying levels which a group of people adopt and integrate behaviors, knowledge, and beliefs from a dominant culture (Lara et al., 2005). In this small study, participants with higher diabetes numeracy scores also had higher levels of acculturation. This further emphasizes that it is our vulnerable patient populations that are at the highest risk of limited skills, and the impact of this may be additive.

Role of numeracy in diabetes health disparities

It has been consistently recognized that racial disparities exist related to glycemic control. A variety of underlying mechanisms have been discussed; however diabetes numeracy has been demonstrated to explain at least in part differences in A1C by race (Osborn et al., 2009). In 383 participants (65% White and 35% Non-White), race was significantly associated with both A1C ($r = 0.12$, $p < 0.01$) and diabetes numeracy ($r = -0.46$, $p < 0.001$). Inclusion of diabetes numeracy in the analysis of the association between race and A1C reduced the effect to non-significance ($r = 0.10$, NS) (Osborn et al., 2009). Additional analyses examined the relationship between numeracy and intermediate health behaviors with a focus on medication adherence and differences by race. Although health literacy was significantly associated with self-reported adherence to diabetes medications, diabetes-related numeracy was not (Osborn et al., 2011). This finding was unexpected given the numeracy burden of diabetes medication management, and inconsistent with previous studies in patients with HIV. The study may have been underpowered to examine this association fully, as the majority of participants reported excellent medication adherence overall. These novel findings advance the understanding of the implications for educational and other social factors as potential targets to bridge the gap and promote health equity for all patients with diabetes, but also leave many questions unanswered.

Summary

Although the total number of patients with diabetes and assessed numeracy skills remains less than desired, the findings support that there is a high prevalence of quantitative skill deficits. This is consistent across both general numeracy and diabetes-specific numeracy assessments. Associations with glycemic control are even more limited, and at times demonstrating mixed results due in part to small sample sizes. However, numeracy compared to health literacy appears to be more closely related to diabetes clinical outcomes. More research is needed to clarify the magnitude of impact that numeracy has on diabetes control. Importantly, preliminary evidence supports the association between numeracy and behavioral mechanisms such as diabetes knowledge and self-efficacy of self-care. The execution of daily diabetes care is dependent upon numeracy skills, highlighting its potential importance as a target for improving delivery of instruction, counseling, and tools to support patients.

Strategies to address barriers due to diabetes-related numeracy

Addressing health literacy has been identified as a national priority in the US Department of Health and Human Services National Action Plan to Improve Health Literacy (US Department of Health and Human Services, 2010). This report promotes research, as well as development, implementation, and evaluation of interventions to improve health literacy and related outcomes. A recent systematic review of trials examining diverse health literacy interventions is available elsewhere (Sheridan et al., 2011). Often, health literacy focused interventions will integrate numeracy strategies rather than address them in isolation. The fundamental principles underlying these programs are often those of clear communication, including assessments of understanding, using plain language in conversation, and employing effective printed materials (Kripalani & Weiss, 2006). See Table 5.3 for a list of other strategies for clear communication.

There is a diverse body of resources available for clinical applications in the care of diabetes. The cornerstone of these resources includes print materials that cover the range of topics necessary for comprehensive patient-centered care. Previous review of diabetes documents including those from advocacy organizations found a range of reading levels, with many at higher levels than suggested to adequately reach patients with low health literacy (Hill-Briggs & Smith, 2008). There are also many statements and concepts throughout these materials that require at least basic numeracy skills to understand, process, and apply to self-care. A review of a

Table 5.3. *Clear communication strategies.*

1) Assess patients' baseline understanding before providing extensive information
   Examples for a patient newly diagnosed with hypertension: "Before we go on, could you tell me what you already know about high blood pressure?"
   This allows educational content to be tailored to the patient's informational needs
2) Explain things clearly using plain language. Avoid medical jargon, vague terms, and terms with different medical and lay meanings
   Example: say "chest pain" instead of "angina"
   Example: say "hamburger" instead of "red meat"
   Example: say "You don't have HIV" instead of "Your HIV test results were negative"
3) Emphasize 1 to 3 key points
   Repeat these points throughout the visit
4) Effectively encourage patients to ask questions. Use an open-ended approach
   Example: ask "What questions do you have?" instead of "Do you have questions?"
5) Use a teach-back to confirm patient understanding
   Place the burden on your shoulders to have explained the information clearly. Normalize the process, and be specific
   Example: "I always ask my patients to repeat things back to make sure I have explained them clearly. I'd like you to tell me how you're going to take the new medicine that we talked about today"
   Example: "When you get home, your [husband/wife] will ask you what the doctor said. What will you tell them?"
   To confirm understanding of a skill ask the patient to demonstrate the behavior (e.g., use of a metered dose inhaler)
6) Write down important instructions
   This lets patients know exactly what they should do after the visit
7) Provide useful educational materials
   This gives patients more time to absorb the information. Such materials are accessible to family members who may be helping patients at home

Reproduced with permission from Kripalani et al., 2006.

sample of 50 diabetes educational documents supplied by five organizations characterized the numerical content as basic, intermediate, or advanced (Joram et al., 2012). Approximately 11 numeracy concepts per 100 words were identified, and interestingly the most advanced mathematical text was more often found within the general information passages. Three recommendations were highlighted: (1) assume that readers will have low numeracy skills overall; (2) use visual support for quantitative concepts including pictures or diagrams; and (3) when using illustrations to represent a concept select objects that will be familiar to the target audience (Joram et al., 2012). Attending to numeracy in educational materials is likely to have similar or perhaps more impact as ensuring reading levels are appropriate.

Many resources are available for use through internet sources as well as diabetes-related organizations. We will highlight two examples that have

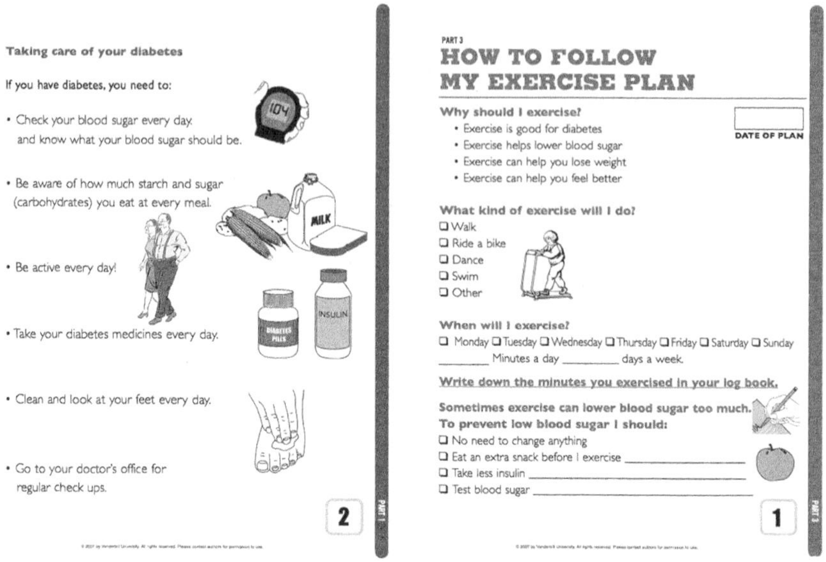

Figure 5.3. Examples of pages from the Diabetes Literacy and Numeracy Education Toolkit (DLNET).

been tested in research trials. The first resource is the Diabetes Literacy and Numeracy Education Toolkit (DLNET), which is a 24-module booklet intended to be used cooperatively between patients and providers to promote engaged and effective diabetes self-care (Wolff et al., 2009). The various modules were designed to be presented by either the patient or the provider during a clinical encounter and to be discussed at that time. Within the pages of the module notations can be made, instructions tailored to the patient's specific needs, on the spot assessments made of a patient's skills to interpret and apply health information, and there is a dedicated space for partnered goal setting. DLNET topics include general information about diabetes, recommendations and instructions for blood glucose monitoring, medication administration, physical activity, self-assessment of symptoms, and also nutritional advice. See a sample page of the booklet in Figure 5.3. Clear communication principles provided the foundation for the content of the DLNET by ensuring a low-grade reading level, images to explain more complex information, color coding, step-by-step instructions, and tools for tracking status of diabetes, medications, and other self-care.

The impact of the DLNET was evaluated in two concurrent randomized controlled trials at two academic medical centers (Cavanaugh et al.,

2009). In 198 patients, use of the DLNET was compared to standard educational materials in an enhanced diabetes care program. This was an existing diabetes educational program that included multidisciplinary visits including services provided by a dietitian, and an advanced practice nurse, in addition to the usual physician encounters. During the trial, these providers did not receive the additional communication training, nor were they permitted to use the tools of the DLNET. Three months after enrollment, at the conclusion of the intervention administration period, a greater reduction in A1C was found in the DLNET group compared to the control (–0.70 (95%CI: –1.10 to –0.20); $p = 0.005$). However, this difference was not sustained after an additional 3-month passive observation period. This study was not powered to examine for differences in the effects of the intervention by either health literacy or numeracy skill level. In adults, ongoing support may be required and the challenge will be identifying the most impactful components of our materials and programs to ensure efficient and cost-effective care. Although the DLNET tools are available for use, they have not been specifically promoted and their uptake is likely limited. At our medical center, a further distilled version of the modules where they have been reduced to interactive worksheets is currently under examination within a federally funded translational cluster randomized controlled trial. We expect findings from that research in the near future to assist with understanding more about the translation of these specific materials to clinical practice.

Created with similar underlying principles, the "Living with Diabetes Guide" of the American College of Physicians Foundation (ACPF) promotes health literacy and numeracy-sensitive goal setting and shared decision making (DeWalt et al., 2009; Wallace et al., 2009). Six topics are highlighted in this resource: diet, physical activity, blood glucose self-monitoring, insulin and oral medication adherence, and foot care. Its 56 pages use clear communication principles highlighting key points, adhering to lower reading levels, use of many pictures, and also dedicated locations for "You Can Do It" goal setting. Evaluation of this resource found that its use translated into more than 90% of patients carrying out a self-identified diabetes care goal (DeWalt et al., 2009). Although this resource and the DLNET are available via the internet, both are traditional printed booklet formats. However, there are a growing number of web-based interactive formats (Table 5.4 for suggested resources) with the goal to even more closely connect patients with educational and practical as well as provider support. Development and use of these format methods also need to be sensitive to the potential complexity and numeracy demands of not only the information delivered within the web

Table 5.4. *List of web resources.*

Tool	Internet address	Target audience	Information provided
Diabetes Numeracy Test (DNT) and DNT-15	www.mc.vanderbilt.edu/diabetes/drtc/preventionandcontrol/tools.php	Health providers	Brief assessment of diabetes-related numeracy
Scientific and technical information: simply put	www.cdc.gov/healthliteracy/pdf/Simply_Put.pdf	Health providers Health systems	Instructions to make useable patient education materials
Diabetes Literacy and Numeracy Educational Toolkit (DLNET)	www.mc.vanderbilt.edu/diabetes/drtc/preventionandcontrol/tools.php	Patients and providers	Complete guide and 24 modules to promote interactive diabetes care
APC Guide to Living with Diabetes	diabetesguide.acponline.org/	Patients	Can be used to aid patients in behavioral goal setting associated with diabetes
American Association of Diabetes Educators Patient Materials	www.diabeteseducator.org/DiabetesEducation/Patient_Resources/	Patients and providers	Brief worksheets on topics relevant to diabetes care
National Diabetes Education Program	ndep.nih.gov/resources/	Patients and providers	Comprehensive group of materials freely available in English and Spanish. Special attention to numeracy

resource, but also as applies to the navigation and use of the site itself. Even in the face of concerns regarding the digital divide and lack of access among vulnerable patient groups, there is promising research to suggest these tools may have a broader reach and impact than anticipated (Sarkar et al., 2010; Osborn et al., 2010b; Mayberry et al., 2011).

Translating and implementing findings of diabetes numeracy research into clinical practice

Assessment of numeracy in patients who have diabetes or other conditions that require application of quantitative information is feasible, although not routinely performed in clinical practice. The American Diabetes Association endorses in their standards of practice considering numeracy to optimize communication and care (American Diabetes Association; Funnell et al., 2012). Over the past 5 years, there have been advances in the methodology of both objective and subjective measures that may permit this potentially highly impactful information to be integrated into practice. Interestingly, it appears that diabetes-related numeracy is more closely aligned with important outcomes such as glycemic control, as compared to that of general numeracy assessments. Items that include practical skills required in the day-to-day management may be more useful in both clinical practice and ultimately research. To promote further ease of administration, the DNT has been reduced to a total of five items that significantly lowers its related burden. Its use is currently being examined in a large translational randomized trial among patients with low socioeconomic status. In addition, the SNS is a relatively short measure to administer and preliminary research suggests it too may be further reduced to only three items. However, its impact related to diabetes care and outcomes is unknown at this time. Administration of these measures is straightforward and does not require significant staff training or time and could be considered for use in nearly any healthcare setting. Low numeracy is a risk for poor outcomes in diabetes, and identification of patients with lower skills may be a powerful tool. Screening of all patients may not be an efficient application; however targeted assessments in those who may have risk factors for low numeracy, or among those who are already struggling to optimize diabetes care may be recommended. Although not specifically reported for numeracy, consideration of elicitation of shame or other anxiety during assessments must always be acknowledged.

Diabetes management programs most likely already include elements directed at addressing health literacy or numeracy barriers. The first step is to recognize that these are important factors in the delivery of patient education, and to review current process of care. Tools are available to perform a self-assessment of the organization's communication culture, although these are not numeracy-specific (Wynia et al., 2010). Evaluation of the processes and materials to ensure they are relevant and accessible to the target audience is the second step. This includes reviewing the suitability of the materials, selecting those components that are most appropriate for the patients and the setting, and then implementing. Evaluation after implementation is critical as programs and content frequently need to evolve as the patients or their needs change. Related to this may be the role of physician or provider numeracy skills. Similar to the patient, the provider must be adept at the quantitative tasks related to diabetes. If the provider does not possess the skills, or is unable to communicate the instructions effectively, the patient may be unable to complete required numeracy tasks. There is no published research in diabetes examining the role of provider numeracy skill independently or in combination with patient numeracy and diabetes care. Gaps related to provider statistical literacy and risk interpretation is discussed in Chapter 3. Additional research is needed to understand the true magnitude of the impact of numeracy in diabetes, and other disease care, including testing of innovative educational and behavioral interventions.

There are other chronic conditions in addition to diabetes that rely on quantitative skills to optimize execution of clinical recommendations. One example is the management of chronic congestive heart failure, where diet must be closely monitored and modified, and complex medication schedules executed often with adjustments for daily weight assessments. Similarly to diabetes, numeracy may be an important factor in successful self-care. A common consequence of diabetes is chronic kidney disease (CKD). This is a condition where the majority of patients are unaware of their disease (Coresh et al., 2005), due to the lack of symptoms and reliance on only an interpretation of quantitative laboratory information for diagnosis. Optimization of care to prevent the progression of CKD in addition to control of diabetes or hypertension also includes adherence to prescribed medications, avoidance of known toxins to the kidney, and healthy dietary and physical activity choices. In kidney failure that requires dialysis therapy, quantitative assessment of a patient's fluid status, blood pressure, weight, and laboratory measures reflecting anemia, nutritional status, and bone health are performed up to 14 times per month. The intensity of this information load is daunting and generally requires more than just basic numeracy skills to process. The influence of numeracy in the care of complex kidney patients is unknown, but improvement in kidney education is likely to be an important novel target to promote understanding and motivate self-care.

Future research

As described throughout this chapter, while there is exciting research and potential applications related to numeracy in the care of patients with diabetes much more work needs to be done. Further refinement of the Diabetes Numeracy Test through item reduction is under evaluation as described. The utility of developing additional diabetes-related measures remains uncertain, and it is only through additional critical evaluation of the DNT and identification of unmet needs may this be determined.

Application of the DNT in larger, more diverse, patient samples would enhance our understanding of its impact. The current studies are small and therefore must be interpreted with caution. Cultural factors are consistently recognized as contributors not only to the assessment of health literacy itself, but also to nearly all of the detailed components of health literacy representing how patients engage with their healthcare systems (Shaw et al., 2012).

The experience from developing a disease-specific measure may serve as a model for other complex chronic conditions. To enhance understanding of the mechanisms by which disease-specific numeracy may impact outcomes, it is recommended to include a disease-specific knowledge measure as well as one of self-efficacy of self-care if available. Assessments of these factors support construct validity of the measure, and may also lead to the specific identification of more influential numeracy intervention targets.

Finally, once efficacy of interventions has been established in clinical trials the next steps in translation and implementation also need to be determined. There is limited existing research in this area, possibly due to the heterogeneous approach to address barriers in health communication generally. It will be important for health systems to collaborate to better inform the underlying common needs of patients, providers, and systems that can be assembled into a more influential program ready for dissemination. Use of information technology platforms will likely contribute to rapid dissemination of successful efforts, and longevity of the program's application will be determined by its value as determined by the balance of its impact on outcomes and resource requirements.

Conclusions

Numeracy, especially applied quantitative skills, is an inherent component of successful diabetes care and warrants consideration, especially when patients may be struggling to optimize care. Tools to assess diabetes-related numeracy are improving and show promise for potential use even in demanding clinical settings. Administration of the instruments in large samples of patients with diabetes is needed to advance our understanding of their utility and how best to use the information gathered from these assessments. Although there are available resources to address numeracy gaps in diabetes, the resources are most often integrated into comprehensive educational programs and it has yet to be determined the impact of specific strategies to communicate and ultimately for patients to translate quantitative information and instructions into best diabetes practices.

References

Al Sayah, F., Williams, B., & Johnson, J. A. (2013). Measuring health literacy in individuals with diabetes: A systematic review and evaluation of available measures. *Health Education Behavior*, 40(1), 42–55.

Apter, A. J., Cheng, J., Small, D., Bennett, I. M., Albert, C., Fein, D. G., et al. (2006). Asthma numeracy skill and health literacy. *Journal of Asthma*, 43, 705–710.

Berkman, N. D., Davis, T. C., & McCormack, L. (2010). Health literacy: what is it? *Journal of Health Communication*, 15 (Suppl 2), 9–19.

Brega, A. G., Jiang, L., Beals, J., Manson, S. M., Action, K. J., & Roubideaux, Y. (2012). Special diabetes program for Indians: reliability and validity of brief measures of print literacy and numeracy. *Ethnicity and Disease*, 22, 207–214.

Cavanaugh, K., Huizinga, M. M., Wallston, K. A., Gebretsadik, T., Shintani, A., Davis, D., et al. (2008). Association of numeracy and diabetes control. *Annals of Internal Medicine*, 148, 737–746.

Cavanaugh, K., Wallston, K. A., Gebretsadik, T., Shintani, A., Huizinga, M. M., Davis, D., et al. (2009). Addressing literacy and numeracy to improve diabetes care: two randomized controlled trials. *Diabetes Care*, 32, 2149–2155.

Chew, L. D., Griffin, J. M., Partin, M. R., Noorbaloochi, S., Grill, J. P., Snyder, A., et al. (2008). Validation of screening questions for limited health literacy in a large VA outpatient population. *Journal of General Internal Medicine*, 23, 561–566.

Coresh, J., Byrd-Holt, D., Astor, B. C., Briggs, J. P., Eggers, P. W., Lacher, D. A., et al. (2005). Chronic kidney disease awareness, prevalence, and trends among U.S. adults, 1999 to 2000. *Journal of the American Society of Nephrology*, 16, 180–188.

Davis, T. C., Crouch, M. A., Long, S. W., Jackson, R. H., Bates, P., George, R. B., et al. (1991). Rapid assessment of literacy levels of adult primary care patients. *Family Medicine*, 23, 433–435.

Davis, T. C., Long, S. W., Jackson, R. H., Mayeaux, E. J., George, R. B., Murphy, P. W., et al. (1993). Rapid estimate of adult literacy in medicine: A shortened screening instrument. *Family Medicine*, 25, 391–395.

DeWalt, D. A., Davis, T. C., Wallace, A. S., Seligman, H. K., Bryant-Shilliday, B., et al. (2009). Goal setting in diabetes self-management: taking the baby steps to success. *Patient Education and Counseling*, 77, 218–223.

Estrada, C. A., Martin-Hryniewicz, M., Peek, B. T., Collins, C., & Byrd, J. C. (2004). Literacy and numeracy skills and anticoagulation control. *American Journal of Medical Science*, 328, 88–93.

Fagerlin, A., Zikmund-Fisher, B. J., Ubel, P. A., Jankovic, A., Derry, H. A., & Smith, D. M. (2007). Measuring numeracy without a math test: development of the Subjective Numeracy Scale. *Medical Decision Making*, 27, 672–680.

Funnell, M. M., Brown, T. L., Childs, B. P., Haas, L. B., Hosey, G. M., Jensen, B., et al. (2012). National standards for diabetes self-management education. *Diabetes Care*, 35 (Suppl 1), S101–S108.

Gazmararian, J. A., Baker, D. W., Williams, M. V., Parker, R. M., Scott, T. L., Green, D. C., et al. (1999). Health literacy among Medicare enrollees in a managed care organization. *JAMA*, 281, 545–551.

Gerber, B. S., Cano, A. I., Caceres, M. L., Smith, D. E., Wilken, L. A., Michaud, J. B., et al. (2010). A pharmacist and health promoter team to improve medication adherence among Latinos with diabetes. *Annals of Pharmacotherapy*, 44, 70–79.

Green, J. K., Rothman, R. L., & Cavanaugh, K. L. (2011). Patient-provider communication in patients with diabetes and depressive symptoms. *Diabetes Research and Clinical Practice*, 95, e10–13.

Hill-Briggs, F., & Smith, A. S. (2008). Evaluation of diabetes and cardiovascular disease print patient education materials for use with low-health literate populations. *Diabetes Care*, 31, 667–671.

Huizinga, M. M., Elasy, T. A., Wallston, K. A., Cavanaugh, K., Davis, D., Gregory, R. P., et al. (2008). Development and validation of the Diabetes Numeracy Test (DNT). *BMC Health Services Research*, 8, 96.

Joram, E., Roberts-Dobie, S., Mattison, S. J., Devlin, M., Herbrandson, K., Hansen, K., et al. (2012). The numeracy demands of health education information: An examination of numerical concepts in written diabetes materials. *Health Communication*, 27, 344–355.

Kandula, N. R., Nsiah-Kumi, P. A., Makoul, G., Sager, J., Zei, C. P., Glass, S., et al. (2009). The relationship between health literacy and knowledge improvement after a multimedia type 2 diabetes education program. *Patient Education and Counseling*, 75, 321–327.

Kirk, J. K., Grzywacz, J. G., Arcury, T. A., Ip, E. H., Nguyen, H. T., Bell, R. A., et al. (2011). Performance of health literacy tests among older adults with diabetes. *Journal of General Internal Medicine*, 27, 534–540.

Kripalani, S., & Weiss, B. D. (2006). Teaching about health literacy and clear communication. *Journal of General Internal Medicine*, 21, 888–890.

Kutner, M., Greenberg, E., Jin, Y., & Paulsen, C. (2006). *The Health Literacy of America's Adults: Results from the 2003 National Assessment of Adult Literacy (NCES 2006-483)*. Washington, DC: US Department of Education, National Center for Education Statistics.

Lara, M., Gamboa, C., Kahramanian, M. I., Morales, L. S., & Bautista, D. E. (2005). Acculturation and Latino health in the United States: a review of the literature and its sociopolitical context. *Annual Review of Public Health*, 26, 367–397.

Lipkus, I. M., Samsa, G., & Rimer, B. K. (2001). General performance on a numeracy scale among highly educated samples. *Medical Decision Making*, 21, 37–44.

Marden, S., Thomas, P. W., Sheppard, Z. A., Knott, J., Lueddeke, J., & Kerr, D. (2012). Poor numeracy skills are associated with glycaemic control in Type 1 diabetes. *Diabetes Medicine*, 29, 662–669.

Mayberry, L. S., Kripalani, S., Rothman, R. L., & Osborn, C. Y. (2011). Bridging the digital divide in diabetes: Family support and implications for health literacy. *Diabetes Technology and Therapeutics*, 13, 1005–1012.

Osborn, C. Y., Weiss, B. D., Davis, T. C., Skripkauskas, S., Rodrigue, C., Bass, P. F., et al. (2007). Measuring adult literacy in health care: Performance of the newest vital sign. *American Journal of Health Behavior*, 31 (Suppl 1), S36–46.

Osborn, C. Y., Cavanaugh, K., Wallston, K. A., White, R. O., & Rothman, R. L. (2009). Diabetes numeracy: An overlooked factor in understanding racial disparities in glycemic control. *Diabetes Care*, 32, 1614–1619.

Osborn, C. Y., Cavanaugh, K., Wallston, K. A., & Rothman, R. L. (2010a). Self-efficacy links health literacy and numeracy to glycemic control. *Journal of Health Communication*, 15 (Suppl 2), 146–158.

Osborn, C. Y., Mayberry, L. S., Mulvaney, S. A., & Hess, R. (2010b). Patient web portals to improve diabetes outcomes: A systematic review. *Current Diabetes Reports*, 10, 422–435.

Osborn, C. Y., Cavanaugh, K., Wallston, K. A., Kripalani, S., Elasy, T. A., Rothman, R. L., et al. (2011). Health literacy explains racial disparities in diabetes medication adherence. *Journal of Health Communication*, 16 (Suppl 3), 268–278.

Rothman, R. L., Housam, R., Weiss, H., Davis, D., Gregory, R., Gebretsadik, T., et al. (2006). Patient understanding of food labels: the role of literacy and numeracy. *American Journal of Preventive Medicine*, 31, 391–398.

Saaddine, J. B., Cadwell, B., Gregg, E. W., Engelgau, M. M., Vinicor, F., Imperatore, G., et al. (2006). Improvements in diabetes processes of care and intermediate outcomes: United States, 1988–2002. *Annals of Internal Medicine*, 144, 465–474.

Sarkar, U., Karter, A. J., Liu, J. Y., Adler, N. E., Nguyen, R., Lopez, A., et al. (2010). The literacy divide: Health literacy and the use of an internet-based patient portal in an integrated health system: Results from the diabetes study of northern California (DISTANCE). *Journal of Health Communication*, 15 (Suppl 2), 183–196.

Schapira, M. M., Walker, C. M., Cappaert, K. J., Ganschow, P. S., Fletcher, K. E., McGinley, E. L., et al. (2012). The numeracy understanding in medicine instrument: A measure of health numeracy developed using item response theory. *Medical Decision Making*, 32, 851–865.

Schwartz, L. M., Woloshin, S., Black, W. C., & Welch, H. G. (1997). The role of numeracy in understanding the benefit of screening mammography. *Annals of Internal Medicine*, 127, 966–972.

Shaw, S. J., Armin, J., Torres, C. H., Orzech, K. M., & Vivian, J. (2012). Chronic disease self-management and health literacy in four ethnic groups. *Journal of Health Communication*, 17 (Suppl 3), 67–81.

Sheridan, S. L., Halpern, D. J., Viera, A. J., Berkman, N. D., Donahue, K. E., & Crotty, K. (2011). Interventions for individuals with low health literacy: A systematic review. *Journal of Health Communication*, 16 (Suppl 3), 30–54.

The Excellence Gateway. Skills for Life Programme. Standard Tools. Initial Numeracy and Literacy Assessments. 2006. Available at www.excellencegateway.org.uk/toolslibrary (accessed 12/4/2012).

US Department of Health and Human Services, Office of Disease Prevention and Health Promotion. (2010). National Action Plan to Improve Health Literacy. Washington, DC. Available at: www.health.gov/communication/hlactionplan/

Wallace, A. S., Seligman, H. K., Davis, T. C., Schillinger, D., Arnold, C. L., Bryant-Shilliday, B., et al. (2009). Literacy-appropriate educational materials and brief counseling improve diabetes self-management. *Patient Education and Counseling*, 75, 328–333.

White, R. O., 3rd, Osborn, C. Y., Gebretsadik, T., Kripalani, S., & Rothman, R. L. (2011). Development and validation of a Spanish diabetes-specific numeracy measure: DNT-15 Latino. *Diabetes Technology and Therapeutics*, 13, 893–898.

Whiting, D. R., Guariguata, L., Weil, C., & Shaw, J. (2011). IDF diabetes atlas: Global estimates of the prevalence of diabetes for 2011 and 2030. *Diabetes Research and Clinical Practice*, 94, 311–321.

Wilkinson, G. S., & Robertson, G. J. (2006). *WRAT4: Wide Range Achievement Test Professional Manual*. Lutz, FL: Psychological Assessment Resources, Inc.

Wolff, K., Cavanaugh, K., Malone, R., Hawk, V., Gregory, B. P., Davis, D., et al. (2009). The Diabetes Literacy and Numeracy Education Toolkit (DLNET): Materials to facilitate diabetes education and management in patients with low literacy and numeracy skills. *Diabetes Education*, 35, 233–236, 238–241, 244–245.

Wynia, M. K., Johnson, M., McCoy, T. P., Griffin, L. P., & Osborn, C. Y. (2010). Validation of an organizational communication climate assessment toolkit. *American Journal of Medical Quality*, 25, 436–443.

Zikmund-Fisher, B. J., Smith, D. M., Ubel, P. A., & Fagerlin, A. (2007). Validation of the Subjective Numeracy Scale: effects of low numeracy on comprehension of risk communications and utility elicitations. *Medical Decision Making*, 27, 663–671.

6 Numeracy and genetic screening

Stephanie Dukhovny & Louise Wilkins-Haug

The necessity for clinicians to understand and interpret genetic tests is moving at a rapid pace. Within the past three decades genetics has changed from the study of individual genes and their resultant disorders to an analysis of the whole genome – the entire gene sequence which governs an organism's development, health, and variation. In 2001 the DNA sequence of a single human genome was decoded at a cost of three billion dollars and required 6 years of work. Ten years later, sequencing a single human genome now costs $10 000 with further price reductions to $1000 or even $100 expected and can be accomplished in weeks (Wetterstrand, 2013).

Facing clinicians now is the challenge of genomic health literacy; the translation of genomic information into healthcare in a format that is understandable to both healthcare providers and their patients. Often, however, neither the physician nor the patient has adequate training to understand the new genomic tests or the numerically based genetic calculations behind them (see Chapters 3 and 4 in this volume).

The field of obstetrics and gynecology is one medical specialty in which both the healthcare providers and patients have been at the forefront of the introduction of genetics into healthcare. Examples in this chapter from obstetric practice and in particular prenatal genetic testing will highlight several themes common to all discussions involving genetic health literacy. A further example from gynecologic care, BRCA1/2 genetic testing for ovarian and breast cancer risk, provides insight into one of the first direct-to-consumer genetic tests. This chapter will first review these genetic tests followed by an assessment of the unique numeracy skills needed for genetic test interpretation. As importantly, the subsequent sections highlight the healthcare providers responsible for these services and the current genetic literacy of these providers and their patients.

Genetic testing examples from obstetrics and gynecology

During pregnancy, prenatal genetic testing is traditionally directed toward conditions resulting in intellectual disability, major health concerns, or life-limiting disease. Screening women for their individual risk of a fetus having one of several such genetic conditions is now an integral part of prenatal care. Several examples below highlight the disorder, genetics, and numeracy skills that are required by patients for these testing paradigms to be completed. In addition to examples from obstetrics, examples from gynecology are provided with testing for breast/ovarian cancer risk. Although healthcare providers routinely assess an individual's risk for cancer, unique to this last testing is the introduction of the direct-to-consumer aspect of genetic testing. For all of these tests, genetic health literacy involves both an understanding of basic genetic concepts, such as inheritance, as well as numeracy. These examples highlight how genetic testing inherently incorporates comparative probability, risk reduction, ratios, and frequencies, all concepts which require a level of numeracy above that needed for typical medical counseling.

Screening for Down syndrome

Down syndrome, trisomy 21, is the most common chromosomal cause of intellectual disability. All women are at risk of having a child with Down syndrome, although the risk increases with advancing maternal age (approximately 1 in 1400 live births at age 25 to 1 in 100 live births at age 40). Down syndrome can be accurately diagnosed by chorionic villus sampling (CVS) or amniocentesis. However these invasive procedures carry a risk of miscarriage (see below). Several approaches to adjust the maternal age risk have been developed which incorporate biomarkers from the mother's blood or structural changes seen on an ultrasound. These associations occur in normal fetuses but all are known to occur more commonly if Down syndrome is present. The first association noted was a lower maternal serum alpha-fetoprotein (MSAFP), a protein made by the fetus and transferred into the maternal circulation. Currently an expanded second trimester screening panel includes MSAFP and three other biomarkers with altered levels when a fetus with Down syndrome is present – human chorionic gonadotropin (hCG), unconjugated estriol, and inhibin A (collectively known as a quadruple screen). Approximately 5% of pregnant women will have a quad screen which indicates a risk of 1 in 250 or greater that the fetus has Down syndrome. The majority of fetuses with Down syndrome (80%) will be detected among women with a positive quad screen (ACOG Committee on Practice Bulletins, 2007). However, only 1–3% of those with a positive quad screen have Down syndrome confirmed in the fetus.

Various other screening programs for Down syndrome exist, though all essentially function in a similar fashion, with either maternal serum markers or ultrasound findings adjusting the background age risk for Down syndrome. First trimester Down syndrome screening incorporates a measurement of a fluid collection at the fetal neck (nuchal translucency) combined with maternal serum free beta hCG and pregnancy associated plasma protein A (PAPP-A). The detection rate for Down syndrome using this method is 82–87% (ACOG Committee on Practice Bulletins, 2007). Again, many fetuses without Down syndrome will screen positive (5% among low risk women), but only 2% will have trisomy 21 (Down syndrome) when fetal cells are tested. Refinements of Down screening programs to include both first and second trimester assessments (integrated, sequential, and contingent screening) each have the advantage of increasing the detection of Down syndrome to above 90 or even 95%, but all still have the limitation that the majority of screen positive women will be found to have chromosomally normal fetuses when invasive testing is performed (Palomaki et al., 2012). Fundamental to Down syndrome and other aneuploidy screening programs is the reliance on provider/patient understanding of a priori risk reduction and the low specificity and poor positive predictive probability of the existing aneuploidy screening programs.

Population based carrier screening

Screening pregnant women for their carrier status for specific genetic disorders is the standard of care in prenatal practice. All individuals are thought to carry 3 to 5 gene mutations which could lead to disease if the mutations were present in a double dose. In the carrier individual, as these mutations occur in combination with a healthy gene, they do not cause the individual ill consequences. However, when the mutation is inherited by a fetus who receives the same specific mutation from the other parent, the presence of both mutations within the gene may lead to disease. These are known as autosomal recessive diseases. For most mutations, the chance that any two random individuals in the population would carry the same mutations is extremely rare. The chances become higher when individuals have a shared ancestry or shared gene pool either due to geography, culture, race, or ethnicity. Several autosomal recessive disorders occur with a high enough frequency that the underlying gene mutations are recognized as specific to certain races or ethnicities. Common examples include the sickle cell mutation in the African-American population, the Tay–Sachs mutation in the Ashkenazi Jewish population, and the hemoglobin mutation in the Mediterranean population. One gene in particular, the gene for cystic fibrosis, in the American population occurs at a rate high enough (1 in 20 individuals) that persons of all races and ethnicities warrant screening.

Guidelines for risk assessment for specific conditions vary but in general are targeted by ethnicity. The American College for Medical Genetics (ACMG) and the American College of Obstetricians and Gynecologists (ACOG) have recommendations for specific disorders for carrier screening for people of Ashkenazi Jewish ancestry. Although the list of disorders is not identical, each College based recommendations on carrier frequency as well as detection rate for testing (ACOG Committee on Genetics, 2009b; Ready et al., 2012). ACOG recommends that individuals of African, Southeast Asian, and Mediterranean ancestry be offered screening for carrier status for hemoglobinopathies (ACOG Committee on Obstetrics, 2007). ACMG recommends carrier screening for spinal muscular atrophy (SMA) for all couples who are considering pregnancy, while ACOG recommends screening only in patients with a family history of SMA (Prior, 2008; ACOG Committee on Genetics, 2009a; Ram & Klugman, 2010). ACOG recommended in 2011 that all women of reproductive age should be offered preconception and prenatal cystic fibrosis carrier screening, regardless of ethnic background (ACOG Committee on Genetics, 2011) (Figure 6.1).

	Recommended by	
Disease	**ACOG**	**ACMG**
Ashkenazi Jewish		
Tay-Sachs	X	X
Canavan disease	X	X
Familial dysautonomia	X	X
Bloom syndrome		X
Gaucher disease		X
Fanconi anemia type C		X
Mucolipidosis IV		X
Niemann-Pick disease type A		X
African		
Sickle cell disease	X	
Asian		
Alpha thalassemia	X	
Beta thalassemia	X	
Panethnic		
Cystic fibrosis	X	X
Spinal muscular atrophy		X

Figure 6.1. A comparison of ethnicity-based carrier screening guidelines between ACOG and ACMG. (Reprinted from *Fertility and Sterility*, 97(2), "Knowledge and attitudes regarding expanded genetic carrier screening among women's healthcare providers," Ready et al., 2012, with permission from Elsevier.)

While current standards for preconception and prenatal genetic screening depend on screening for specific genetic conditions in populations considered to be at risk, newer genetic technologies permit a broad search for genetic disease carrier states untied to ethnicity. Recently introduced technology offers a panethnic universal carrier test for 100 mendelian disorders, mostly autosomal recessive disorders. The disorders tested range from uncommon to extremely rare, and the conditions included can encompass those with life-limiting implications to those with the possibility of no discernible medical impact. Similar, however, to current genetic carrier testing directed by ethnicity, once a carrier is identified by this expanded panel, the partner's genetic status for the same disorder becomes important if the disorder has implications for their prenatal planning. Importantly, though, while individual disorders may be uncommon, once screening tests combine multiple rare disorders into a large panel of 100, the likelihood an individual is identified as a carrier for any one of the 100 disorders is approximately 1 in 3 (Lazarin et al., 2013). Providers and patients will need heightened genetic health literacy not only for the numerous disorders tested but also for the underlying probability principles of mendelian genetics as described below.

Invasive prenatal diagnosis

Currently, when a definitive chromosome or genetic diagnosis of a fetus is desired, an invasive prenatal procedure is performed to obtain a sample of DNA. One avenue to an invasive prenatal test may be a positive screen for Down syndrome such as described above. Or an ultrasound may reveal a structural anomaly in the developing fetus suggesting an increased risk of aneuploidy. Alternatively if both parents are carriers of a gene mutation, invasive testing may be the only option for assessing fetal DNA for the specific DNA mutations.

Amniocentesis involves the removal of amniotic fluid from around the fetus and is generally performed at 15 weeks' gestation or later. The amniotic fluid can be examined for fetal DNA, fetal cells cultured for chromosome analysis, and the fluid studied for alpha-fetoprotein for spinal defects. Chorionic villus sampling, available in experienced centers, provides an opportunity for DNA and karyotype evaluation at an earlier gestation (>10 weeks). Chorionic villus sampling removes a small specimen of placental tissue. Amniocentesis has an approximate risk of pregnancy loss of 1/300 and risk of rupture of membranes of 1/100. CVS has a risk of miscarriage of 1/100 (Rhoads et al., 1989). The choice between amniocentesis or CVS may be further impacted by such complexities as the time required to obtain results (can vary from 24 hours to

4 weeks), the potential need for additional studies, and the current gestational age.

Regardless of the option chosen, medical decision making at this juncture is a multistep process for the patient and provider:

1. understanding of the disease process suspected in the fetus (whether of a chromosomal or gene nature as detailed above)
2. comprehension as to how the risk to the fetus was ascertained
3. expectations as to risk associated with diagnostic testing
4. balance of risk to fetus against risk of diagnostic test (numerical and relative to outcome)

While these steps are inherent to all medical decision making, when invasive prenatal testing is considered, numeracy and health literacy play a central role given the underlying themes of genetic testing, which include probability, statistical reasoning, and problem solving.

Once the diagnostic testing method is determined, newer molecular techniques with their own unique genetic health literacy challenges are now being applied to the analyses of invasive testing. Chromosome analysis was traditionally performed through microscopic assessment of a metaphase spread with visualization of numerical changes of whole chromosomes, large deletions or duplications, inversions, and balanced translocations (Bianci, 2012). Newer array technology allows application of fetal DNA to a slide printed with high density, known DNA segments, which is then interpreted by a scanner. Arrays can detect whole chromosome aneuploidy, as well as much smaller duplications and deletions than traditional karyotype. These changes in the genome have many different terms and are referred to as microdeletions, microduplications, copy number variants, and copy number changes, amongst others (Friedman, 2009; Bianci, 2012). With increased resolution has come an increased recognition of variance within the human genome. With greater variance comes a component of numeracy in which adjustment for uncertainty plays a role. The incorporation of uncertainty into genetics, which is viewed to be highly infallible, may be particularly difficult for individuals to understand (Gigerenzer, Mata & Frank, unpublished data).

Non-invasive prenatal genetic testing

Isolation of fetal DNA from the maternal plasma provides a non-invasive method to identify pregnancies with Down syndrome as well as other non-invasive genetic studies of the fetus. Fetal DNA in the maternal circulation is present early in pregnancy, is relatively unaltered during pregnancy, is removed within hours of delivery of the placenta, and is derived mostly from the placenta (Lo et al., 1997, 1998b; Lun et al., 2008). With recently developed "next generation sequencing" techniques, the fetal fraction of DNA can also be quantified. If a fetus has a disproportionately larger amount of DNA material from chromosome 21, the analysis will reflect a higher percentage of fetal chromosome 21 than expected (Palomaki et al., 2011). Studies from women at high risk for aneuploidy have demonstrated 99–100% sensitivity and 98–99.7% specificity for the fetal Down syndrome (Chiu et al., 2008, 2010; Fan et al., 2008; Ehrich et al., 2011). These same analyses have been extended to trisomy 13 and 18 and the sex chromosome aneuploides.

Non-invasive prenatal testing for aneuploidy is now offered commercially in the USA. Guidelines currently recommend limiting these tests to high risk women and emphasize confirmatory testing with CVS or amniocentesis for positive results (Benn et al., 2012). As neither the sensitivity nor specificity is 100%, fetal DNA in the maternal circulation is considered an advanced form of screening and not diagnostic for aneuploidy (ACOG Committee on Genetics, 2012). The impact of introducing non-invasive prenatal screening for Down syndrome as a secondary test for patients who screen positive using traditional screening methods requires complex comparative numeracy skills on part of both the patient and the providers.

Non-invasive genetic diagnostic applications include Rh determination, fetal sex determination, and on a research basis, some single gene disorders. Maternal Rh alloimmunization, despite widespread implementation of Rh(D) immune globulin prophylaxis, remains an important cause of fetal stillbirth. Women without the D antigen on their erythrocytes are RhD negative and without prophylaxis, at risk of developing antibodies if their fetus is Rh positive. RhD positive men, who are heterozygotic, have a 50% chance of an RhD positive fetus. Invasive procedures can ascertain the fetal RhD status but put the pregnancy at risk for miscarriage, and if the fetus is RhD positive, increase the risk of transplacental hemorrhage and the risk for hemolytic disease (Daniels et al., 2012). Non-invasive diagnosis for fetal RhD can assist in the management of RhD isoimmunization and also screen for the need for RhD immunoglobulin, which is considered a blood product (Lo et al., 1998a). Programs applying these technologies have been implemented for use in England and Denmark (Finning et al., 2002; Clausen et al., 2012).

Genetic testing for breast and ovarian cancer risk (BRCA1/2)

Among gynecology patients, BRCA1/2 studies are the most commonly encountered genetic studies obtained. Typically a gynecologist would obtain a family history positive for breast or ovarian cancer and following the US Preventive Services Task Force (USPSTF) refer the patient for genetic counseling and consideration for BRCA1/2 testing. Three specific mutations within BRCA1/2 are associated with up to a 35–84% risk of developing breast cancer and 10–50% of ovarian by age 70 years (US Preventive Services Task Force, 2005). However, these BRCA1/2 mutations are infrequent among the general population, occur among only 1–2% of all breast cancer patients, and occur with greater frequency among the Ashkenazi population. Counseling would include risk assessment, pedigree analysis, and guiding of informed decisions about genetic testing (US Preventive Services Task Force, 2005). Such discussion would include the nuances of the ethnic distribution of BRCA1/2 and the implications of effect size (see below). However, consumers can also order a kit online which includes a tube for a saliva sample. The sample is then sent back to the company for analysis. At least one company is offering testing for three mutations in the BRCA1/2 genes. Board certified genetic counselors are available to discuss results, and their website does state that absence of these three mutations does not rule out the possibility of a mutation present that increases the risk for breast or ovarian cancer (23 and Me, 2012). A number of professional societies including ACOG, the National Society of Genetic Counselors, and the American Society of Clinical Oncology recommend pre- and post-test counseling when considering BRCA testing (Dohany et al., 2012). Not all companies offer genetic counseling, but do charge an additional fee to discuss results with a staff doctor (Wolfber, 2006).

Numeracy skills (genetic literacy) needed by healthcare providers to interpret and counsel

Physicians have a range of genetic health literacy which they acquire during their medical education and importantly must maintain through ongoing education. The major medical societies offer guidelines, as do the American College of Medical Genetics and the National Society of Genetic Counselors. While patients may have access to direct-to-consumer marketing, studies show that they prefer their physician's opinion on these studies. Physicians also have a role as gate keepers for genetic testing in many situations. A recent study of internists at an academic medical center found that almost half (44%) had ordered genetic tests in the past month which was significantly correlated to whether the patient had inquired concerning the test. This association had been previously reported (Sifri et al., 2003). Of concern is that the majority of these responders rated their knowledge concerning genetics as poor (73.7%) and awareness of guidelines as poor (87.1%) (Klitzman et al., 2013).

What follows are four areas of healthcare providers' genetic health literacy integral to their translation of genomic technology into patient care. These areas require ongoing attention as they are particularly relevant to genetic technology and will impact health literacy as genomic medicine continues to advance.

"A priori" risk reduction

An aspect of genetic health literacy essential to physician counseling is a familiarity with "a prior" genetic risk and adjustment of risk. In prenatal counseling, understanding of the risk of aneuploidy during pregnancy requires understanding of "a priori risk" (aneuploidy risk by maternal age) and risk adjustment (by serum screening or ultrasound). Maternal age (expressed as 1 in XXX) was the initial screening tool for risk of aneuploidy although it inherently functioned poorly as it screened positive a large portion of the population (15% of women are over 35 years of age and pregnant), detected only a fraction of the pregnancies complicated by trisomy 21 (approximately 30%), and has a poor positive predictive value (all the women undergoing amniocentesis for maternal age over 35 years have only a 1–2% risk of having a trisomy 21 fetus). The addition of nuchal lucency and serum markers described above refine an individual woman's "a prior" risk based on her maternal age and the results are reported to the clinician as "1 in n." This format was in keeping with the prior tradition of reporting a woman's risk based on her maternal age of a fetus with Down syndrome being presented as "1 in n."

This specific type of genetic counseling involves two numeracy concepts which are known to present difficulties for patients as well as their providers. First, conditional probabilities are presented which are known to be less transparent and more difficult for both patients and providers to follow. A typical explanation of aneuploidy screening is that 5% of women will have a positive Down syndrome screen, 80% of Down syndrome fetuses will be detected within the quad screen positive group, and within the group of women with a positive quad screen, the chance of Down syndrome is about 2–3%. Translation of conditional probabilities into natural frequencies has been proposed as a more transparent and less computationally driven approach (Hoffrage & Gigerenzer, 1998). For example, Down screening comparative probabilities stated as natural frequencies would be 17 of 10 000 women carry a pregnancy with Down syndrome, 500 women screen positive for Down syndrome, and 10 of the 500 will have a pregnancy with Down syndrome. Obstetricians/gynecologists have demonstrated greater ease with a translational approach with application to mammography risk reduction counseling. Greater facility with natural frequency presentation of data as compared to conditional probabilities has been shown in other medical risk assessments such as screening for cancer (Hoffrage & Gigerenzer, 1998). The ability to calculate a positive predictive probability (Bayesian calculation) is fundamental to much risk assessment in genetic disease calculation although this is a calculation which requires numeracy skills beyond that of most patients and many physicians (Ghosh & Ghosh, 2005; Hoffrafe & Gigerenzer, 1998). For patients and providers, conversion from a conditional probability and positive predictive probability calculation to a natural frequency format markedly improves comprehension of the risks presented (Gigerenzer et al., 2008).

Furthermore, to complete Down syndrome screening, additional numerical complexity occurs for patients and providers as they consider the patient's risk for Down syndrome, traditionally expressed as a frequency – 1 in XXX. For example her risk of a fetus with Down syndrome based on her screening is 1 in 500 compared to the risk of miscarriage from an invasive prenatal test, for example amniocentesis, 1 in 300. This format of comparison of two frequencies with differing denominators is a difficult comparison and often misinterpreted even among those with higher numeracy skills (Reyna, 2004; Reyna et al., 2003; ACOG Committee on Practice Bulletins, 2007). Conversion of frequencies (1/500 vs. 1/300) to percents (0.2% vs. 0.3%) in order to represent the comparisons in a different format is generally not helpful as this numeracy skill is the most difficult and beyond the basic numeracy skills of many patients and even inaccurately completed by 1 in 4 physicians (Schwartz et al., 1999). Studies have demonstrated that physicians who perceive themselves as comfortable with numeracy tasks are more likely to use numbers when describing Down syndrome risks to patients, than to present results as "low risk" or "high risk" (Anderson et al., 2011).

Genetic variance

Variance in the human genome is also being encountered to a greater degree by physicians. As advanced genetic technologies provide greater resolution of the human genome, a greater degree of variance between individuals is being recognized. The ability of patients to successfully incorporate uncertainty into medical decision making and risk counseling often reflects their underlying numeracy skills. An acceptance of uncertainty is considered to be an essential requirement for numeracy skills. Uncertainty or variance revealed on genetic testing may be particularly difficult for people to understand as DNA testing in particular is associated inherently in peoples' minds with one of the highest degrees of certainty (Gigerenzer et al., 2008). One example of this is the incorporation of chromosomal microarray testing. In pediatrics, the chromosome microarray with its greater resolution for microduplication and microdeletion of DNA now replaces the standard karyotype in which the chromosomes were stained and counted. The microarray is likewise gaining utility in the prenatal setting especially when anomalies on ultrasound are identified (ACOG Committee on Genetics, 2009c; Wapner et al., 2012b).

Microarray analysis, however, is associated with the identification of potentially unknown copy number variants (CNV) – DNA segments which do not have a known effect on the individual. While some CNVs or changes in the length of DNA are known to be associated with specific malformations or genetic syndromes, others are thought not to affect the individual's health as they are present in the normal parent, are small in size, or do not contain known harmful genes. However, others of unknown significance remain and leave the potential for deleterious impact on the developing fetus. When a copy number variant of unknown significance is detected in the prenatal setting, a major counseling dilemma is encountered. In the postnatal setting, copy number variants can be correlated with the clinical exam, such as structural or developmental abnormalities. In the prenatal setting, an inherent uncertainty of the complete phenotype is present, and is limited to ultrasound only. While labs will report previously described and well characterized variants, for variants of uncertain clinical significance, it is left to the clinician to know the next steps for interpretation (Wapner et al., 2012a). There are also publically available references online that can be used to interpret microarray results. The frequency of these unknown CNVs increase with the density of the microarray which is ordered and the level of expertise to determine the level of array density needed for a specific indication typically requires in depth genetic health literacy. In cases of an identified ultrasound malformation, a more in depth array may be chosen in order to ascertain a possible association of a copy number variant with the identified fetal structural malformations (Bianci, 2012).

Mendelian genetics

Genetic health literacy with regard to computation of risk for autosomal recessive/dominant and sex-linked disorders among physicians has typically remained solid. This is likely due to the traditional teaching of this subject in medical schools. For carrier testing, obstetrician gynecologists have demonstrated an understanding about basic genetic concepts. In one recent study 94% of physicians surveyed understood the definition of a "carrier," and 93–98% were able to identify the potential range of severity of genetic disorders (Ready et al., 2012). In contrast, prior studies had shown that obstetrician gynecologists were more familiar with genetic concepts surrounding aneuploidy screening and neural tube defect risk than mendelian genetics (Wilkins-Haug et al., 1999). However, genetic testing for mendelian disorders has grown to encompass more than straightforward mendelian genetics with interpretation of the testing results requiring a further degree of genetic literacy. For example, using a 23 mutation panel for cystic fibrosis screening, the detection rate varies depending on the ethnic group tested. The detection rate for cystic fibrosis in an Asian American is 49%, while in a woman of Ashkenazi Jewish background the detection rate is 94%. Thus, negative test results in these women have very different implications. There are more than 1700 mutations that have been identified in the CFTR gene, the gene responsible for cystic fibrosis. There are panels available that will screen for more mutations. Sequencing of the entire CFTR gene is also clinically available. A clinician who is performing carrier screening for cystic fibrosis must have an understanding as to which test has been ordered and, importantly, how to interpret the results if a more extensive panel has been tested (ACOG Committee on Genetics, 2011). Because carrier screening in more specific populations, such as the Ashkenazi Jewish population, is more likely to detect ethnicity specific mutations, the detection rate for these patients is much higher (95–99%) and thus, a negative test is easier for the clinician to interpret (ACOG Committee on Genetics, 2009b).

Carrier screening is expanding with inherent changes in genetic health literacy needed to interpret the results. Panethnic application of these panels removes identification of a patient's ethnicity, which can be inaccurate if determined solely by the MD's assessment of physical characteristics and likely admixed within the USA (Tayo et al., 2011). Of relevance to the ordering physician, these large panels will identify 1 in 3 people as a carrier for at least one disease. Thus, clinicians who order these tests must be prepared to perform pre- and post-test counseling, offer testing to partners, and consider issues surrounding counseling to family members. However, a recent voluntary survey of physician and non-physician providers in reproductive medicine and obstetrics and gynecology concerning genetic carrier screening raised some concerns regarding baseline knowledge. While basic knowledge was strong, understanding of inheritance once a carrier state was identified was less robust and incorrect in a third of responders. Not surprisingly, this same survey identified a substantial reliance on post-test consultation with a genetic counselor (78% essential, 83% helpful). This represents a significant workforce dilemma as 77.7% of respondents reported that if the costs were the same, their preference would be testing for a larger number of genetic disorders than a smaller number (Ready et al., 2012).

Large vs. small effect genetic determinants

The expansion of molecular technologies has transformed genetics from the study of specific gene mutations leading to single diseases to the incorporation of the genetics into practically all aspects of human health and disease. Along with this transformation, physicians will have to incorporate a range of genetic effects into their understanding within any particular disease. This requires an understanding of effect size of a reported gene change and the implications for their patient's health.

Perhaps the best example of a large effect genetic determinant are the genes increasing the risk for breast cancer and ovarian cancer (Weaver & Pollin, 2012). Three specific mutations within BRCA1 and BRCA2 are associated with substantial risks of breast and ovarian cancer by age 70 years (US Preventive Services Task Force, 2005). However, these BRCA1/2 mutations are infrequent among the general population, occur among only 1–2% of all breast cancer patients but do occur with greater frequency among the Ashkenazi population. While associated with a large genetic effect on breast cancer, the medical provider of women's healthcare should have genetic health literacy and numeracy to establish a paradigm for offering BRCA1/2 to their patients. Based on the provided information, women of Ashkenazi Jewish ancestry in whom a first-degree relative has breast and/or ovarian cancer should be screened. In other individuals, various combinations of multiple first- and second-degree relatives with breast/ovarian and other cancers might prompt testing. Given this understanding of large effect within a smaller population, general screening of all women for BRCA1/2 is not recommended (US Preventive Services Task Force, 2005). Despite these guidelines, primary care providers in several studies continue to order BRCA1/2 screening in low risk women likely due to their misunderstanding of the effect size in the general population (Van Riel et al., 2010; Bellcross et al., 2011; Trivers et al., 2011).

There is growing information concerning the small effect genetic changes which occur in common conditions such as diabetes, hypertension, and dementia. Much of this genetic information has been retrieved from gene-wide association studies in which single nucleotide polymorphism (SNPs) have served as markers for possible associations between candidate genes and the condition in question. These gene-wide association studies (GWAS) bring fresh reports of association between a candidate gene or SNP almost daily and a range of common disorders leaving the impression that genetic testing will soon unravel the basis for most of health and disease. Unfortunately, most GWAS findings are specific only to the population in which they were ascertained and typically are responsible for only a low level (generally less than 10%) of a disease's effect (Weaver & Pollin, 2012). Whether sequencing will increase the fidelity of these studies remains to be seen.

An example of the genetic literacy which would be required from a MD to understand small effect size can be seen in the GWAS studies related to type 2 diabetes. Over 40 genes have been associated with type 2 diabetes and in total account for only 10% of the heritable risk of the disorder (Voight et al., 2010; Ahlqvist et al., 2011). While panels using these SNPs have been designed to help predict whether an individual will develop type 2 diabetes, and are indeed marketed for this purpose, a recent analysis revealed no clinical utility (Mihaescu et al., 2011). The lack of clinical utility likely reflects the inherent issues raised with the GWAS studies noted above and the small effect of inheritance on type 2 diabetes. Concerns remain that inappropriate utilization of such panels by physicians and patients may lead to a negating of their risk as well as an avoidance of interventions which may be more appropriate such as diet and weight loss (Weaver & Pollin, 2012). Despite the lack of published clinical utility, 79% of primary care physicians and endocrinologists would likely order such testing. The level of genetic health literacy required for physicians to remain abreast of these changes is challenging.

Healthcare providers who perform genetic testing

Counseling surrounding genetic risks is provided by a range of individuals depending upon the situation. Genetic counselors have completed post-graduate, master level course work in the intricacies of risk interpretation, genetic theory, and the non-numerical complexities of counseling. A national board certifies genetic counselors and maintains ongoing continued education (National Society of Genetic Counselors; www.NSGC.org). Genetic counselors often choose to become specialized in areas undergoing rapid change such as prenatal genetics, cancer genetics, and personalized medicine so they can remain current for patient care and knowledgeable as educators for other healthcare providers. NSGC publishes guidelines for counseling for genetic carrier states as well as position statements related to genetic screening.

Genetic screening may be initiated by a physician, a physician's nurse, or by the individual themselves through direct-to-consumer marketing. For example, as mentioned, ACOG recommends screening and invasive diagnostic testing for aneuploidy for all pregnant women who present for prenatal care prior to 20 weeks' gestation (ACOG Committee on Practice Bulletins, 2007). Given the scope of the population covered by this recommendation, referral of all pregnant women to a genetic counselor is not possible. Such counseling for aneuploidy screening often occurs by a variety of providers, including physicians, nurses, and midwives. A survey of voluntary ACOG responders concerning their aneuploidy assessment routine noted overall consistency of their practices as within guidelines. However, less than half were correctly knowledgeable concerning numerical information related to Down syndrome likely being discussed by themselves and their patients in the office. Whether this reflects lack of recall or an inherent trend to counsel without numbers by the physician was not addressed (ACOG Committee on Genetics, 2009c). Although non-invasive prenatal screening for aneuploidy is still in its infancy, this is likely true for this new generation of testing as well.

Physicians generally perform definitive aneuploidy testing on amniocytes or placental villi, often with consultation with genetic counselors. Genetic counselors are particularly needed for chromosomal microarrays, as interpretation and communication with the laboratory often requires genetic counselor support. ACOG states that if chromosomal microarray is used in settings of abnormal fetal anatomy, that testing occurs in concert with pre- and post-test genetic counseling (ACOG Committee on Genetics, 2009c).

An increasing range of providers are faced with the numerical challenges of counseling for autosomal recessive genetic diseases. In each individual, among the thousands of genes contained in that person's genetic code are three to four genes which if paired with the same recessive gene from the partner, could lead to a child with an inherited disorder. When one copy of an autosomal recessive gene is disrupted no ill effects are produced and the individual is a "carrier." However, children of this individual and another "carrier" of the same genetic autosomal recessive disease face a 25% chance of inheriting both abnormal genes and having the disease in question. For several decades, attention was focused on the specific populations in which the specific autosomal recessive disorders clustered. Successful counseling and screening programs were initiated through a combination of community leaders, specialized clinics, and physicians knowledgeable within these communities. The best examples are the increased rate of Tay–Sachs among individuals of Ashkenazi Jewish ancestry and beta thalassemia among people with a Mediterranean background. Within these communities, non-medical and medical providers became skilled at the presentation of specific carrier frequencies, and the mendelian risks.

On a larger scale, carrier screening for cystic fibrosis is now recommended as a panethnic screen by ACOG. At this level, referral to genetic counselors for all patients is not possible and incorporation of screening into the physician's office is paramount. Ideally as these carrier tests should be performed preconception, increased knowledge attainment for the providers both in the gynecologic and obstetric office was needed. Two years after these recommendations were made a survey of obstetricians and gynecologists demonstrated that physicians who had reviewed the guidelines for screening were significantly more likely to demonstrate correct understanding about knowledge of cystic fibrosis and screening recommendations (Morgan et al., 2005). However, while carrier screening is initiated by the primary provider, interpretation of results often requires the expertise of genetic counselors or geneticists, particularly in the case of complicated carrier screening, such as cystic fibrosis (ACOG Committee on Genetics, 2011). In one study, 83.7% of obstetrician gynecologists surveyed felt that post-test consultation with a genetic counselor after carrier screening was performed would be beneficial (Ready et al., 2012).

As DNA costs of testing have lowered, carrier screening is moving from specific genes identified based on ethnicity to wide screens for numerous genes. Panels of testing for over 100 genes are now available. Medical care providers in the office will likely be the primary counselors for these patients and while initial voluntary studies show they support these tests, a third to half possessed incorrect factual knowledge on questions related to correctly counseling regarding autosomal recessive inheritance (Wolfber, 2006).

Genetic health literacy of patients

The public is continually being informed of the newest progress of genetics and a challenge remains as to whether they are prepared to understand the implications for their own health. Technology has reduced the price for seemingly once impossible tasks such as learning the DNA composition of your pet, your ancestry, or the sex of your unborn child without having to leave home. Such direct-to-consumer marketing (DTC) can be extended to learning your own individual risks of developing a variety of common adult disorders (diabetes, hypertension), a risk of developing cancer, or your athletic prowess. Currently these companies operate without FDA regulation and provide a variable degree of genetic counseling support often with the recommendation to consult with your primary physician.

Direct-to-consumer marketing continues to have supporters though several concerns have been raised. In 1990 there were 100 DTC studies available and in 2011 this has increased to 1000 (Langford et al., 2012). DTC should increase access and lead to lower costs although much of the lowering of cost is being driven by the technology itself. DTC allows the public to retain its right to their medical information without involvement of their medical record. However concerns arise with splintering of information between multiple sources and lack of integration of information with a primary provider if DTC information is not disclosed. Lastly, the extent to which an individual will alter their lifestyle based on their identified risk profile (for example an identified risk of developing diabetes) and whether this intervention significantly alters their risk of disease over other lifestyle interventions, which could be initiated without the genetic information, such as diet and exercise, remains speculative.

Direct-to-consumer testing with regard to comprehension from a genetic health literacy standpoint has been assessed in at least one study. In a recent comparison study regarding DTC genetic testing, results were understood correctly by about 60% of the general public as compared to 90% of genetic counselors. The majority of the general public considered the results easy to understand though interpreted them incorrectly and had a strong belief the results would be beneficial to their providers (Leighton et al., 2012). In 2007, the Health Information National Trends study assessed the role of access to DTC genetic tests and the parameters affecting confidence in interpretation. African Americans were significantly less likely than Whites to know about DTC genetic testing even when age, gender, income, and education were taken into consideration. However, the significance was lost when numeracy was added to the model. In other words, those who strongly agreed that they relied on numbers were more likely to seek out information on DTC regardless of race (Langford et al., 2012). The interesting implication is the strong cotracking of numeracy and race irrespective of age, income, or education implying different perhaps cultural aspects of importance among genetic health literacy.

Alternatively, genetic knowledge is gained by patients when provided to them by healthcare providers and has been assessed typically through specialty clinics such as sickle cell, cystic fibrosis, or a prenatal setting. In these directed settings, most patients recognize genetic language and the terms genes and heredity. However the majority has difficulty explaining how genes work, how they are passed from one generation to another, and where they are located in the body. Many admit they had little knowledge of genetics (Christensen et al., 2010).

To understand the current genetic knowledge of the US population in 2001, a telephone survey of over a thousand individuals (N = 1200), mostly in their mid 40s, with more than 20% having a college education was conducted. From eight agree/disagree questions, the majority understood mendelian genetics but only a minority understood further concepts (where genes were located, genetic determination of race). The findings were not influenced by race though did show an expected relationship with education and age (Christensen et al., 2010). In general, the public seems to understand that genetics is one aspect of multifactorial disease although there are gaps in their knowledge surrounding basic genetics and DNA. Their knowledge also appears to be influenced by their personal experience and they tend to overestimate their genetic knowledge base (Lea et al., 2011). This trend to overestimate understanding despite poor actual quantitative performance appears not to be unique to genetic health literacy as similar findings are noted across numeracy testing studies (Sheridan et al., 2003).

Future research

As research in the field of numeracy advances benefits will likely also accrue in genomic health literacy of patients and providers. However, what is unstudied is whether improved numeracy skills will easily translate into the unique skills underlying the tasks required for genetic medical decision making. Work is needed not only on how individuals process numbers in genetic scenarios but additionally on how they incorporate this information into genomic medical decision making. In contrast to other areas of medical decision making, discussions involving genetics may have implications for other than one's own health with considerations for a child's or a family member's well-being. Little is known regarding how the larger perceived burden of obtaining the genetic information interacts with the numerical interpretation required for genomic testing.

A question also exists as to whether genetic health literacy is sufficiently numerically dependent that identification of numeracy skills should be incorporated into general genetic counseling. Physicians themselves have limited skills at estimates of patients' numeracy and patients' self assessments are often inflated (Reyna et al., 2009; also see Chapter 8 in this volume). Some evidence suggests that there are cultural differences in approaches to numeracy separate from education and age and whether there are similar differences in genetic health literacy independent of education should be explored. Evidence from other areas of numeracy research suggests individuals with lower numeracy skills rely more greatly on narrative presentations (Reyna et al., 2009). Examination of these trends in genomic health literacy would be important given the almost exclusive use of numbers currently noted in most genetic counseling programs. Additionally those with low numeracy appear to have greater difficulty with weighing of choices, a key skill inherent in much of the genetic counseling (Reyna et al., 2009). Attention to this aspect of health literacy is important as genetic health decision making will involve decisions which may impact not only the individual's health but the health of the family.

Conclusion

Genetic health literacy and its substantial component of numeracy represent a significant challenge for healthcare providers and patients as genetic technologies continue to advance. Genomics is but one aspect of an individual's health and medical care and the incorporation of this increasing knowledge into a paradigm which will involve the patient and the provider is challenging. Individuals are gaining increasing access to their own medical information and genetic testing. They will remain confronted, though, by an array of options available and the incorporation of their results within the framework of their health profile.

Physicians are increasingly being asked to integrate genetic tests into their medical practice and undertake counseling for genetic risk profiles of common disorders. As has been seen in carrier screening for cystic fibrosis, clinical practice guidelines have been shown to be effective education tools for obstetrician gynecologists (Farquhar et al., 2002). Lessons can be learned from the arena of obstetrics and gynecology and the complexities of patient comprehension of a priori risk, risk reduction, variance, mendelian inheritance, and effect size.

Numeracy is a major contributor to the understanding of genetics and genomics. The ability of an individual, whether they are a healthcare provider or a patient, to understand the rationale for obtaining a genetic test or interpret the result is influenced by numeracy skills. Only preliminary research exists which suggest that individuals avoid genetic tests due to their reluctance with numeracy tasks and further research is needed across a broad spectrum to equalize this barrier. For medical care providers and patients, numeracy skills are essential to the successful incorporation of genomic information into medicine in the twenty-first century. These skills need to be assessed, avenues found to improve specific skills, and ongoing evaluations of educational interventions established.

References

23 and Me. (2012, September). BRCA Cancer Mutations (Selected). www.23andme.com/health/BRCA-Cancer/

ACOG Committee on Genetics. (2009a). ACOG Committee Opinion No. 432: Spinal muscular atrophy. *Obstetrics and Gynecology*, 113(5), 1194–1196.

ACOG Committee on Genetics. (2009b). ACOG Committee Opinion No. 442: Preconception and prenatal carrier screening for genetic diseases in individuals of Eastern European Jewish descent. *Obstetrics and Gynecology*, 114(4), 950–953.

ACOG Committee on Genetics. (2009c). ACOG Committee Opinion No. 446: Array comparative genomic hybridization in prenatal diagnosis. *Obstetrics and Gynecology*, 114(5), 1161–1163.

ACOG Committee on Genetics. (2011). ACOG Committee Opinion No. 486: Update on carrier screening for cystic fibrosis. *Obstetrics and Gynecology*, 117(4), 1028–1031.

ACOG Committee on Genetics. (2012). Committee Opinion No. 545: Noninvasive prenatal testing for fetal aneuploidy. *Obstetrics and Gynecology*, 120(6), 1532–1534.

ACOG Committee on Obstetrics. (2007). ACOG Practice Bulletin No. 78: Hemoglobinopathies in pregnancy. *Obstetrics and Gynecology*, 109(1), 229–237.

ACOG Committee on Practice Bulletins. (2007). ACOG Practice Bulletin No. 77: Screening for fetal chromosomal abnormalities. *Obstetrics and Gynecology*, 109(1), 217–227.

Ahlqvist, E., Ahluwalia, T. S., & Groop, L. (2011). Genetics of type 2 diabetes. *Clinical Chemistry*, 57(2), 241–254.

Anderson, B. L., Obrecht, N. A., Chapman, G. B., Driscoll, D. A., & Schulkin, J. (2011). Physicians' communication of Down syndrome screening test results: The influence of physician numeracy. *Genetics in Medicine*, 13(8), 744–749.

Bellcross, C. A., Kolor, K., Goddard, K. A., Coates, R. J., Reyes, M., & Khoury, M. J. (2011). Awareness and utilization of BRCA1/2 testing among U.S. primary care physicians. *American Journal of Preventive Medicine*, 40(1), 61–66.

Benn, P., Borrell, A., Cuckle, H., Dugoff, L., Gross, S., Johnson, J. A., et al. (2012). Prenatal detection of Down syndrome using Massively Parallel Sequencing (MPS): A rapid response statement from a committee on behalf of the Board of the International Society for Prenatal Diagnosis, 24 October 2011. *Prenatal Diagnosis*, 32(1), 1–2.

Bianci, D. W. (2012). From prenatal genomic diagnosis to fetal personalized medicine: progress and challenges. *Nature Medicine*, 18(7), 1041–1051.

Chiu, R. W., Chan, K. C., Gao, Y., Lau, V. Y., Zheng, W., Leung, T. Y., et al. (2008). Noninvasive prenatal diagnosis of fetal chromosomal aneuploidy by massively parallel genomic sequencing of DNA in maternal plasma. *Proceedings of the National Academy of Sciences USA*, 105(51), 20458–20463.

Chiu, R. W., Sun, H., Akolekar, R., Clouser, C., Lee, C., McKernan, K., et al. (2010). Maternal plasma DNA analysis with massively parallel sequencing by ligation for noninvasive prenatal diagnosis of trisomy 21. *Clinical Chemistry*, 56(3), 459–463.

Christensen, K. D., Jayaratne, T. E., Roberts, J. S., Kardia, S. L., & Petty, E. M. (2010). Understandings of basic genetics in the United States: Results from a national survey of black and white men and women. *Public Health Genomics*, 13(7–8), 467–476.

Clausen, F. B., Christiansen, M., Steffensen, R., Jørgensen, S., Nielsen, C., Jakobsen, M. A., et al. (2012). Report of the first nationally implemented clinical routine screening for fetal RHD in D- pregnant women to ascertain the requirement for antenatal RhD. *Transfusion*, 52(4), 752–758.

Daniels, G., Finning, K., & Martin, P. (2010). Noninvasive fetal blood grouping: present and future. *Clinics in Laboratory Medicine*, 30(2), 431–442.

Dohany, L., Gustafson, S., Ducaine, W., & Zakalik, D. (2012). Psychological distress with direct-to-consumer genetic testing: A case report of an unexpected BRCA positive test result. *Journal of Genetic Counseling*, 21(3), 399–401.

Ehrich, M., Deciu, C., Zwiefelhofer, T., Tynan, J. A., Cagasan, L., Tim, R., et al. (2011). Noninvasive detection of fetal trisomy 21 by sequencing of DNA in maternal blood: A study in a clinical setting. *American Journal of Obstetrics and Gynecology*, 204(3), 205.e1–205.e11.

Fan, H. C., Blumenfeld, Y. J., Chitkara, U., Hudgins, L., & Quake, S. R. (2008). Noninvasive diagnosis of fetal aneuploidy by shotgun sequencing DNA from maternal blood. *Proceedings of the National Academy of Sciences USA*, 105(42), 16266–16271.

Farquhar, C. M., Kofa, E., Power, M. L., Zinberg, S., & Schulkin, J. (2002). Clinical practice guidelines as educational tools for obstetrician-gynecologists. *Journal of Reproductive Medicine*, 47(11), 897–902.

Finning, K. M., Martin, P. G., Soothill, P. W., & Avent, N. D. (2002). Prediction of fetal D status from maternal plasma: Introduction of a new noninvasive fetal RHD genotyping service. *Transfusion*, 42(8), 1079–1085.

Friedman, J. M. (2009). High-resolution array genomic hybridization in prenatal diagnosis. *Prenatal Diagnosis*, 29(1), 20–28.

Ghosh, A. K., & Ghosh, K. (2005). Translating evidence-based information into effective risk communication: current challenges and opportunities. *Journal of Laboratory and Clinical Medicine*, 145(4), 171–180.

Gigerenzer, G., Mata, J., & Frank, R. (2008). A survey of health knowledge in seven European countries. Unpublished manuscript.

Hoffrage, U., & Gigerenzer, G. (1998). Using natural frequencies to improve diagnostic inferences. *Academic Medicine*, 73(5), 538–540.

Klitzman, R., Chung, W., Marder, K., Shanmugham, A., Chin, L. J., Stark, M., et al. (2013). Attitudes and practices among internists concerning genetic testing. *Journal of Genetic Counseling*, 22(1), 90–100.

Langford, A. T., Resnicow, K., Roberts, J. S., & Zikmund-Fisher, B. J. (2012). Racial and ethnic differences in direct-to-consumer genetic tests awareness in HINTS 2007: Sociodemographic and numeracy correlates. *Journal of Genetic Counseling*, 21(3), 440–447.

Lazarin, G. A., Haque, I. S., Nazareth, S., Iori, K., Patterson, A. S., Jacobsen, J. L., et al. (2013). An empirical estimate of carrier frequencies for 400+ causal Mendelian variants: Results from an ethnically diverse clinical sample of 23,453 individuals. *Genetics in Medicine*, 15(3), 178–186.

Lea, D. H., Kaphingst, K. A., Bowen, D., Lipkus, I., & Hadley, D. W. (2011). Communicating genetic and genomic information: Health literacy and numeracy considerations. *Public Health Genomics*, 14(4–5), 279–289.

Leighton, J. W., Valverde, K., & Bernhardt, B. A. (2012). The general public's understanding and perception of direct-to-consumer genetic test results. *Public Health Genomics*, 15(1), 11–21.

Lo, Y. M., Corbetta, N., Chamberlain, P. F., Rai, V., Sargent, I. L., Redman, C. W., et al. (1997). Presence of fetal DNA in maternal plasma and serum. *Lancet*, 350(9076), 485–487.

Lo, Y. M., Hjelm, N. M., Fidler, C., Sargent, I. L., Murphy, M. F., Chamberlain, P. F., et al. (1998a). Prenatal diagnosis of fetal RhD status by molecular analysis of maternal plasma. *New England Journal of Medicine*, 339(24), 1734–1738.

Lo, Y. M., Tein, M. S., Lau, T. K., Haines, C. J., Leung, T. N., Poon, P. M., et al. (1998b). Quantitative analysis of fetal DNA in maternal plasma and serum: Implications for noninvasive prenatal diagnosis. *American Journal of Human Genetics*, 62(4), 768–775.

Lun, F. M., Chiu, R. W., Allen Chan, K. C., Yeung Leung, T., Kin Lau, T., & Dennis Lo, Y. M. (2008). Microfluidics digital PCR reveals a higher than expected fraction of fetal DNA in maternal plasma. *Clinical Chemistry*, 54(10), 1664–1672.

Mihaescu, R., Meigs, J., Sijbrands, E., & Janssens, A. C. (2011). Genetic risk profiling for prediction of type 2 diabetes. *PLoS Currents*, 3, RRN1208.

Morgan, M. A., Driscoll, D. A., Zinberg, S., Schulkin, J., & Mennuti, M. T. (2005). Impact of self-reported familiarity with guidelines for cystic fibrosis carrier screening. *Obstetrics and Gynecology*, 105(6), 1355–1361.

Palomaki, G. E., Kloza, E. M., Lambert-Messerlian, G. M., Haddow, J. E., Neveux, L. M., Ehrich, M., et al. (2011). DNA sequencing of maternal plasma to detect Down syndrome: An international clinical validation study. *Genetics in Medicine*, 13(11), 913–920.

Palomaki, G. E., Deciu, C., Kloza, E. M., Lambert-Meserlian, G. M., Haddow, J. E., Neveux, L. M., et al. (2012). DNA sequencing of maternal plasma reliably identifies trisomy 18 and trisomy 13 as well as Down syndrome: An international collaborative study. *Genetics in Medicine*, 14(3), 296–305.

Prior, T. W. (2008). Carrier screening for spinal muscular atrophy. *Genetics in Medicine*, 10(11), 840–842.

Ram, K. T., & Klugman, S. D. (2010). Best practices: Antenatal screening for common genetic conditions other than aneuploidy. *Current Opinion in Obstetrics and Gynecology*, 22(2), 139–145.

Ready, K., Haque, I. S., Srinivasan, B. S., & Marshall, J. R. (2012). Knowledge and attitudes regarding expanded genetic carrier screening among women's healthcare providers. *Fertility and Sterility*, 97(2), 407–413.

Reyna, V. F. (2004). How people make decisions that involve risk: A dual-processes approach. *Current Directions in Psychological Science*, 13(2), 60–66.

Reyna, V. F., Lloyd, F. J., & Brainerd, C. J. (2003). Memory, development, and rationality: An integrative theory of judgment and decision-making. In: S. Schneider & J. Shanteau (Eds.), *Emerging Perspectives on Judgment and Decision Research*. New York, NY: Cambridge University Press; pp. 201–245.

Reyna, V. F., Nelson, W. L., Han, P. K., & Dieckmann, N. F. (2009). How numeracy influences risk comprehension and medical decision making. *Psychological Bulletin*, 135(6), 943–973.

Rhoads, G. G., Jackson, L. G., Schlesselman, S. E., de la Cruz, F. F., Desnick, R. J., Golbus, M. S., et al. (1989). The safety and efficacy of chorionic villus sampling for early prenatal diagnosis of cytogenetic abnormalities. *New England Journal of Medicine*, 320(10), 609–617.

Schwartz, L. M., Woloshin, S., & Welch, H. G. (1999). Risk communication in clinical practice: Putting cancer in context. *Journal of the National Cancer Institute Monographs*, (25), 124–133.

Sheridan, S. L., Pignone, M. P., & Lewis, C. L. (2003). A randomized comparison of patients' understanding of number needed to treat and other common risk reduction formats. *Journal of General Internal Medicine*, 18(11), 884–892.

Sifri, R., Myers, R., Hyslop, T., Turner, B., Cocroft, J., Rothermel, T., et al. (2003). Use of cancer susceptibility testing among primary care physicians. *Clinical Genetics*, 64(4), 355–360.

Tayo, B. O., Teil, M., Tong, L., Qin, H., Khitrov, G., Zhang, W., et al. (2011). Genetic background of patients from a university medical center in Manhattan: implications for personalized medicine. *PLoS ONE*, 6(5), e19166.

Trivers, K. F., Baldwin, L. M., Miller, J. W., Matthews, B., Andrilla, C. H., Lishner, D. M., et al. (2011). Reported referral for genetic counseling or BRCA 1/2 testing among United States physicians: A vignette-based study. *Cancer*, 117(23), 5334–5343.

US Preventive Services Task Force. (2005). Genetic risk assessment and BRCA mutation testing for breast and ovarian cancer susceptibility: Recommendation statement. *Annals of Internal Medicine*, 143(5), 355–361.

Van Riel, E., Wárlám-Rodenhuis, C. C., Verhoef, S., Rutgers, E. J., & Ausems, M. G. (2010). BRCA testing of breast cancer patients: Medical specialists' referral patterns, knowledge and attitudes to genetic testing. *European Journal of Cancer Care (England)*, 19(3), 369–376.

Voight, B. F., Scott, L. J., Steinthorsdottir, V., Morris, A. P., Dina, C., Welch, R. P., et al. (2010). Twelve type 2 diabetes susceptibility loci identified through large-scale association analysis. *Nature Genetics*, 42(7), 579–589.

Wapner, R. J., Driscoll, D. A., & Simpson, J. L. (2012a). Integration of microarray technology into prenatal diagnosis: Counselling issues generated during the NICHD clinical trial. *Prenatal Diagnosis*, 32(4), 396–400.

Wapner, R. J., Martin, C. L., Levy, B., Ballif, B. C., Eng, C. M., Zachary, J. M., et al. (2012b). Chromosomal microarray versus karyotyping for prenatal diagnosis. *New England Journal of Medicine*, 367, 2175–2184.

Weaver, M., & Pollin, T. I. (2012). Direct-to-Consumer genetic testing: What are we talking about? *Journal of Genetic Counseling*, 21(3), 361–366.

Wetterstrand, K. A. (2013). DNA sequencing costs: Data from the NHGRI Genome Sequencing Program (GSP). From *National Human Genome Research Institute*. Retrieved from: http://www.genome/gov/sequencingcosts (accessed 2/21/13).

Wilkins-Haug, L., Schmidt, L., Holzman, G. B., & Schulkin, J. (1999). Genetics in obstetricians' offices: A survey study. *Obstetrics and Gynecology*, 93(5 Pt 1), 642–647.

Wolfber, A. J. (2006). Genes on the Web – Direct-to-consumer marketing of genetic testing. *New England Journal of Medicine*, 355(6), 543–545.

7 Using visual aids to help people with low numeracy make better decisions

Rocio Garcia-Retamero & Edward T. Cokely

To effectively participate in decision making, patients and healthcare professionals need to understand the risks and benefits of different medical treatments, screenings, and lifestyle choices (Garcia-Retamero & Galesic, 2013). Unfortunately, research indicates that people often struggle to grasp numerical concepts that are essential for understanding and communicating health-relevant information (Reyna et al., 2009; Peters, 2012; Garcia-Retamero & Galesic, 2013; Chapters 2 and 4 in this volume). Even highly educated individuals tend to have difficulties understanding and manipulating a host of elementary probability expressions (Ancker & Kaufman, 2007). In short, the general public lacks basic numeracy, which limits their risk literacy (i.e., the ability to accurately interpret and make good decisions based on information about risk; Galesic & Garcia-Retamero, 2010; Cokely et al., 2012). (For major assessments of risk literacy in large adult and student samples see Kutner et al., 2006 and OECD, 2012.)

Over the past 20 years, numerical reasoning skills have become increasingly necessary for navigating the modern healthcare environment (Fagerlin et al., 2007; Apter et al., 2008; Keller & Siegrist, 2009). For example, people with low numeracy have less accurate perceptions of the risks and benefits of screenings and medical treatments (Schwartz et al., 1997; Davids et al., 2004; Donelle et al., 2008), which reduces their medication compliance and impairs risk communication (Reyna et al., 2009). People with low numerical ability are also especially vulnerable to having difficulty with following a complicated dosing regimen (Estrada et al., 2004), they have more hospitalizations (Apter et al., 2006), they have more deficits in understanding nutrition labels necessary

The studies presented in this chapter are part of the projects "How to Improve Understanding of Risks about Health (PSI 2008-02019)" funded by the Ministerio de Ciencia e Innovación (Spain) and "Helping Doctors and Their Patients Make Decisions About Health (PSI 2011-22954)," funded by the Ministerio de Economía y Competitividad (Spain). The authors declare independence from these funding agencies.

to following dietary recommendations (Rothman et al., 2006), and they are more susceptible to being influenced by the way the health information is framed in problems involving probabilities (Peters et al., 2006). Moreover, people with low numeracy are generally less willing to participate in decision making about their health (Galesic & Garcia-Retamero, 2011a; Garcia-Retamero et al., in press).

Visual aids are simple graphical representations of numerical expressions of probability and include bar and line charts and icon arrays, among others (Paling, 2003; Spiegelhalter et al., 2011). Visual aids have long been known to confer benefits when communicating risk information. However, not all visual aids are equally effective. Visual aids tend to provide an effective means of risk communication when they are *transparent* (Garcia-Retamero & Cokely, 2013) – that is, when their elements are well defined and they accurately and clearly represent the relevant risk information by making part-to-whole relationships in the data visually available (Ancker et al., 2006; Reyna & Brainerd, 2008). (For good practices for designing transparent visual aids, see the guidelines of the Human Factors and Ergonomics Society; Gillan et al., 1998). For example, appropriately designed visual aids improve comprehension of risks associated with different medical treatments, screenings, and lifestyles, and they promote consideration of beneficial treatments despite side effects (Paling, 2003; Lipkus, 2007; Waters et al., 2007; Zikmund-Fisher et al., 2008a). Visual aids also increase appropriate risk-avoidance behaviors, they promote healthy behaviors, they reduce errors induced by anecdotal narratives (Fagerlin et al., 2005; Schirillo & Stone, 2005; Cox et al., 2010), and they can aid comprehension of complex concepts such as incremental risk (Zikmund-Fisher et al., 2008b). Risk information presented visually is also judged as easier to understand and recall, and requires less viewing time than the same information presented numerically (Feldman-Stewart et al., 2007b; Goodyear-Smith et al., 2008; Gaissmaier et al., 2012). Nevertheless, the benefits of visual aids are different for different people. Our hypothesis is that visual aids might be especially useful for people with low numeracy. In the following sections, we describe the results of a series of studies supporting this hypothesis and provide some guidelines for transparent risk communication by using visual aids.

Using visual aids to improve risk understanding in people with limited numeracy

People with high numeracy can often understand health risks even if visual aids are not provided (Galesic et al., 2009; Keller & Siegrist, 2009). The challenge is to reach vulnerable people with low numeracy as they are likely to make errors or avoid decision making altogether (Hawley et al., 2008; Peters et al., 2009). Recently, Galesic and Garcia-Retamero (2011b) revealed that people, regardless of their numeracy skills, differ substantially in their ability to understand graphically presented quantitative information. The authors developed a graph literacy scale and investigated the distribution of graph literacy in probabilistic national samples in the USA and Germany. The graph literacy scale consists of 13 items and measures several abilities of graph comprehension (Friel et al., 2001); covers four frequently used graph types – line plots, bar charts, pies, and icon arrays; and includes items dealing with the communication of medical risks, treatment efficiency, and prevalence of diseases.

In a related study, Garcia-Retamero and Galesic (2010b) showed that well designed visual aids can improve risk understanding in people with limited numerical skills to the level of those who are more skilled in understanding risks as long as they have relatively high graph literacy. In particular, the authors investigated whether numeracy and graph literacy affect the efficacy of visual aids reporting information about treatment risk reduction. Participants were probabilistic national samples in the USA and Germany, and completed the graph literacy scale of Galesic and Garcia-Retamero (2011b) and a numeracy scale consisting of nine items selected from Schwartz et al. (1997) and Lipkus et al. (2001). Participants were classified in four groups depending on whether their numerical and graph literacy skills were above or below the median scores of their group. The authors compared the efficacy of different types of visual aids (i.e., icon arrays and bar graphs), representing either affected individuals only or the entire population at risk (see Figure 7.1). In addition, they tested the efficacy of visual aids when the numerical information added to the visual aids was presented either as absolute or relative risk reduction. When the information was presented in absolute terms, participants were told: "Of the patients who took a placebo, 20 had a stroke. Compared to the group that took a placebo, 5 fewer patients had a stroke in the group that took Vitarilen." When the information was presented in relative terms, participants were told: "Compared to the group that took a placebo, the relative reduction in risk of having a stroke in the group that took Vitarilen was 25%."

Results were clear: Garcia-Retamero and Galesic (2010b) observed similar increases in accuracy with icon arrays and bar graphs; visual aids were useful additions when the numerical information was presented both in terms of absolute and relative risk reductions; and they were especially useful when they represented the entire population at risk. Importantly, results showed that visual aids were most beneficial for individuals who

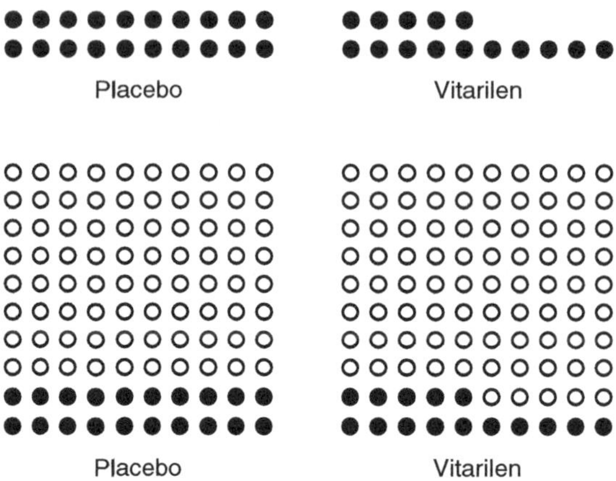

Figure 7.1. Icon arrays presented in addition to numerical information about risk reduction when they represent affected individuals only (top) or the entire population at risk (bottom). (Reprinted from *Social Science & Medicine*, 70(7), April 2010, "Who profits from visual aids: Overcoming challenges in people's understanding of risks" by Rocio Garcia-Retamero and Mirta Galesic, with permission from Elsevier.)

had low numeracy but relatively moderate-to-high graph literacy, especially when the visual aids presented the entire population at risk (see Figure 7.2). Among this group of people, accuracy increased from less than 20% to nearly 80% when visual aids were used. In fact, providing visual aids about the effectiveness of medical treatments eliminated the differences between these people and those with high numeracy. Unfortunately, people with both low numeracy and low graph literacy did not benefit from visual aids (see also Gaissmaier et al., 2012).

Visual aids are also helpful to other vulnerable populations with limited numerical skills. Due to age-related cognitive decline and other cohort effects, older adults often struggle with numerical concepts (Finucane et al., 2002). Given that older adults more frequently suffer chronic diseases and confront health-related decision making, the challenges when dealing with health risks are magnified (Peters et al., 2000, 2007). A study by Garcia-Retamero et al. (2010) showed that visual aids can help less numerate, older adults make accurate assessments of the effectiveness of medical treatments. However, visual aids confused rather than helped some older adults. Again, those people who were both low in numeracy and low in graph literacy did not benefit from the visual aids (Ruiz et al., 2013). Garcia-Retamero and Dhami (2011) showed similar results in immigrants with limited language and numerical skills.

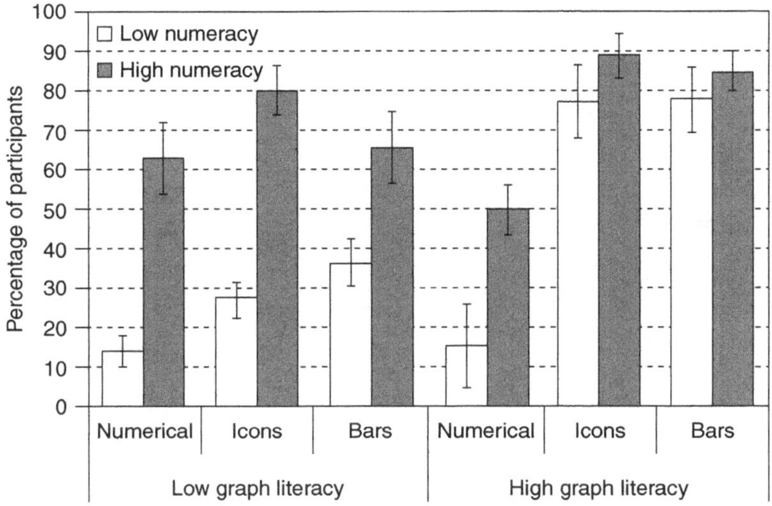

Figure 7.2. Percentage of participants with low and high graph literacy and numeracy who correctly inferred treatment risk reduction, by visual aids condition. In the visual aids conditions, icon arrays and bars reported the entire population at risk. Error bars represent one standard error.

Using visual aids to reduce biases in people with limited numeracy

Visual aids can also reduce or eliminate several biases with important consequences for decision making. A prominent example is *denominator neglect* – the tendency to focus on the number of times a target event has happened (i.e., the numerator), while ignoring the overall number of opportunities for it to happen (i.e., the denominator; Reyna, 2004). To illustrate, in clinical trials the number of patients who receive a certain drug is often smaller than the number of those who do not. If people disregard denominators, neglecting the overall number of treated and non-treated patients (e.g., 100 and 800, respectively), they might perceive the drug to be more effective than it actually is. In other words, they might only compare absolute numbers of treated and non-treated patients who do not recover or die (e.g., 5 versus 80, respectively) rather than the proportion of treated and non-treated patients who do not recover or die (e.g., 5 of 100 and 80 of 800 for a treatment risk reduction of 50%; see Figure 7.3).

Past laboratory research examining perceptions of treatment risk reduction has often employed samples of treated and non-treated patients of the same size. However, this research is not representative of the type of

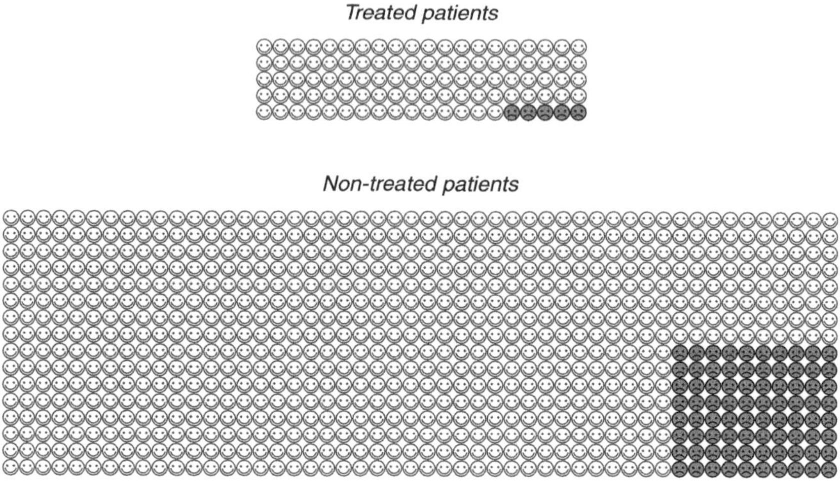

Figure 7.3. Icon arrays representing a treatment risk reduction of 50% with unequal samples of treated and non-treated patients (i.e., 100 and 800, respectively). Patients who died are represented in dark gray; healthy patients are represented in light gray.

information that people normally encounter when they assess the effectiveness of medical treatments (Garcia-Retamero et al., 2012). To address this concern of ecological validity, Garcia-Retamero and Galesic (2009) conducted a study reporting numerical information about the effectiveness of medical treatments using unequal samples of treated and non-treated patients. In particular, the overall numbers of treated and non-treated patients (i.e., the sizes of the denominators) were manipulated to be either 800 or 100 (see Table 7.1). To keep treatment risk reduction constant (i.e., 50%), the sizes of the numerators (i.e., the number of treated and non-treated patients who died) varied within conditions depending on the sizes of the denominators. Independently of this manipulation, half of the participants received – in addition to the numerical information about risk reduction – two icon arrays presenting such information (Figure 7.3 shows the icon arrays of the 100–800 condition). Again, participants were probabilistic national samples in the USA and Germany, and completed a numeracy scale consisting of nine items selected from Schwartz et al. (1997) and Lipkus et al. (2001). They were then classified in two groups depending on whether their numerical skills were above or below the median scores of their group.

Garcia-Retamero and Galesic (2009) showed that participants exhibited denominator neglect when the information about the medical treatment

Table 7.1. *Number of treated and non-treated patients who died in the scenarios with different denominator sizes.*

	Treated patients		Non-treated patients	
Sizes of denominators[a]	Dead patients	Population size	Dead patients	Population size
800–800	40	800	80	800
100–800	5	100	80	800
800–100	40	800	10	100
100–100	5	100	10	100

Treatment risk reduction is 50% in all conditions.
[a] Treated and untreated patients, respectively.

was provided only numerically. That was especially the case in participants with relatively low numeracy. In particular, 71% of these participants *overestimated* treatment risk reduction when the overall number of treated patients was lower than the overall number of patients who did not receive the treatment (i.e., in the 100–800 condition), whereas only 25% of the participants with high numeracy provided a lower estimate than the exact value in that condition (see Figure 7.4). Note that in such a case, the number of patients who received the treatment and died (N = 5) is much lower than the number of patients who did not receive the treatment and died (N = 80; see Table 7.1). It seems likely that many participants – especially those with low numeracy – did not take proportions into account but only absolute numbers in the numerators, which would have led them to believe that the treatment had a larger effect than it actually did.

In contrast, 67% of the participants with low numeracy *underestimated* risk reduction when the number of treated patients was higher than the number of patients who did not receive treatment (i.e., in the 800–100 condition), whereas only 19% of the participants with high numeracy provided a higher estimate than the exact value in that condition. In such a case, the number of patients who received the treatment and died (N = 40) is higher than the number of patients who did not receive the treatment and died (N = 10; see Table 7.1). This might have led participants – especially those with low numeracy – to believe that the treatment had a smaller effect than it actually did.

Finally, results showed that denominator neglect was effectively eliminated by using visual aids representing the risk information. This was particularly the case among participants who were less skilled in using numerical information. When the sizes of the denominators were different

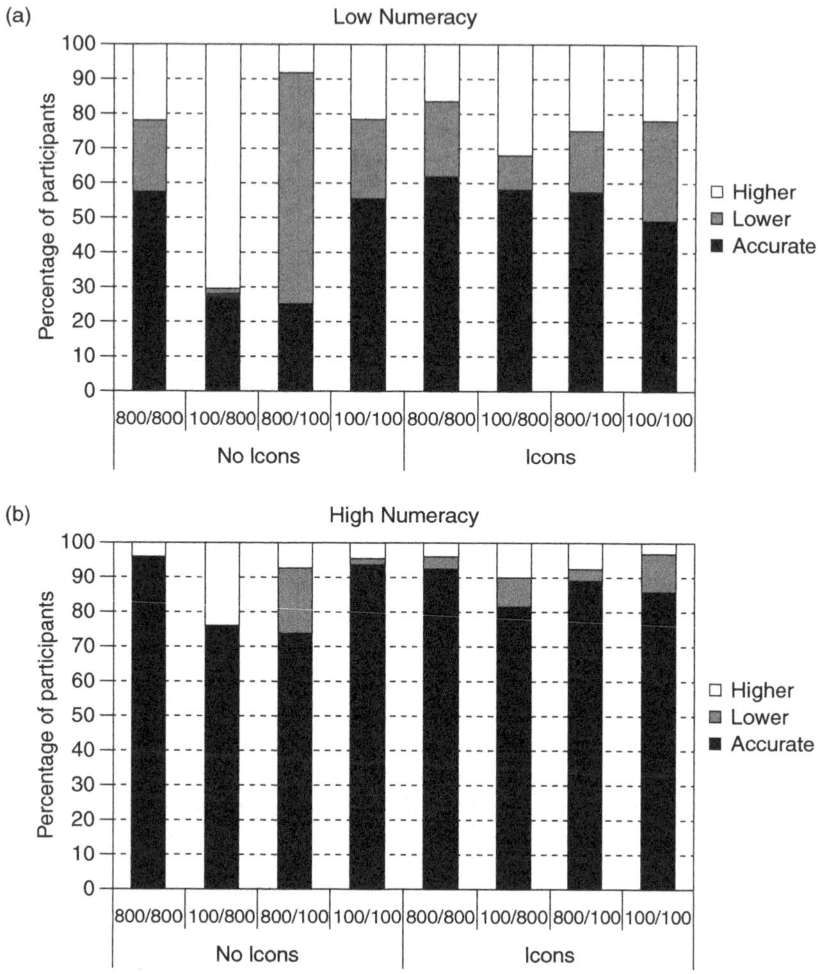

Figure 7.4. Percentage of participants with low (a) and high (b) numeracy whose estimates of risk reduction were either accurate or lower or higher than the exact value as a function of the sizes of the denominators and icon arrays. (Reprinted from *American Journal of Public Health*, 99(12), December 2009, "Communicating treatment risk reduction to people with low numeracy skills: A cross-cultural comparison" by Rocio Garcia-Retamero and Mirta Galesic, with permission from The Sheridan Press on behalf of The American Public Health Association.)

and icon arrays were added to the numerical information, the percentage of low numeracy participants who estimated the treatment risk reduction incorrectly decreased from 74 to 42%, and from 26 to 15% in participants with high numeracy. These percentages (i.e., 42 and 15%) are similar to those when the sizes of the denominators were equal (i.e., 45 and 22% for high and low numeracy participants). Thus, participants' estimates of risk reduction were not influenced by the sizes of the denominators when icon arrays were provided. Okan et al. (2012a) conducted a similar study in a large sample of undergraduate students in Spain. Participants completed the graph literacy scale of Galesic and Garcia-Retamero (2011b) and were classified in two groups depending on whether their graph literacy skills were above or below the median scores of their group. The authors showed that visual aids were effective for reducing denominator neglect in participants with relatively high – but not low – graph literacy.

Visual aids also reduce the influence of other errors and biases in populations with limited numerical skills, including the effect of message framing. Garcia-Retamero and Galesic (2010a) examined the effect of framed messages in perceptions of the effectiveness of medical surgery. The surgery was described in positive (i.e., "991 in 1000 people survive this surgery") or negative (i.e., "9 in 1000 people die from this surgery") terms. As in some of the studies described above, participants were probabilistic national samples in the United States and Germany, and completed a numeracy scale consisting of nine items selected from Schwartz et al. (1997) and Lipkus et al. (2001). They were classified in two groups depending on whether their numerical skills were above or below the median scores of their group. All participants answered a question about the effectiveness of the surgery. Half of the participants answered the question when the surgery was described in negative terms first, while the remaining participants answered the question when the surgery was described in positive terms first. Between the two questions, all participants answered a set of unrelated problems. The provision of visual aids – in addition to the numerical information about the effectiveness of the surgery – was manipulated between subjects across five conditions. In the four visual aids conditions, the number of patients who died and survived from surgery was represented using an icon array, a horizontal bar graph, a vertical bar graph, or a pie chart (see Figure 7.5). Participants in the numerical condition did not receive visual aids but received only the numerical information.

Garcia-Retamero and Galesic (2010a) showed that participants with low numeracy were more susceptible to framing than those with high numeracy (see also Peters & Levin, 2008, and Peters et al., 2006 for similar results in other unrelated topics). When only numerical information was provided,

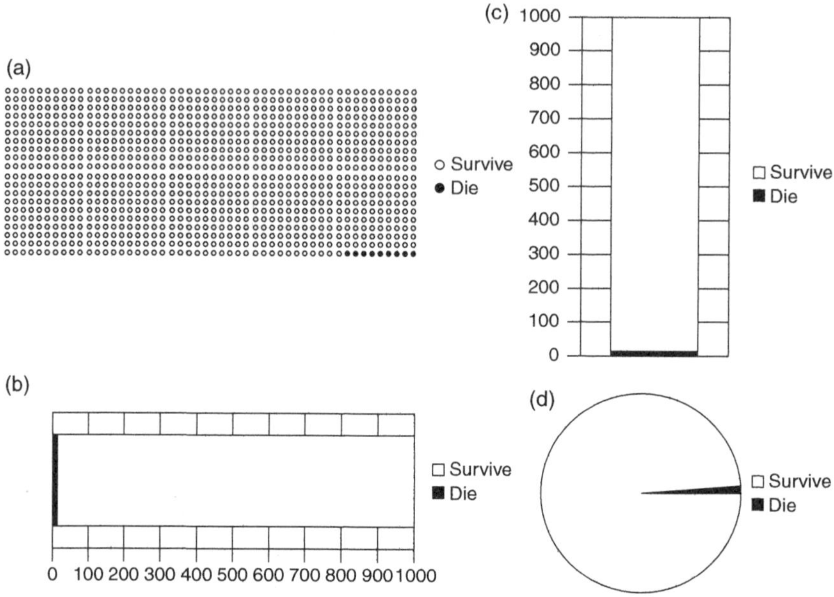

Figure 7.5. (a) Icon array presented in Condition 1; (b) horizontal bar graph presented in Condition 2; (c) vertical bar graph presented in Condition 3; and (d) pie chart presented in Condition 4. All figures represented the number of people who died (i.e., 9) and survived (i.e., 991) from the surgery. (Reprinted from *Journal of General Internal Medicine*, 25(12), January 1, 2010, "How to reduce the effect of framing on messages about health" by Rocio Garcia-Retamero and Mirta Galesic, with kind permission from Springer Science and Business Media.)

participants with low numeracy often perceived the surgical procedure as less risky when the associated risk was presented in positive terms (i.e., chances of surviving) than in negative terms (i.e., chances of dying). In contrast, participants with high numeracy often provided equal estimates when the risks were expressed in positive and negative terms. Accordingly, the average difference between perceptions of the risk of the surgery expressed in positive and negative terms in the numerical condition was 0.90 (SEM = 0.12) and 0.10 (SEM = 0.06) for participants with low and high numeracy, respectively. When visual aids were added to the numerical information, the effect of framing was reduced in low-numeracy participants. The average difference between perceptions of the risk of the surgery expressed in positive and negative terms in the visual conditions was 0.16 (SEM = 0.09) for participants with low numeracy. In contrast, participants more skilled in using quantitative information benefited less from visual aids. For these participants, the average difference between perceptions of the risk expressed in positive and negative terms was similar when they received (0.21; SEM = 0.08) and did not receive visual aids (0.10; SEM = 0.06). Recent behavioral interventions involving visual aids indicate that these aids can also reduce the effect of framed messages promoting health behaviors in patients with low numeracy.

Behavioral interventions involving visual aids

Messages promoting a health behavior can be framed in terms of the benefits afforded by adopting the behavior (a gain-framed appeal) or in terms of the costs associated with failing to adopt the behavior (a loss-framed appeal; see Rothman et al., 1999). To illustrate, a message promoting condom use can emphasize the benefits of this practice (e.g., using condoms helps prevent sexually transmitted diseases or STDs) or the costs of avoiding this practice (e.g., failing to use condoms increases the risk of STDs – a loss-framed appeal; see Garcia-Retamero & Cokely, 2012 for a review). In a longitudinal study, Garcia-Retamero and Cokely (2011) examined the effects of a brief risk awareness intervention (i.e., a sexual health information brochure) in a large sample of sexually active young adults in Spain. These participants had very limited numerical skills according to the nine-item numeracy scale described above. Garcia-Retamero and Cokely (2011) showed that gain-framed messages induced greater adherence for a prevention behavior (e.g., condom use), whereas loss-framed messages were more effective for promoting an illness-detecting behavior (e.g., STD screening; see Figure 7.6). This was the case even if the two types of framed messages were comparable. However, when visual aids reporting numerical information about STDs were added to the health information, both the gain- and loss-framed messages became equally and highly effective (i.e., the framing bias was eliminated). Providing the same information in numbers did not reduce the effect of the framed messages.

Follow-up interventions conducted in large samples of sexually active young adults in Spain showed that well-constructed visual aids were as effective as an extensive 8–10 hour "best practices" educational program for promoting condom use (Garcia-Retamero & Cokely, in press a). Young adults disadvantaged by their lack of numerical skills benefitted more from the visual aids than those who had higher numeracy as long as they were moderately graph literate (Garcia-Retamero & Cokely, in press b).

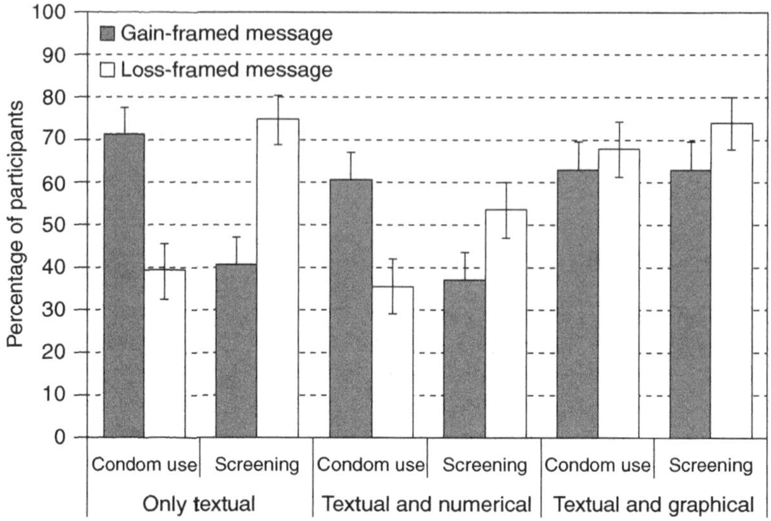

Figure 7.6. Percentage of participants who reported performing the promoted behavior (condom use or STD screening) when the health information brochure was framed as gains or losses as a function of message format (text only, text and numerical information, and text and graphical information). Error bars represent one standard error.

Ongoing research indicates that visual aids can also encourage patients' trust in their own physician and their willingness to participate in decision making about their health. Visual aids seem particularly beneficial for patients who have relatively low numeracy – a group that generally tends to be more passive in health decision making (Galesic & Garcia-Retamero, 2011a). Visual aids have also been found to boost accuracy above and beyond the effect of other transparent information formats. For instance, doctors and their patients often have difficulties inferring the predictive value of medical tests from information about the prevalence of diseases and the sensitivity and false-positive rate of the tests (Gigerenzer & Hoffrage, 1995; Hoffrage & Gigerenzer, 1998). Communicating information about the tests in natural frequencies as compared to conditional probabilities improves diagnostic inferences (Hoffrage et al., 2000a, 2000b). However, our research shows that visual aids improve these inferences in doctors and their patients beyond the effect of natural frequencies (Garcia-Retamero & Hoffrage, 2013). This research also indicates that doctors tend to be more accurate in their diagnostic inferences than their patients – a difference in accuracy that disappeared when differences in numerical skills were controlled for.

What have we learned so far?

The research reviewed in this chapter shows that well designed visual aids can be especially useful for people with limited numerical skills as long as they have moderate-to-high levels of graph literacy. Although less numerate people typically have problems understanding risks, visual aids confer benefits and can raise their performance to the level of those who are more skilled in using numerical information. In short, our research converges to suggest that well-constructed visual aids offer a highly effective, transparent, and ethically desirable means of risk communication.

Although our studies take center stage in the current chapter, it is important to note that this work contributes to a large, active interdisciplinary field (see Ancker et al., 2006; Lipkus, 2007; Zikmund-Fisher et al., 2008a, 2008b; Keller & Siegrist, 2009; Reyna et al., 2009; Peters, 2012). In addition, our conclusions are likely to be robust as they are based on a variety of studies conducted in the general public (e.g., large, probabilistic national samples) and in diverse groups of patients from a wide range of countries (e.g., the USA, Germany, Great Britain, and Spain). These studies examined risk communication in different ecologically valid tasks that accurately reproduce the problems that people commonly encounter when they face health decisions. These ecological studies covered diverse topics including estimates of risk and risk reduction; diagnostic inferences and perceptions of treatment effectiveness; confidence and accuracy; and changes in attitudes, behavioral intentions, actual behaviors, and decision making. In addition, the general findings hold across different types of visual aids (e.g., icon arrays, bar charts, and line plots, presenting either affected individuals only or these individuals and the entire population at risk); when visual aids differ in iconicity (i.e., when they are more or less abstract; see also Gaissmaier et al., 2012); when visual aids are provided either in addition to or instead of numerical information; and when the numerical information is presented using different information formats (e.g., absolute or relative risks; see Garcia-Retamero & Galesic, 2013 and Garcia-Retamero & Cokely, 2013).

Our research adds to the literature by showing that problems associated with risk illiteracy are not simply the result of limited capacities or inherent cognitive biases that prevent good decision making (see also Gigerenzer et al., 2007; Gigerenzer & Gray, 2011). Instead, errors occur because ineffective information formats can complicate and mislead adaptive decision makers. Good decision making results when there is an appropriate fit between people's skills, processes, and environments. To the extent that information formats leverage people's inherent capacity to recognize and contextualize relationships in naturally occurring tasks, they are likely to confer benefits. In this regard, transparent visual aids can improve risk understanding in people who are less skilled in using numerical information by making part-to-whole relations in the data visually available (Ancker et al., 2006) and helping them understand and represent superordinate classes (Reyna & Brainerd, 2008). Visual aids have also been shown to be suited best to convey essential aspects of information (Feldman-Stewart et al., 2000; Zikmund-Fisher et al., 2010) and bottom line meaning (e.g., patterns in the data; Reyna, 2004). Superior decisions also often follow from elaborative encoding of contextual and relevant risk information (Woller-Carter et al., 2012; see also Cokely & Kelley, 2009; Ghazal et al., 2014). By influencing encoding and representation, visual aids give rise to enduring changes in attitudes and behavioral intentions, which in turn affect actual behavior and risky decision making (Garcia-Retamero & Cokely, 2011).

We have also learned ways in which visual aids are limited or can be misused, so some caution is warranted (Stone et al., 2003; Kurz-Milcke et al., 2008; Ancker et al., 2011). For example, visual aids can increase overestimates of low probabilities and underestimates of high probabilities (i.e., the magnifier effect; Gurmankin et al., 2005). However, the opposite effect (i.e., less overestimation) on low probabilities and no effect on high probabilities have also been described (Woloshin et al., 2000). In addition, numerical representations can be better suited than visual aids to convey precise aspects of the information (e.g., detailed-level information), whereas visual aids have been shown to be best suited to convey essential aspects of the information (i.e., gross-level information; Feldman-Stewart et al., 2000). Thus, a potential concern when using visual aids is that people might focus more on the pattern of data than the precise values. Finally, specific graphs are better suited for certain tasks (e.g., line graphs for trends over time and bar graphs for comparison across groups; Lipkus, 2007; Lipkus & Hollands, 1999). Therefore, developers should avoid using misleading visual aids by pilot testing their graphs before conducting an intervention (Trevena et al., 2012).

Where do we go next?

Although our work and that of others sheds some light on why visual aids improve decision making in people with limited numerical skills, more research is needed. Future studies should investigate the cognitive processes that underlie differences in risk understanding in people with different levels of numeracy and graph literacy (Okan et al., 2012b). Theories of mathematical cognition (Dehaene, 1997; Gallistel & Gelman, 2005; Nelson et al., 2008) and graph comprehension (e.g., Carpenter & Shah, 1998; Friel et al., 2001; Cooper et al., 2003) can provide a foundation for this understanding. To model underlying individual differences in cognitive processing of visually represented health risks, studies recording people's eye movements while exploring graphs can be particularly useful (see Okan et al., 2010; Woller-Carter et al., 2012).

Future research can also explore age-related changes in numeracy and graph literacy throughout the life span (Siegler & Booth, 2004; Siegler & Opfer, 2003), as well as the role of cultural factors in the development of these skills (Garcia-Retamero & Galesic, 2013). What are the developmental precursors of limited numeracy and graph literacy? Is the nature of limited numeracy in older adults different from that in younger populations? More studies are also needed on the effectiveness of interventions aimed at increasing numeracy or reducing its impact for different age groups (see Wolf et al., 2005). Future studies should also identify suitable strategies for communicating health risks to people who are neither graph literate nor numerate. For example, ongoing work using analogies from people's everyday lives shows that these analogies are relatively undemanding in terms of numeracy and may be useful for promoting more custom-tailored risk communication (Galesic & Garcia-Retamero, 2013). In order to identify strategies for communicating health risks to people who are neither graph literate nor numerate, we will need to refine our theoretical understanding of the underlying cognitive mechanisms of risk perception (Volz & Gigerenzer, 2012; Slovic & Peters, 2006).

Modifying risky behavior is difficult. To the extent that our results generalize, visual aids offer a relatively efficient means of reaching other vulnerable individuals, including children, adolescents, people in the criminal justice system, people with mental illnesses, and people in rural and inner-city areas. For example, visual aids could provide low-cost supplements for individual, community-based, or school-based interventions with potentially long-lasting effects. To maximize potential benefits, more research on these groups and other applications of visual aids is needed, as are more prospective studies investigating the comparative effects of visual aids in the long run (e.g., years after interventions). Future studies can also investigate whether health professionals possess adequate communication skills for adapting to the communication needs of patients with limited numerical skills (Anderson et al., 2014; Donelle et al., 2008). What is the impact of the lack of these skills on adherence to health recommendations, engagement in healthcare, and use of health technologies other than visual aids (see Estrada et al., 2004; Apter et al., 2006; Amalraj et al., 2009 for some preliminary results)? Research should also determine what healthcare system designs support the information needs of patients with different levels of numeracy (see Chapter 9 of this volume).

Looking forward, risk communication will increasingly be integrated with information technology. There are well established standards for the construction of decision aids (IPDAS; see Feldman-Stewart et al., 2007a; for more information see ipdas.ohri.ca/), and theories of risk literacy and graph literacy are now starting to be embodied in adaptive instruments and software. Some such programs provide free online tools allowing anyone to build better graphs (e.g., www.iconarray.com). Other online programs provide fast, free, validated assessments of risk literacy for use by researchers and the public alike (e.g., www.RiskLiteracy.org; see also GraphLiteracy.org available summer 2014). The use of similar instruments may eventually help healthcare professionals quickly assess individual differences in risk literacy, with only a couple of questions. Adaptive, internet-based tutoring programs and custom-tailored educational brochures are also under development. These interactive educational and decision aid technologies hold great promise for leveraging what we already know about communicating risk and supporting informed decision making.

Conclusion

The ideal of informed and shared decision making requires that patients understand health risks. Unfortunately, most patients are not sufficiently risk literate and thus are easily biased by commonly used risk communication formats. In this chapter, we reviewed a collection of studies investigating the benefits of visual aids for communicating health risks to individuals with different levels of numeracy. Results indicate that well-constructed visual aids are often highly effective, transparent, fast, memorable, and ethically desirable risk communication tools.

Recommended online resources

www.iconarray.com. Create tailored, embeddable icon-based risk graphics for use in risk communications, free of charge for all academic and non-commercial uses.

www.RiskLiteracy.org. With this adaptive test, in about 3 minutes, you can assess your ability to accurately interpret risk as compared to educated people from around the world.

References

Amalraj, S., Starkweather, C., Nguyen, C., & Naeim, A. (2009). Health literacy, communication, and treatment decision-making in older cancer patients. *Oncology*, 23, 369–375.

Ancker, J. S., & Kaufman, D. (2007). Rethinking health numeracy: A multidisciplinary literature review. *Journal of the American Medical Informatics Association*, 14, 713–721.

Ancker, J. S., Senathirajah, Y., Kukafka, R., & Starren, J. B. (2006). Design features of graphs in health risk communication: A systematic review. *Journal of the American Medical Informatics Association*, 13, 608–618.

Ancker, J. S., Weber, E. U., & Kukafka, R. (2011). Effect of arrangement of stick figures on estimates of proportion in risk graphics. *Medical Decision Making*, 31, 143–150.

Anderson, B. L., Gigerenzer, E., Parker, S., & Schulkin, J. (2014). Statistical literacy in obstetricians and gynecologists. *Journal for Healthcare Quality*, 36, 5–17.

Apter, A. J., Cheng, J., Small, D., Bennett, I. M., Albert, C., Fein, D. G., et al. (2006). Asthma numeracy skill and health literacy. *Journal of Asthma*, 43, 705–710.

Apter, A. J., Paasche-Orlow, M. K., Remillard, J. T., Bennett, I. M., Ben-Joseph, E. P., Batista, R. M. et al. (2008). Numeracy and communication with patients: They are counting on us. *Journal of General Internal Medicine*, 23, 2117–2124.

Carpenter, P. A., & Shah, P. (1998). A model of the perceptual and conceptual processes in graph comprehension. *Journal of Experimental Psychology: Applied*, 4, 75–100.

Cokely, E. T., & Kelley, C. M. (2009). Cognitive abilities and superior decision making under risk: A protocol analysis and process model evaluation. *Judgment and Decision Making*, 4, 20–33.

Cokely, E. T., Galesic, M., Schulz, E., Ghazal, S., & Garcia-Retamero, R. (2012). Measuring risk literacy: The Berlin Numeracy Test. *Judgment and Decision Making*, 7, 25–47.

Cooper, R. J., Schriger, D. L., Wallace, R. C., Mikulich, V. J., & Wilkes, M. S. (2003). The quantity and quality of scientific graphs in pharmaceutical advertisements. *Journal of General Internal Medicine*, 18, 294–297.

Cox, D. S., Cox, A. D., Sturm, L., & Zimet, G. (2010). Behavioral interventions to increase HPV vaccination acceptability among mothers of young girls. *Health Psychology*, 29, 29–39.

Davids, S. L., Schapira, M. M., McAuliffe, T. L., & Nattinger, A. B. (2004). Predictors of pessimistic breast cancer risk perceptions in a primary care population. *Journal of General Internal Medicine*, 19, 310–315.

Dehaene, S. (1997). *The Number Sense: How the Mind Creates Mathematics*. New York: Oxford University Press.

Donelle, L., Arocha, J. F., & Hoffman-Goetz, L. (2008). Health literacy and numeracy: Key factors in cancer risk comprehension. *Chronic Diseases in Canada*, 29, 1–8.

Estrada, C. A., Martin-Hryniewicz, M., Peek, B. T., Collins, C., & Byrd, J. C. (2004). Literacy and numeracy skills and anticoagulation control. *The American Journal of the Medical Sciences*, 328, 88–93.

Fagerlin, A., Wang, C., & Ubel, P. A. (2005). Reducing the influence of anecdotal reasoning on people's health care decisions: Is a picture worth a thousand statistics? *Medical Decision Making*, 25, 398–405.

Fagerlin, A., Ubel, P. A., Smith, D. M., & Zikmund-Fisher, B. J. (2007). Making numbers matter: Present and future research in risk communication. *American Journal of Health Behavior*, 31, 47–56.

Feldman-Stewart, D., Kocovski, N., McConnell, B. A., Brundage, M. D., & Mackillop, W. J. (2000). Perception of quantitative information for treatment decisions. *Medical Decision Making*, 20, 228–238.

Feldman-Stewart, D., Brennenstuhl, S., McIsaac, K., Austoker, J., Charvet, A., Hewitson, P., et al. (2007a). A systematic review of information in decision aids. *Health Expectations*, 10, 46–61.

Feldman-Stewart, D., Brundage, M. D., & Zotov, V. (2007b). Further insight into the perception of quantitative information: Judgments of gist in treatment decisions. *Medical Decision Making*, 27, 34–43.

Finucane, M. L., Slovic, P., Hibbard, J. H., Peters, E., Mertz, C. K., & Macgregor, D. G. (2002). Aging and decision-making competence: An analysis of comprehension and consistency skills in older versus younger adults considering health-plan options. *Journal of Behavioral Decision Making*, 15, 141–164.

Friel, S. N., Curcio, F. R., & Bright, G. W. (2001). Making sense of graphs: Critical factors influencing comprehension and instructional implications. *Journal for Research in Mathematics Education*, 32, 124–158.

Gaissmaier, W., Wegwarth, O., Skopec, D., Müller, A., Broschinski, S., & Politi, M. C. (2012). Numbers can be worth a thousand pictures: Individual differences in understanding graphical and numerical representations of health-related information. *Health Psychology*, 31, 286–296.

Galesic, M., & Garcia-Retamero, R. (2010). Statistical numeracy for health: A cross-cultural comparison with probabilistic national samples. *Archives of Internal Medicine*, 170, 462–468.

Galesic, M., & Garcia-Retamero, R. (2011a). Do low-numeracy people avoid shared decision making? *Health Psychology*, 30, 336–341.

Galesic, M., & Garcia-Retamero, R. (2011b). Graph literacy: A cross-cultural comparison. *Medical Decision Making*, 31, 444–457.

Galesic, M., & Garcia-Retamero, R. (2013). Using analogies to communicate information about medical treatments and screenings. *Applied Cognitive Psychology*. doi: 10.1002/acp.2866.

Galesic, M., Garcia-Retamero, R., & Gigerenzer, G. (2009). Using icon arrays to communicate medical risks: Overcoming low numeracy. *Health Psychology*, 28, 210–216.

Gallistel, C. R., & Gelman, R. (2005). Mathematical cognition. In: K. J. Holyoak & R. G. Morrison (Eds.), *The Cambridge Handbook of Thinking and Reasoning*. New York, NY: Cambridge University Press; pp. 559–588.

Garcia-Retamero, R., & Cokely, E. T. (2011). Effective communication of risks to young adults: Using message framing and visual aids to increase condom use and STD screening. *Journal of Experimental Psychology: Applied*, 17, 270–287.

Garcia-Retamero, R., & Cokely, E. T. (2012). Advances in efficient health communication: Promoting prevention and detection of STDs. *Current HIV Research*, 10, 262–270.

Garcia-Retamero, R., & Cokely, M. (2013). Communicating risks to vulnerable populations: Improving decision making with visual aids. *Current Directions in Psychological Science*, 22, 392–399.

Garcia-Retamero, R., & Cokely, E. T. (in press a). Simple but powerful health messages for increasing condom use in young adults. *Journal of Sex Research*. doi:10.1080/00224499.2013.806647.

Garcia-Retamero, R., & Cokely, E. (in press b). The influence of skills, message frame, and visual aids on prevention of sexually transmitted diseases. *Journal of Behavioral Decision Making*. doi: 10.1002/bdm.1797.

Garcia-Retamero, R., & Dhami, M. K. (2011). Pictures speak louder than numbers: On communicating medical risks to immigrants with limited non-native language proficiency. *Health Expectations*, 14, 46–57.

Garcia-Retamero, R., & Galesic, M. (2009). Communicating treatment risk reduction to people with low numeracy skills: A cross-cultural comparison. *American Journal of Public Health*, 99, 2196–2202.

Garcia-Retamero, R., & Galesic, M. (2010a). How to reduce the effect of framing on messages about health. *Journal of General Internal Medicine*, 25, 1323–1329.

Garcia-Retamero, R., & Galesic, M. (2010b). Who profits from visual aids: Overcoming challenges in people's understanding of risks. *Social Science & Medicine*, 70, 1019–1025.

Garcia-Retamero, R., & Galesic, M. (2013). *Transparent Communication of Health Risks: Overcoming Cultural Differences*. New York, NY: Springer.

Garcia-Retamero, R., & Hoffrage, U. (2013). Visual representation of statistical information improves diagnostic inferences in doctors and their patients. *Social Science & Medicine*, 83, 27–33.

Garcia-Retamero, R., Galesic, M., & Gigerenzer, G. (2010). Do icon arrays help reduce denominator neglect? *Medical Decision Making*, 30, 672–684.

Garcia-Retamero, R., Okan, Y., & Cokely, E. T. (2012). Using visual aids to improve communication of risks about health: A review. *The Scientific World Journal*, 2012. Article ID 562637.

Garcia-Retamero, R., Wicki, B., Cokely, E. T., & Hanson, B. (in press). Factors predicting surgeons' preferred and actual roles in interactions with their patients. *Health Psychology*, doi:10.1037/hea0000061.

Ghazal, S., Cokely, E. T., & Garcia-Retamero, R. (2014). Predicting biases in very highly educated samples: Numeracy and metacognition. *Judgment and Decision Making*, 9, 15–34.

Gigerenzer, G., & Gray, J. A. M. (2011). *Better Doctors, Better Patients, Better Decisions: Envisioning Health Care 2020*. Strüngemann Forum Report, Vol. 6. Cambridge, MA: MIT Press.

Gigerenzer, G., & Hoffrage, U. (1995). How to improve Bayesian reasoning without instruction: Frequency formats. *Psychological Review*, 102, 684–704.

Gigerenzer, G., Gaissmaier, W., Kurz-Milcke, E., Schwartz, L. M., & Woloshin, S. (2007). Helping doctors and patients make sense of health statistics. *Psychological Science in the Public Interest*, 8, 53–96.

Gillan, D. J., Wickens, C. D., Hollands, J. G., & Carswell, C. M. (1998). Guidelines for presenting quantitative data in HFES publications. *Human Factors*, 40, 28–41.

Goodyear-Smith, F., Arroll, B., Chan, L., Jackson, R., Wells, S., & Kenealy, T. (2008). Patients prefer pictures to numbers to express cardiovascular benefit from treatment. *Annals of Family Medicine*, 6, 213–217.

Gurmankin, A. D., Helweg-Larsen, M., Armstrong, K., Kimmel, S. E., & Volpp, K. G. M. (2005). Comparing the standard rating scale and the magnifier scale for assessing risk perceptions. *Medical Decision Making*, 25, 560–570.

Hawley, S. T., Zikmund-Fisher, B., Ubel, P., Jancovic, A., Lucas, T., & Fagerlin, A. (2008). The impact of the format of graphical presentation on health-related knowledge and treatment choices. *Patient Education and Counseling*, 73, 448–455.

Hoffrage, U., & Gigerenzer, G. (1998). Using natural frequencies to improve diagnostic inferences. *Academic Medicine*, 73, 538–540.

Hoffrage, U., Gigerenzer, G., Krauss, S., & Martignon, L. (2000a). Representation facilitates reasoning: What natural frequencies are and what they are not. *Cognition*, 84, 343–352.

Hoffrage, U., Lindsey, S., Hertwig, R., & Gigerenzer, G. (2000b). Communicating statistical information. *Science*, 290, 2261–2262.

Keller, C., & Siegrist, M. (2009). Effect of risk communication formats on risk perception depending on numeracy. *Medical Decision Making*, 29, 483–490.

Kurz-Milcke, E., Gigerenzer, G., & Martignon, L. (2008). Transparence in risk communication: Graphical and analog tools. *Annals of the New York Academy of Sciences*, 1128, 18–28.

Kutner, M., Greenberg, E., Jin, Y., & Paulsen, C. (2006). *The Health Literacy of America's Adults: Results from the 2003 National Assessment of Adult Literacy (NCES 2006–483)*. Washington, DC: National Center for Education Statistics.

Lipkus, I. M. (2007). Numeric, verbal, and visual formats of conveying health risks: Suggested best practices and future recommendations. *Medical Decision Making*, 27, 696–713.

Lipkus, I. M., & Hollands, J. G. (1999). The visual communication of risk. *Journal of the National Cancer Institute Monographs*, 25, 149–163.

Lipkus, I. M., Samsa, G., & Rimer, B. K. (2001). General performance on a numeracy scale among highly educated samples. *Medical Decision Making*, 21, 37–44.

Nelson, W., Reyna, V. F., Fagerlin, A., Lipkus, I., & Peters, E. (2008). Clinical implications of numeracy: Theory and practice. *Annals of Behavioral Medicine*, 35, 261–274.

OECD (2012). *PISA 2009 Technical Report*. Paris: OECD Publishing. Retrieved May 18, 2012 from http://dx.doi.org/10.1787/9789264167872-en

Okan, Y., Galesic, M., & Garcia-Retamero. (2010). Graph comprehension in medical contexts: An eye-tracking study. 13th Biennial European Conference of the Society for Medical Decision Making. Hall in Tyrol, Austria.

Okan, Y., Garcia-Retamero, R., Cokely, E. T., & Maldonado, A. (2012a). Individual differences in graph literacy: Overcoming denominator neglect in risk comprehension. *The Journal of Behavioral Decision Making*, 25, 390–401.

Okan, Y., Garcia-Retamero, R., Galesic, M., & Cokely, E. (2012b). When higher bars are not larger quantities: On individual differences in the use of spatial information in graph comprehension. *Spatial Cognition and Computation*, 12, 195–218.

Paling, J. (2003). Strategies to help patients understand risks. *British Medical Journal*, 327, 745–748.

Peters, E. (2012). Beyond comprehension: The role of numeracy in judgment and decisions. *Current Directions in Psychological Science*, 21, 31–35.

Peters, E., & Levin, I. P. (2008). Dissecting the risky choice framing effect: Numeracy as an individual difference factor in weighting risky and riskless options. *Judgment and Decision Making*, 3, 435–448.

Peters, E., Finucane, M. L., MacGregor, D. G., & Slovic, P. (2000). The bearable lightness of aging: Judgment and decision processes in older adults. In: P. C. Stern & L. L. Carstensen (Eds.), *The Aging Mind: Opportunities in Cognitive Research*. Washington, DC: National Research Council, National Academy Press; pp. 144–165.

Peters, E., Vastfjall, D., Slovic, P., Mertz, C. K., Mozzocco, K., & Dickert, S. (2006). Numeracy and decision making. *Psychological Science*, 17, 406–413.

Peters, E., Hess, T. M., Västfjäll, D., & Auman, C. (2007). Adult age differences in dual information processes: Implications for the role of affective and deliberative processes in older adults' decision making. *Perspectives on Psychological Science*, 2, 1–23.

Peters, E., Dieckmann, N. F., Västfjäll, D., Mertz, C. K., Slovic, P., & Hibbard, J. (2009). Bringing meaning to numbers: The impact of evaluative categories on decisions. *Journal of Experimental Psychology: Applied*, 15, 213–227.

Reyna, V. F. (2004). How people make decisions that involve risk. *Current Directions in Psychological Science*, 13, 60–66.

Reyna, V. F., & Brainerd, C. J. (2008). Numeracy, ratio bias, and denominator neglect in judgments of risk and probability. *Learning and Individual Differences*, 18, 89–107.

Reyna, V. R., Nelson, W. L., Han, P., & Dieckmann, N. F. (2009). How numeracy influences risk comprehension and medical decision making. *Psychological Bulletin*, 135, 943–973.

Rothman, A. J., Martino, S. C., Bedell, B. T., Detweiler, J. B., & Salovey, P. (1999). The systematic influence of gain- and loss-framed messages on interest in and use of different types of health behavior. *Personality and Social Psychology Bulletin*, 25, 1355–1369.

Rothman, R. L., Housam, R., Weiss, H., Davis, D., Gregory, R., Gebretsadik, T., et al. (2006). Patient understanding of food labels: The role of literacy and numeracy. *American Journal of Preventive Medicine*, 31, 391–398.

Ruiz, J. G., Andrade, A. D., Garcia-Retamero, R., Anam, R., Rodriguez, R., & Sharit, J. (2013). Communicating global cardiovascular risk: Are icon arrays better than numerical estimates in improving understanding, recall and perception of risk? *Patient Education and Counseling*, 93, 394–402.

Schirillo, J. A., & Stone, E. R. (2005). The greater ability of graphical versus numerical displays to increase risk avoidance involves a common mechanism. *Risk Analysis*, 25, 555–566.

Schwartz, L. M., Woloshin, S., Black, W. C., & Welch, H. G. (1997). The role of numeracy in understanding the benefit of screening mammography. *Annals of Internal Medicine*, 127, 966–972.

Siegler, R. S., & Booth, J. L. (2004). Development of numerical estimation in young children. *Child Development*, 75, 428–444.

Siegler, R. S., & Opfer, J. (2003). The development of numerical estimation: Evidence for multiple representations of numerical quantity. *Psychological Science*, 14, 237–243.

Slovic, P., & Peters, E. (2006). Risk perception and affect. *Current Directions in Psychological Science*, 15, 322–325.

Spiegelhalter, D., Pearson, M., & Short, I. (2011). Visualizing uncertainty about the future. *Science*, 333, 1393–1400.

Stone, E. R., Sieck, W. R., Bull, B. E., Yates, J. F., Parks, S. C., & Rush, C. J. (2003). Foreground: background salience: Explaining the effects of graphical displays on risk avoidance. *Organizational Behavior and Human Decision*, 90, 19–36.

Trevena, L., Zikmund-Fisher, B., Edwards, A., Gaissmaier, W., Galesic, M., Han, P., et al. (2012). Presenting probabilities. In: R. Volk & H. Llewellyn-Thomas (Eds.), *Update of the International Patient Decision Aids Standards (IPDAS) Collaboration's Background Document*. Chapter C. Retrieved from ipdas.ohri.ca/resources.html

Volz, K. G., & Gigerenzer, G. (2012). Cognitive processes in decision under risk are not the same as in decision under uncertainty. *Frontiers in Neuroscience*, 6, 105.

Waters, E. A., Weinstein, N. D., Colditz, G. A., & Emmons, K. M. (2007). Reducing aversion to side effects in preventive medical treatment decisions. *Journal of Experimental Psychology: Applied*, 13, 11–21.

Wolf, M. S., Gazmararian, J. A., & Baker, D. W. (2005). Health literacy and functional health status among older adults. *Archives of Internal Medicine*, 165, 1946–1952.

Woller-Carter, M., Okan, Y., Cokely, E. T., & Garcia-Retamero, R. (2012). Communicating risks with graphs: An eye-tracking study. *Proceedings of the Human Factors and Ergonomics Society Annual Meeting*, 56, 1723–1727.

Woloshin, S., Schwartz, L. M., Byram, S., Fischhoff, B., & Welch, H. G. (2000). A new scale for assessing perceptions of chance: A validation study. *Medical Decision Making*, 20, 298–307.

Zikmund-Fisher, B. J., Fagerlin, A., & Ubel, P. A. (2008a). Improving understanding of adjuvant therapy options by using simpler risk graphics. *Cancer*, 113, 3382–3390.

Zikmund-Fisher, B. J., Ubel, P. A., Smith, D. M., Derry, H. A., McClure, J. B., Stark, A. T., et al. (2008b). Communicating side effect risks in a tamoxifen prophylaxis decision aid: The debiasing influence of pictographs. *Patient Education & Counseling*, 73, 209–214.

Zikmund-Fisher, B. J., Fagerlin, A., & Ubel, P. A. (2010). A demonstration of "less can be more" in risk graphics. *Medical Decision Making*, 30, 661–671.

8 Anticipating barriers to the communication of critical information

Ellen Peters

A psychological approach to understanding barriers in health communication can point towards reasons why both basic research and applied research in communication are critical. These barriers also highlight opportunities to conduct research in areas that can have a positive impact on improving health and well-being. In the present chapter, I focus on what is needed to make a good decision, highlighting the importance of effective communication and the multiple barriers that exist to attaining it.

Making good decisions

In health decisions, effective communication of information is one step towards patients and consumers making good decisions about prevention and treatment. For example, US healthcare costs have skyrocketed in recent years, and recent healthcare policy has focused on controlling costs and improving quality (see Chapter 9 in this volume). The success of these policies depends, to a large extent, on the public's ability to make informed choices because choosing better options can influence the quality of individual care as well as the efficacy of the healthcare system itself. The idea is that actively involved consumers who understand and demand high-quality clinical care can be potent agents for change (Frosch & Kaplan, 1999; Hibbard & Peters, 2003). Data are increasingly available to the US public including comparative performance data on providers, health plans, nursing homes, and hospitals as well as recommended clinical guidelines for treatment or screening of many conditions. If consumers access, understand, and use this information, they can increase control over their healthcare experiences and health outcomes.

Informed health decision making is a process in which patients and consumers (and sometimes their loved ones) receive sufficient information about risks, benefits, limitations, alternatives, and uncertainties to make a value-concordant decision and participate in decision making at a desired level (Braddock et al., 1997, 1999). Research has demonstrated that more informed, involved, and activated patients are healthier patients. Ward et al. (2003), for example, found that women with lupus who participate more actively in their visits have less morbidity than those who participate less actively.

Decision aids are often used to assist informed decision making and research demonstrates that they are of value. In one recent study, a decision aid was developed for screening colorectal cancer (CRC), the second leading cause of US cancer-related death and third most commonly diagnosed cancer. Fifty percent of eligible Americans have not had appropriate screening (United States Department of Health and Human Services, 2005). The decision aid study was conducted at an urban, academic hospital and community health center between 2005 and 2010. Participants were asymptomatic, average risk patients aged 50 to 75 years who were due for CRC screening. With exposure to the decision aid (compared to no exposure), knowledge, satisfaction with choice, and intentions to get screened were all higher. Intentions to get screened were also higher when the test recommended by the physician reflected patient preferences (Schroy et al., 2011; see Table 8.1). In a follow-up with these same patients, Schroy et al. (2012) further found that those in the decision aid group were more likely to complete a screening test than control patients within 12 months of the study visit. These effects, however, were modest (43% vs. 35%, respectively, $p = 0.05$). A decision aid plus personalized risk assessment tool was no more effective than the decision aid alone (37% vs. 43%, $p = 0.15$). Informing choices with decision aids often helps as has been demonstrated in numerous studies that show

Table 8.1. *Decision aids inform decisions about colorectal cancer screening.*

	Decision aid only	Decision aid plus Your Disease Risk	Control group
Post-test knowledge (0–12)	10.9	10.7	8.6
Change in knowledge from pre- to post-	3.2	3.0	0.8
Satisfaction with decision process (0–60)	50.7	50.5	46.7
Intentions to get screened (1–5)	4.4	4.3	3.9
Received screening test within 12 months	43.1%	37.1%	34.8%

Means and frequencies between the two decision aid groups were similar to one another and significantly greater than those for the control group.
From Schroy et al., 2011; Schroy et al., 2012.

increased knowledge and decreased decisional conflict with the use of a decision aid (O'Connor et al., 2003).

Decision aids, when well designed, help to target a number of factors necessary to making good decisions (Hibbard & Peters, 2003). To make good decisions, for example, decision makers must have information, and this information can be provided by a decision aid. The information has to be available, accurate, and provided in a timely fashion for the decision at hand. Individuals have to attend to the information (i.e., they have to look at it). They also have to be able to comprehend the information; this is a basic building block of good decision making that information providers usually recognize. But good decision making requires more than simple comprehension of information. Simple comprehension of numbers often involves assessing whether an individual can repeat back a fact such as 6% of smokers will die in the next 10 years from cancer (a simple unweighted average of the risks posed by smoking to 35–75-year-old men; Woloshin et al., 2008). Decision makers need to be able to understand more than just the facts, however. They have to be able to understand the meaning of those facts as well. What does 6% mean? How good or bad is that? The next step is that the decision maker has to be able to determine meaningful differences between options. Continuing the previous example, the smoker would need to determine the meaning of a number comparison. How good or bad is it that 6% of smokers will die in the next 10 years from cancer compared to 1% of non-smokers? The decision maker then needs to weight factors to match his or her own needs and values (and this process requires understanding one's own needs and values within the specific concrete situation, a difficult process in and of itself; Peters, 2009). Finally, the decision maker has to make trade-offs such as between risks, benefits, and costs, and ultimately make a choice. What appears at face value to be a simple task ("just pick one") is actually a complex cognitive process that requires motivation and ability.

Barriers to effective communication

In an ideal world, of course, this would all be quite easy. We could simply tell patients and consumers exactly what they need to know and understand and leave it to them to take charge and make choices that are in their best interests. It sounds so easy, but multiple barriers exist to obtaining and using information effectively in choices. Some of the barriers are systemic; other barriers emerge from either the communicators or from the patient or consumer who receives the communications. See Table 8.2.

Table 8.2. *Types of barriers to effective communication of health information.*

A. Systemic barriers	B. Barriers from the communicators	C. Barriers from the patient or consumer
Information is insufficient (e.g., missing information)	Failure to identify communication goals and to prioritize information	Lack of comprehension (due to numeracy, literacy, or motivational issues) undermines informed choice
Information is uncertain (e.g., the benefits are probabilistic and may or may not help me)	Overestimation of what patients and consumers know (e.g., the curse of knowledge)	Lack of affective meaning means that information is not used
Information is ambiguous (e.g., the results of two studies are in conflict)	Hindsight bias ("I knew it all along")	Preferences for information formats do not maximize comprehension
Information changes rather than staying fixed (e.g., new data emerges as additional studies are conducted)	Overestimation of the effectiveness of communications	The inverse relation between perceptions of risks and benefits
	Communicator intuitions about how best to present information do not always maximize patient and consumer comprehension	Greater patient autonomy may lead to increased risk perceptions and decreased willingness for treatments

Systemic barriers

Information in health decisions unfortunately is often insufficient, uncertain, and changing. For example, information can change as new data emerges about the risks of a class of pharmaceuticals, or the benefits of a preventive. Vioxx is one such example. It was considered at first a very effective pain reliever without the usual side effects. However, new data came out about its risk profile, and Vioxx, a once popular drug, was removed from the market. To some extent, this changing information is a byproduct of the scientific process, in which scientists take two steps forward (with study number one) and then one step back (as results from study number two emerge).

Breast self exam is an example where conflicting evidence exists. A meta-analysis conducted by Hackshaw and Paul (2003) demonstrated no mortality benefit from breast self exam, and yet medical professionals often recommend them nonetheless. In another example of conflicting information, eating salmon is recommended for everyone because of its nutritional benefits, but salmon also contains traces of mercury that could harm an unborn baby or young child's developing nervous system.

As a result, pregnant women and parents are faced with conflicting information about both risks and benefits from eating salmon. The US Food and Drug Administration tries to decrease perceived conflict in this choice by providing simple rules for eating fish (www.fda.gov/food/resourcesforyou/consumers/ucm110591.htm). Well-intended government advice is not always enough, however. Downs et al. (2008) found that parents wanted more information about the risks and benefits of vaccines, but they did not necessarily find the best information. In their study, parents intuitively chose search terms that led them to vaccine-skeptics websites, rather than to websites of proponents. They trusted the pro-vaccination websites more, but even parents who were generally in favor of vaccines were sometimes confused by the ongoing debate.

Another major systemic barrier to effective communication emerges from the variety of sources of uncertainty and ambiguity that exist in health, including uncertainty about future outcomes, ambiguity or uncertainty about the strength or validity of evidence about risks, uncertainty about the personal significance of particular risks (e.g., their severity, timing), uncertainty arising from the complexity of risk information (e.g., the multiplicity of risks and benefits or the instability of risks and benefits over time), and uncertainty resulting from lack of knowledge (Politi et al., 2007). Ambiguity aversion can emerge as a result of this inherent uncertainty. For example, studies have shown that, with missing information about the risks of adverse events from flu vaccination, decision makers are less likely to intend to get vaccinated (Ritov & Baron, 1990); similar effects occur when the ambiguity is due to expert disagreement regarding the advisability of getting a vaccine (Meszaros et al., 1996). With conflicting expert risk estimates from two independent studies, perceptions of an environmental risk of cancer increased (Viscusi et al., 1991). Finally, use of confidence intervals to display uncertainty on top of a precise risk estimate also produced greater cancer worry (Han et al., 2011). Systemic barriers exist and have impacts on consumer and patient perceptions of provided information.

Barriers from the communicators

Barriers to effective communication also emerge from the communicators themselves. For example, communicators may fail to properly identify the goal or goals of a communication and what information the decision maker needs to receive to meet communication goals. Without this identification of what matters and to whom, communication efforts may be inadequate.

Second, communicators tend to overestimate what other people know (Nickerson, 1999, 2001). This overestimation is important because communicators tend to adapt communications to intended recipients to improve its effectiveness. To do this adaption, information providers have to have a model of what the "other person" knows. For large agencies such as the FDA to do this adaptive communication, they need a model of what "most people" know since they usually communicate to the public at large. Physicians and other healthcare providers, who communicate more often one-on-one with patients, need models of what "this patient" knows. Research demonstrates, however, that the default model humans use to figure out what the "other" knows is to consider, first, one's own perspective and knowledge and to use this knowledge to estimate what others know. This approach often works because others are similar enough. The problem is that we then insufficiently adjust for those who lack the same specialized knowledge, especially when the information is familiar as it is to an expert in that field. To the expert, the information seems much simpler and more straightforward than it does to someone seeing it for the first time, and the expert cannot put herself in the position of that naïve person. This "curse of knowledge" causes communicators to overestimate what others know and is a barrier to effective communication because we cannot adapt communication to the appropriate level if we do not know what that level is. It is not entirely clear to what extent this is true of physicians, genetic counselors, and other health professionals and information providers who attempt to communicate with patients and consumers.

Communicators also show hindsight bias, also called the "I knew it all along effect." After an event has occurred, people tend to exaggerate the extent to which they think they could have predicted it beforehand (Fischhoff, 1975). It appears to be due to memory for complex events being a reconstructive process. Ultimately, we are "insufficiently surprised" by experience (Fischhoff cited in Hastie & Dawes, 2010, p. 133). Physicians demonstrate hindsight bias in ways that are similar to nonphysicians. Arkes et al. (1981) found that physicians asked to estimate the likelihood of each of four diagnoses for a patient gave much greater estimates for the least likely diagnosis when they were told ahead of time that that diagnosis was correct compared to when they were not told anything. The authors concluded that such hindsight biases, similar to the curse of knowledge above, leads to a lack of learning that could be used to improve communications. Among physicians, in particular, it would likely lead to "overconfident second opinions, overconfidence in diagnostic accuracy, and inadequate appreciation of the original difficulty of diagnoses" (p. 252).

Fourth, communicators tend to overestimate how effectively they communicate. This is important because if we overestimate our effectiveness, we lose opportunities to improve communication. Communicators speak from their own perspective (remember the "curse of knowledge") while listeners interpret from their own perspective. As communicators, we are somewhat sensitive to these differences in perspective, but not as much as we could be. A simple study by Boaz Keysar (Keysar & Henly, 2002) illustrates this point. Participants, run two-at-a-time were assigned to be either a Speaker or a Listener. The Speaker was told that the sentence "Angela killed the man with the gun" had two meanings: (1) the man holding the gun is the one Angela killed, and (2) Angela killed him with the gun she was holding. The Speaker was then supposed to say this simple sentence to the Listener and disambiguate the meaning of the sentence to match one of the two meanings. Among Speakers who were asked to do this task and who reported that the Listener did understand, about half the time the Listener did not understand. The Speakers used their intuitions to clarify communication, but intuition was not enough. Given that the Speaker had a 50% random chance of being understood, this result tells a powerful story about how well communicators can assess the effectiveness of their own communications.

Health communication is, of course, infinitely more complicated than the simple sentence above. To what extent do physicians, the FDA, and other information providers overestimate their effectiveness in communicating health information? A study with outgoing pediatric interns at a shift change is illuminating (Chang et al., 2010). In it, the most important information about a patient was not successfully communicated 60% of the time despite the outgoing physician thinking that it was. What aspects of the situation, the patient, or other factors make this overestimation more and less likely? How can we overcome this tendency to overestimate our effectiveness in order to become better communicators?

Finally, communicators' intuitions about how best to provide information do not always maximize patient and consumer comprehension. In one example from work out of our laboratory, we wanted to help consumers better understand a new and more complex consumer-directed health insurance plan that was emerging on the market. We had the intuition that providing a framework that broadly explained how the new plan differed from a more familiar plan (that was also offered) would help consumers understand the more detailed information that followed (Greene et al., 2008). The framework's key messages were that the consumer-directed health plan had lower monthly premiums, but enrollees might have higher out-of-pocket costs if they used a lot of

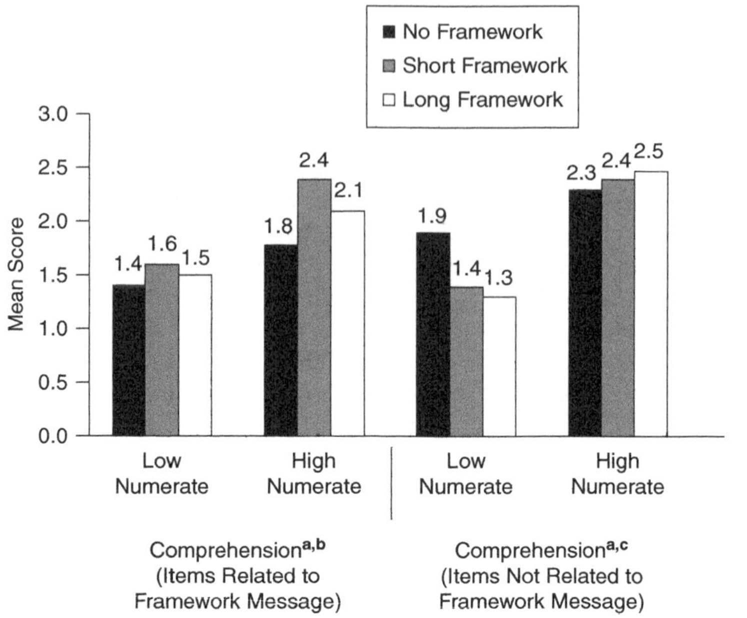

[a]$P < 0.05$ for relationship with numeracy.
[b]$P < 0.05$ for relationship with framework.
[c]$P < 0.05$ for interaction between framework and numeracy.

Figure 8.1. Providing a framework increased understanding of related information that follows, but decreased understanding of unrelated information among the less numerate. (Reprinted from Greene et al., 2008, *The American Journal of Managed Care* with permission from Ascend Media and Intellisphere, LLC.)

medical services. Overall, we found that providing an overarching framework to highlight the differences between the two plans worked to some extent. It boosted comprehension of highly numerate individuals (those who scored higher on a math test focused on probabilistic understanding). Among the less numerate, the framework helped them to better understand items related to the framework message. However, it reduced their comprehension of items not related to the framework (see Figure 8.1). The study results highlighted the difficulty many consumers have in understanding comparative information and in making informed healthcare choices. It also highlighted the difficulty that information providers face when asked to use their intuition to choose best formats and the opportunities to improve communications that exist when information providers conduct focused tests with appropriate populations. We have also examined more generally the notion that intuitions about effective public policy can lead to unintended consequences without such focused tests (Peters et al., 2013).

Barriers from the patient or consumer

The last type of barrier to effective communication is those from the patients or consumers themselves. Although these barriers are often mentioned first when communications fail (the public does not care; they were too uneducated to understand), the sections above hopefully have made it apparent that communication issues do not emerge only due to a lack of ability or motivation from the individuals who need the information.

A critical barrier to effective communication is, nonetheless, patient ability. Patients and consumers do not always understand provided information, suggesting that communicators cannot count on even this simple building block of good decisions when they provide information. In fact, even identifying a dominant option in a large set can be difficult for some individuals (Hibbard et al., 2001). Results from health plan choice studies demonstrate that decision makers do not always comprehend even fairly simple information, and this lack of comprehension is exacerbated with older adult age. Hibbard et al. (2001) presented employment-aged adults (18–64 years old; n = 239) and older adults (65–94 years old; n = 253) with 33 decision tasks that involved interpretation of numbers from tables and graphs. Participants, for example, were asked to identify the health insurance plan with the lowest copayment from a table that included four plans with information about monthly premiums and copayments. A comprehension index reflected the total number of errors made across the 33 tasks. The youngest participants (aged 18–35) averaged 8% errors; the oldest participants (aged 85–94) averaged 40% errors; the correlation between age and the number of errors was 0.31 ($p < 0.001$). Having more formal education was somewhat protective of these age declines.

But a lack of comprehension is by no means limited to older age. Research has demonstrated that people of all ages tend to comprehend more and make better-informed decisions when the presentation format makes the most important information cognitively easier to process and evaluate (Peters et al., 2007). In three experiments concerning comparative hospital performance, the results were particularly strong for those with lower numeracy skills and support the idea that "less is more." In one study, respondents who were given only the most relevant information about hospital quality (e.g., the percentage of patients receiving recommended care) were better able to comprehend that information and were more likely to choose a higher quality hospital compared with respondents who received the same quality information plus less relevant information (e.g., the number of general care beds). In a second study, making only a more important quality measure easier to evaluate through the use of evaluative symbols (e.g., ●, ◐, ○ means that a hospital scored better than average, average, and worse than average, respectively, on that quality indicator) rather than making all indicators easier to evaluate led to more choices of higher quality hospitals. In a third study, less cognitive effort was more; presenting quality information in a format in which a higher number means better (the number of registered nurses per 100 patients) compared to one where a lower number means better (the number of patients per registered nurse) facilitated comprehension and helped respondents make better choices.

Less was also more in women's choices among adjuvant treatments for breast cancer (Zikmund-Fisher et al., 2008). They tested the impact of providing risk information about only the two more appropriate treatment options (compared to all four options) and found that, when fewer options were presented, women reported incremental risk reduction more accurately, responded more quickly to that question, and reported liking the graph more. Requiring more cognitive effort (e.g., by providing more information) appears to result in less comprehension and use of important health information.

A second barrier is that decision makers can comprehend *what* information is (they can identify a cost as $120) without understanding its *meaning* for the decision at hand. This "meaning" is operationalized in research on the affect heuristic as experienced good and bad feelings concerning a likelihood, an attribute, an outcome, or an option in a decision situation. These feelings then guide judgments and decisions (Slovic & Peters, 2006). Oftentimes, however, consumers do not experience a feeling about provided information because they are not able to interpret its meaning (e.g., how good or bad a 6% risk is of developing breast cancer over the next 5 years; Zikmund-Fisher et al., 2010). As a result, the information is not weighed much in decisions. For example, a man may not understand what the experience would be like of an adverse event from a prostate biopsy or cancer treatment such as hormone therapy. Alternatively, he may demonstrate understanding of its precise likelihood by rehearsing the 40% chance of the adverse event, but not understand the meaning of that 40%.

Peters et al. (2009) highlighted the notion that consumers are often quite poor at using numeric information in decisions precisely because they do not understand its meaning. They further demonstrated that providing this meaning can have a marked influence on judgments and choices. In their studies, they provided labels to help consumers evaluate the meaning of provided numeric quality-of-care information about

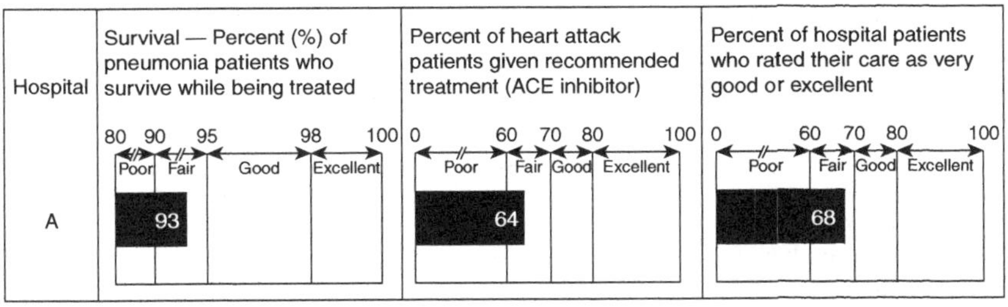

Hospital	Survival — Percent (%) of pneumonia patients who survive while being treated	Percent of heart attack patients given recommended treatment (ACE inhibitor)	Percent of hospital patients who rated their care as very good or excellent
A	93	64	68

Figure 8.2. Hospital quality information is provided in an evaluative categories format (top) or with numbers only (bottom) in Study 1 of Peters et al. (2009).

health insurance plans (e.g., labels such as "excellent" and "poor"; see Figure 8.2). The provision of evaluative labels resulted in greater use of numeric quality-of-care information in judgments in general and less reliance on an irrelevant affective state among the less numerate in particular. In testing possible mechanisms for these effects, it appeared that consumers given evaluative labels, in fact, did process the numeric information (they did not ignore it due to the presence of labels). Memory for precise quality-of-care numbers or their gist did not differ between the conditions. Instead, the evaluative labels appeared to increase the relative accessibility of valenced feelings about the choice options over valenced thoughts about the same options (see Table 8.3). Zikmund-Fisher et al. (2007) further demonstrated that providing interpretive labels for test results (telling patients that a test came back "positive" or "abnormal") induced larger changes to risk perceptions and behavioral intentions than did numeric results alone. Although evaluative labels improved judgments by assisting participants to use more of the provided numeric information, their normative status in choices is not as clear since providing labels alters choices even in the absence of a dominant alternative. Thus, evaluative labels present some ethical issues (at what level of the quality indicator should a hospital be deemed "excellent" as opposed to "very good") and should be applied thoughtfully.

Table 8.3. *Memory for precise numbers (Study 3) and accessibility of feelings versus thoughts (Study 4) in Peters et al. (2009).*

	Evaluative categories	Bar chart only	Significance
Memory for precise patient satisfaction numbers for Plan A (Study 3)	26%	22%	$p = 0.51$
Memory for precise patient satisfaction numbers for Plan B (Study 3)	25%	14%	$p = 0.09$
Average accessibility of feelings about health plans in milliseconds (Study 4)	1266	1545	
Accessibility of thoughts about a simple health plan in milliseconds (Study 4)	1382	1460	Feelings were accessed faster than thoughts with evaluative categories; no difference existed with bar charts only

Ideally, we could simply ask the individuals receiving the information about their preferences for how information should be presented. However, a third barrier is that the intuitions of information recipients can misfire just as the intuitions of communicators are not always perfect. Hawley et al. (2008), for example, demonstrated that the preferences expressed by patients and consumers may not necessarily maximize comprehension of information. In particular, they found that participants across numeracy groups rated a table format as the most effective, trustworthy, and scientific compared to the other formats even though both pictographs and pie charts led to greater understanding (at least among less numerate individuals).

A fourth barrier that emerges from patients and consumers is that communicating risks influences benefit perceptions and vice versa. As suggested earlier, to make a good decision, we want people to tradeoff risks and benefits. Research suggests, however, that communicating about only the risks of a treatment will influence benefit perceptions just as communicating about only its benefits will alter perceived risks. In the real world, risks and benefits are positively correlated, whether risk is defined as severity or likelihood. For example, a medication with serious side effects would have to have benefits that were also quite high to stay on the market as a viable product that people will purchase. But in people's minds, perceptions of risks and benefits are inversely related (Fischhoff et al., 1978). Things that are perceived as high in benefit are simultaneously perceived as low in risk whereas objects perceived as highly risky tend to be perceived at the same time as low in benefit. And the strength of this negative correlation between perceived risks and perceived benefits depends on affect – how good or bad the object feels to the individual (Alhakami & Slovic, 1994). Things that feel good tend to be perceived as high in benefit and low in risk whereas things that feel bad are perceived as high in risk and low in benefit. The inverse relationship can be explained by the affect heuristic (Slovic et al., 2002). Research suggests that we use these often subtle experienced feelings as information to guide perceptions of information, judgments, and choices. The affect heuristic explains how good and bad feelings about nuclear waste repositories or prescription drugs, for example, are associated with perceptions of their risks and benefits. In particular, it predicts that we will look to our good and bad feelings as information to judge perceptions of whether something is risky or beneficial. For example, we found that across a set of 32 pharmaceuticals, a strong correlation existed between perceived risk and perceived benefit, $r = -0.46$ (Slovic et al., 2007). Some drugs were perceived as high benefit and low risk (e.g., osteoporosis drugs) while others were perceived as low in benefit and high in risk (e.g., diet drugs). Most prescription medications fell into the low risk/high benefit quadrant and people had positive affect toward them.

Most affect-heuristic research has been correlational, but experimental studies support the causal link between affect and risk and benefit perceptions. For example, Finucane et al. (2000) conducted a simple experiment in which they provided only information about the risk of a technology or only information about the benefit of a technology. As predicted by the affect heuristic, providing only increased risk information led to an inference of lower benefit whereas providing only increased benefit information led to lower risk perceptions. Government agencies such as the Food and Drug Administration or Homeland Security sometimes choose to provide only risk information (about an emerging security risk to airplanes, for example) without any information about the benefits of air travel. Affect-heuristic research predicts that perceptions of the benefits of air travel will decline nonetheless and people will tend to choose other, and sometimes riskier, forms of transportation instead (see Gigerenzer, 2006, for a possible example). To what extent does this happen in health? Some research suggests that physicians may be better at communicating the benefits of new medications than their possible adverse events (Tarn et al., 2006) although even the benefits may not be provided in much depth (Siminoff et al., 1989).

A final barrier to effective communication is tied up in the reasons why communicators provide information in the first place. The provision of information is intended to increase how often and how well consumers make active choices that (hopefully) reflect their own values and result in superior individual choices, reduced liability for healthcare providers, and improvements in the efficacy of the health system itself. This latter point might be expected because consumers recognize and choose based on quality and their actions drive further quality improvements in the health system. This opportunity to make a more informed decision, however, may result in unintended consequences, a topic that has received little study (Peters et al., 2013). Fraenkel and Peters (2009) conducted one proof-of-concept experiment in which they varied whether a patient made a hypothetical treatment choice with more or less autonomy. They concluded that greater patient autonomy in choice may not inevitably lead to better outcomes. In particular, they demonstrated that highlighting the responsibility of having a choice increased patients' worry about the risks of adverse events and decreased their willingness to accept treatment. Fraenkel and Peters' study, however, was limited in that it used extremes of volition in a within-participant design (their patient participants made the same choice twice, once when told that "the doctor decides" and again when told that "the doctor tells you that it is completely up to you" (order was counterbalanced and did not influence responses)). In clinical practice, the extent of patient involvement (and therefore choice autonomy) varies greatly, and would be expected to be strongly related to patient preferences and experience, the patient–physician relationship, the specific clinical context, and the physicians' recommendation.

Conclusions and next steps

Life is a balance between risks and benefits, but benefits and risks are not always as simple as patients expect. And communication about risks and benefits is not always as easy as experts expect. How do we get patients to finally understand disclosure labels? We can do better than to tell them that the fried stuff on a stick won't kill you, not right away anyhow. How can we communicate health information so that people can understand it and can use it effectively? Understanding the barriers to effective communication is one step in this direction.

Communication in health needs to be considered as a strategic process that is considered early on rather than being tacked on at the end when someone says "oh, now we have to communicate this. Do we have any money left?" If risk information is provided, benefit information should be provided as well; if benefit information is provided so should risk. With pharmaceuticals and similar products, the numeric likelihood of those risks and benefits should be provided as well (Knapp et al., 2004; Peters et al., in press; Steiner et al., 2003).

The communicator needs to ask the question of whether provided information is comprehensible and useable. Dominick Frosch and colleagues, for example, recently examined evidence for the understanding and impact of direct-to-consumer (DTC) pharmaceutical advertising (Frosch et al., 2010). They concluded that DTC ads provide some benefits but could be substantially improved (e.g., DTC ads appear to cause some questionable prescribing practices). In cases like these where identifiable problems exist, the communicator needs to look for ways to improve communications. In fact, one of the most important aspects of communication that result from the fallibility of all of our intuitions is that communications need to be tested prior to use in appropriate populations and including vulnerable populations (literacy, numeracy, age) of individuals who may have more difficulty with the information.

Provided information in health is often abstract and it can be difficult to understand, both in terms of exactly what the information is and what it means. Informing decisions is not about "just the facts." Instead, communicators need to make thoughtful and defensible choices of data presentation. They may need to highlight the affective meaning of information to guide processing and facilitate decisions. Having more knowledgeable and engaged patients is requisite to decreasing variability and disparities in healthcare, but we do not know enough about how to inform decisions and what unintended effects might emerge. A psychological approach is key to developing general principles to guide communications to patients and to setting up appropriate systems to assist them. Risk communication needs to be a strategic process considered as health information develops and it needs to be modified based on the barriers that exist in the particular health situation.

References

Alhakami, A. S., & Slovic, P. (1994). A psychological study of the inverse relationship between perceived risk and perceived benefit. *Risk Analysis*, 14, 1085–1096.

Arkes, H. R., Wortmann, R. L., Saville, P. D., & Harkness, A. R. (1981). Hindsight bias among physicians weighing the likelihood of diagnoses. *Journal of Applied Psychology*, 66(2), 252–254.

Braddock, C. H., Edwards, K. A., Hasenberg, N. M., Laidley, T. L., & Levinson, W. (1999). Informed decision making in outpatient practice: Time to get back to basics. *Journal of the American Medical Association*, 282(24), 2313–2320.

Braddock, C. H., Fihn, S. D., Levinson, W., Jonsen, A. R., & Pearlman, R. A. (1997). How doctors and patients discuss routine clinical decisions: Informed decision making in the outpatient setting. *Journal of General Internal Medicine*, 12(6), 339–345.

Chang, V. Y., Arora, V. M., Lev-Ari, S., D'Arcy, M., & Keysar, B. (2010). Interns overestimate the effectiveness of their hand-off communication. *Pediatrics*, 125(3), 491–496.

Downs, J. S., Bruine de Bruin, W., & Fischhoff, B. (2008). Parents' vaccination comprehension and decisions. *Vaccine*, 26(12), 1595–1607.

Finucane, M. L., Alhakami, A., Slovic, P., & Johnson, S. M. (2000). The affect heuristic in judgments of risks and benefits. *Journal of Behavioral Decision Making*, 13, 1–17.

Fischhoff, B. (1975). Hindsight not equal to foresight: Effect of outcome knowledge on judgment under uncertainty. *Journal of Experimental Psychology: Human Perception and Performance*, 1(3), 288–299.

Fischhoff, B., Slovic, P., Lichtenstein, S., Reid, S., & Coombs, B. (1978). How safe is safe enough? A psychometric study of attitudes towards technological risks and benefits. *Policy Sciences*, 9, 127–152.

Fraenkel, L., & Peters, E. (2009). Patient responsibility for medical decision making and risky treatment options. *Arthritis Care and Research*, 61(12), 1674–1676.

Frosch, D. L., & Kaplan, R. M. (1999). Shared decision making in clinical medicine: Past research and future directions. *American Journal of Preventative Medicine*, 17(4), 285–294.

Frosch, D. L., Grande, D., Tarn, D. M., & Kravitz, R. L. (2010). A decade of controversy: Balancing policy with evidence in the regulation of prescription drug advertising. *American Journal of Public Health*, 100(1), 24–32.

Gigerenzer, G. (2006). Out of the frying pan into the fire: Behavioral reactions to terrorist attacks. *Risk Analysis*, 26(2), 347–351.

Greene, J., Peters, E., Mertz, C. K., & Hibbard, J. H. (2008). Comprehension and choice of a consumer-directed health plan: An experimental study. *The American Journal of Managed Care*, 14(6), 369–376.

Hackshaw, A. K., & Paul, E. A. (2003). Breast self-examination and death from breast cancer: a meta-analysis. *British Journal of Cancer*, 88, 1047–1053.

Han, P. K. J., Klein, W. M. P., Lehman, T., Killam, B., Massett, H., & Freedman, A. N. (2011). Communication of uncertainty regarding individualized cancer risk estimates: Effects and influential factors. *Medical Decision Making*, 31(2), 354–366.

Hastie, R., & Dawes, R. (2010). *Rational Choice in an Uncertain World: The Psychology of Judgment and Decision Making*. Thousand Oaks, CA: Sage Publications.

Hawley, S. T., Zikmund-Fisher, B., Ubel, P., Jancovic, A., Lucas, T., & Fagerlin, A. (2008). The impact of the format of graphical presentation on health-related knowledge and treatment choices. *Patient Education and Counseling*, 73(3), 448–455.

Hibbard, J. H., & Peters, E. (2003). Supporting informed consumer health care choices: Data presentation approaches that facilitate the use of information in choice. *Annual Review of Public Health*, 24, 413–433.

Hibbard, J. H., Peters, E., Slovic, P., Finucane, M. L., & Tusler, M. (2001). Making health care quality reports easier to use. *Joint Commission Journal on Quality Improvement*, 27(11), 591–604.

Keysar, B., & Henly, A. S. (2002). Speakers' overestimation of their effectiveness. *Psychological Science*, 13(3), 207–212.

Knapp, P., Raynor D. K., & Berry, D. C. (2004). Comparison of two methods of presenting risk information to patients about the side effects of medicines. *Quality & Safety in Health Care*, 13(3), 176–180.

Meszaros, J. R., Asch, D. A., Baron, J., Hershey, J. C., Kunreuther, H., & Schwartz-Buzaglo, J. (1996). Cognitive processes and the decisions of some parents to forego pertussis vaccination for their children. *Journal of Clinical Epidemiology*, 49, 697–703.

Nickerson, R. S. (1999). How we know – and sometimes misjudge – what others know: Imputing one's own knowledge to others. *Psychological Bulletin*, 125(6), 737–759.

Nickerson, R. S. (2001). The projective way of knowing: A useful heuristic that sometimes misleads. *Current Directions in Psychological Science*, 10(5), 168–172.

O'Connor, A. M., Stacey, D., Entwistle, V., Llewellyn-Thomas, H., Rovner, D., Holmes-Rovner, M., et al. (2003). Decision aids for people facing health treatment or screening decisions. *Cochrane Database of Systematic Reviews*, 2, CD001431.

Peters, E. (2009). A perspective on eating behaviors from the field of judgment and decision making. *Annals of Behavioral Medicine*, 38, S81–S87, special supplement on Decision Making in Eating Behavior: Interacting Perspectives from the Individual, Family and Environment. doi 10.1007/s12160-009-9121-8.

Peters, E., Dieckmann, N., Dixon, A., Hibbard, J. H., & Mertz, C. K. (2007). Less is more in presenting quality information to consumers. *Medical Care Research & Review*, 64(2), 169–190.

Peters, E., Dieckmann, N. F., Västfjäll, D., Mertz, C. K., Slovic, P., & Hibbard, J. H. (2009). Bringing meaning to numbers: The impact of evaluative categories on decisions. *Journal of Experimental Psychology: Applied*, 15(3), 213–227.

Peters, E., Hart, S., Tusler, M., & Fraenkel, L. (in press). Numbers matter to informed patient choices: The effects of age and numeracy. *Medical Decision Making*.

Peters, E., Klein, W. M., Kaufman, A., Meilleur, L., & Dixon, A. (2013). More is not always better: Intuitions about public policy can lead to unintended health consequences. *Social Issues and Policy Review*, 7(1), 114–148.

Politi, M. C., Han, P. K. J., & Col, N. F. (2007). Communicating the uncertainty of harms and benefits of medical interventions. *Medical Decision Making*, 27(5), 681–695.

Ritov, I., & Baron, J. (1990). Reluctance to vaccinate: Omission bias and ambiguity. *Journal of Behavioral Decision Making*, 3, 263–277.

Schroy, P. C., Emmons, K., Peters, E., Glick, J. T., Robinson, P. A., Lydotes, M. A., et al. (2011). The impact of a novel computer-based decision aid on shared decision-making for colorectal cancer screening: A randomized trial. *Medical Decision Making*, 31(1), 93–107.

Schroy, P. C., Emmons, K. M., Peters, E., Glick, J. T., Robinson, P. A., Lydotes, M. A., et al. (2012). Aid-assisted decision making and colorectal cancer screening: A randomized controlled trial. *American Journal of Preventive Medicine*, 43(6), 573–583.

Siminoff, L. A., Fetting, J. H., & Abeloff, M. D. (1989). Doctor-patient communication about breast-cancer adjuvant therapy. *Journal of Clinical Oncology*, 7(9), 1192–1200.

Slovic, P., & Peters, E. (2006). Risk perception and affect. *Current Directions in Psychological Science*, 15(6), 322–325.

Slovic, P., Finucane, M., Peters, E., & MacGregor, D. G. (2002). The affect heuristic. In: T. Gilovich, D. Griffin, & D. Kahneman (Eds.), *Heuristics and Biases: The Psychology of Intuitive Judgment*. New York: Cambridge University Press; pp. 397–420.

Slovic, P., Peters, E., Grana, J., Berger, S., & Dieck, G. S. (2007). Risk perception of prescription drugs: Results of a national survey. *Drug Information Journal*, 41, 81–100.

Steiner, M. J., Dalebout, S., Condon, S., Dominik, R., & Trussell, J. (2003). Understanding risk: A randomized controlled trial of communicating contraceptive effectiveness. *American Journal of Obstetrics and Gynecology*, 102(4), 709–717.

Tarn, D. M., Heritage, J., Paterniti, D. A., Hays, R. D., Kravitz, R. L., & Wenger, N. S. (2006). Physician communication when prescribing new medications. *Archives of Internal Medicine*, 166(17), 1855–1862.

United States Department of Health and Human Services. (2005). National Health Interview Survey. *National Center for Health Statistics*.

Viscusi, W. K., Magat, W. A., & Huber, J. (1991). Communication of ambiguous risk information. *Theory and Decision*, 31(2–3), 159–173.

Ward, M. M., Sundaramurthy, S., Lotstein, D., Bush, T. M., Neuwelt, C. M., & Street, R. L., Jr. (2003). Participatory patient– physician communication and morbidity in patients with systemic lupus erythematosus. *Arthritis and Rheumatism*, 49(6), 810–818.

Woloshin, S., Schwartz, L. M., & Welch, H. G. (2008). The risk of death by age, sex, and smoking status in the United States: Putting health risks in context. *Journal of the National Cancer Institute*, 100(12), 845–853.

Zikmund-Fisher, B. J., Fagerlin, A., Keeton, K., & Ubel, P. A. (2007). Does labeling prenatal screening test results as negative or positive affect a woman's responses? *American Journal of Obstetrics and Gynecology*, 197(5), 528e1–528e6.

Zikmund-Fisher, B. J., Fagerlin, A., & Ubel, P. A. (2008). Improving understanding of adjuvant therapy options via simpler risk graphics. *Cancer*, 113(12), 3382–3390.

Zikmund-Fisher, B. J., Fagerlin, A., & Ubel, P. A. (2010). Risky feelings: Why a 6% risk of cancer does not always feel like 6%. *Patient Education and Counseling*, 81, S87–S93.

9 Rational healthcare

Ronald Paulus & Walter F. Stewart

The US healthcare system has struggled for decades against seemingly intractable problems: safety concerns, including more than 100 000 unexpected hospital deaths annually (Committee on Quality of Healthcare in America, 2000), incomplete and unequal access to care; perverse payment incentives that reward volume rather than excellent outcomes; fragmented, uncoordinated, and highly variable care processes that result in both harm and significant waste; a disconnect between quality and price; costs rising consistently greater than inflation or gross domestic product; inadequate consumer engagement and empowerment; and the absence of productivity and efficiency gains common in other industries. As one example, healthcare spending per capita in the US greatly exceeds other developed countries without apparent benefit in common measures such as life expectancy.

For example, in 2003 McGlynn and colleagues showed that typical patients received just over half of recommended care and a subsequent study focused on children showed they received recommended care even less consistently at just under half (McGlynn et al., 2003; Mangione-Smith et al., 2007). These problems have resulted in various reform proposals including significant, and often emotional, dialogue during each of the 2008 and 2012 US Presidential political campaigns. Most proposals have focused on providing greater access to care, with intermittent focus on controlling the costs of care. While understandable, this approach ignores the fundamental problem: healthcare value (defined here as health outcomes relative to input costs) simply must increase. Sustainable healthcare value is created only when care becomes evidence-based, is continuously improved, and is accountable for the outcomes (both cost and quality) produced; said another way, when healthcare becomes rational.

Philosophically, "rationality" can be defined as "...a matter of consistency in action: people act rationally to the extent they do what is likely to bring about the best state of affairs, given both their preferences over the outcomes that may be brought about through their agency and their beliefs about the probability of those outcomes" (Wallace, 2009). It is a normative concept of reasoning in that "rational people" should derive conclusions in a consistent way given equal access to information and common goals. In that sense, approaches to rational healthcare would be focused on innovations and approaches to continuous improvement that ensure evidence-based practice, an informed patient, and the power of the patient to exercise choice.

Effective communication is central to these endeavors. Inadequate advice, misinformation, mistaken decisions, missed opportunities, and "poor adherence," among other gaps in care, are the product of the numerous barriers to physicians understanding patients and vice versa. As noted in the chapter by Peters (Chapter 8), communication of comparative information is critical if patients are going to make appropriate decisions given treatment choices. To be effective, patients must understand the meaning of that information to make meaningful comparisons and choices. Many barriers exist to this understanding, including biased perceptions and weighting of numerical data. We agree with Peters' view that communication needs to be a strategic process and must be modified based on the barriers that exist in the particular health situation.

In this chapter, we consider the role of performance improvement in consistently evolving rational approaches to healthcare and note areas where effective communication is particularly important. Performance improvement methods may be particularly relevant to improving patient literacy and numeracy during encounters and to improving patient–provider communication and, importantly, moving exploration of barriers from the "laboratory" to mitigation of these barriers in clinical practice. The challenges to practice-based improvement in communication and health literacy are complex. Meaningful advances will require more rapid and lower-cost means of testing ideas in the settings of intended use.

Since the early observations of Shewhart and Juran, quality improvement efforts have been used across numerous industries. Over time, insights from these activities have evolved into a broader group of methodologies and underlying philosophies such as: Total Quality Management, Continuous Quality Improvement, Six Sigma, Lean, Re-engineering, Microsystems, and other models (Juran, 1995). More recently, these models have been adopted within many healthcare organizations (collectively, referred to in this chapter as "Performance Improvement" or "PI") in an attempt to optimize outcomes. In healthcare, the PI process involves an ongoing cycle of change in organization, care process, decision management, workflow, communications, or other components of care (Shojania et al., 2004). As in other business sectors, PI practice (or science) evolved as healthcare matured from a predominant culture of blame and fault-finding (e.g., peer and utilization review) to a focus on "systems" of care that became increasingly complex and fragmented. Improving such care systems typically relies on one of two primary thematic approaches based either upon "planning" or "experimentation."

Planning models, like Total Quality Management (TQM), incorporate several foundational philosophies including a commitment to: identifying, meeting, and exceeding stakeholder needs; continuously improving while escalating standards of performance; applying structured, problem-solving processes using statistical and related tools such as benchmarking, cause-and-effect diagrams and control charts; and empowering all employees to drive quality improvements. TQM is further characterized by an initial analysis phase used to "diagnose" the cause(s) of a process with less than ideal outcomes. This analytic phase often involves observation and new data (frequently gathered manually). It seeks to establish important performance attributes for ongoing measurement to determine if the new process is improved from baseline. By virtue of this approach and the often limited access to existing (or adequate) data, the planning phase often takes months and the critical steps (e.g., evidence gathering) are generally repeated with each successive initiative but with minimal reusability, scalability, or leverage. Despite its proponents, this elaborate process has been criticized for its length, labor intensiveness, frequent detachment from current reality, and failure to disseminate successful changes.

"Experimentation" models, whether viewed alone or in combination with planning models, have relied on techniques derived from Shewhart's "Plan-Do-Study-Act" ("PDSA") model (Shewhart, 1939) (Langley et al., 2009). The purpose of the PDSA model is to modify an existing process in an attempt to achieve an explicit "aim" (outcome) without necessarily worrying about an explanation for the cause of the underlying problem. More recently, the PDSA model has seen increasing use as a rapid, iterative change technique. Presently, PDSA "cycles" are generally considered to be the core of healthcare performance improvement "experimentation" models. While use of this model is rapidly expanding in healthcare, the research community and, in particular, health services researchers or communications experts, do not rely on means to rapidly, sequentially, and continuously explore pragmatic solutions to persistent health literacy or numeracy challenges.

Limitations of current PDSA approach

Despite the underlying logic, success in other industries and hope for these PI methods in healthcare, actual outcome improvement has often been negligible or unsustainable (Van de Ven & Ferry, 1980; Blumenthal & Kilo,

1998; Shortell et al., 2000; Solberg et al., 2000). Reasons for the gap between PI theory and practice are multifactorial, and the consequences are significant.

First, in most PI initiatives the measured outcome may be only distantly or indirectly related to meaningful change in patient health or to a concrete measure of ROI (return on investment). For example, even when PI is applied to an important problem (e.g., slowing progression of diabetes) in a manner that improves a chosen outcome metric (e.g., ordering HbA1c lab test), the effort may have no effect on more relevant outcomes (e.g., fewer complications or reductions in hospital admissions) as a limitation of the PDSA paradigm in that one is forced to choose surrogates that are only distantly related to meaningful outcomes. Second, outcomes are not usually evaluated in real time or at frequent intervals, limiting the timeliness, ease, or speed of innovation, as well as the dynamism of the process itself. When change and the associated process unfold in slow motion, participants' (or authorizing leaders') energy levels may not rise to or maintain the threshold required to institutionalize new standards of practice. This is particularly challenging when exploring means of improving patient–physician communication during encounters, as real time access to data means, in part, that high throughput processes are required to both record and evaluate conversations. Further, when human processes are required to maintain change, regression to baseline performance is common without real time feedback. Lastly, if a PI endeavor is not the product of a broader strategic focus, these efforts can be perceived as the "initiative of the month," leading to temporary improvements that are quickly lost due to inadequate hardwiring, support systems, vigilance, or PI integration across an organization.

Another primary limitation of most PDSA-based improvement efforts is absence of rich data required to inform the original hypothesis or plan for change and the integrated data collection systems needed to provide rapid post-intervention feedback. When available at all, data are often limited in scope and consist of simple administrative and/or manually collected elements that are not generated as part of the routine course of care delivery. By contrast, robust electronic health records ("EHR"), particularly when used in conjunction with an integrated data warehouse or knowledge system that provides for more extensive, longitudinal, normalized electronic information, provide for a quantum shift in the PDSA paradigm. Such data contains clinical test results, vital signs, flow information, and perhaps most important, explicit information regarding the intent of the clinical decision maker (e.g., reason codes for medication orders). In these settings, PI practitioners have access to a wealth of relevant data that allows for pre-intervention hypothesis testing and refinement, business case generation, and post-intervention, contemporaneous comparisons.

A rational alternative – experimental-grade performance improvement

An experimental performance improvement model would ensure that any unnecessary process steps are eliminated, simple but necessary steps are automated, or appropriately delegated to lower-cost but capable staff. At the same time, a rational approach seeks to actively engage consumers in behaviors that mitigate disease or improve purchasing; ensure that clinicians deliver more rapid, appropriate, and reliable care; eliminate unnecessary tests and therapies; and systematically lower supply chain costs. It would be built upon an integrated platform consisting of an electronic health record, an advanced analytics platform, and a tailored communication process. Aggregated patient data along with associated analytic models are the foundation of Geisinger's Clinical Decision Intelligence System ("CDIS").

At Geisinger, data are increasingly viewed as a core asset. A very heavy emphasis is placed on the collection, normalization, and application of clinical, financial, operational, claims, and other data to inform, guide, measure, refine, and document the results of PI efforts. These data are combined with other inputs (e.g., evidence-based guidelines, third-party benchmarks) and leveraged via decision support applications.

From a distance, EHR data appear to be a promising source for the creation of evidence that is more relevant to every day practice needs. However, a closer look reveals many challenges with the use of such data for this purpose. Compared to the standards established for research data collection, EHR data suffer from many limitations in both quality and completeness. For example, in research settings, specialized staff may have been hired to focus on following protocols while in routine care; simple measures such as blood pressure or smoking status are measured with many more sources of variability. In routine care, questions about smoking history differ and responses to even the very same question can be documented in different ways. The completeness of data is likely to be correlated with disease burden and the need for care rather than collected in the same way on all patients. Further, physicians may select a medication within a class based on the perceived severity of a patient's disease, resulting in a complex form of bias (i.e., confounding by indication) that is difficult to eliminate from data. In the near term, these and other limitations will raise questions about the credibility of evidence derived from EHR data. That said, the credibility of EHR-based findings can be mitigated through replication (i.e., multiple independent EHR-based studies) and, more importantly, practice-based randomized controlled trial.

Like guideline-based evidence, PI initiatives today are similarly limited due to the nature of the evidence base. No two patients are alike. When doctors care for patients, the very essence of the interaction requires extrapolation from knowledge and experience to tailor care for the particular circumstances at hand (i.e., bridging the "inferential gap") (Stewart et al., 2007). While a certain level of "experimentation" is a part of good care, the knowledge base required for such experimentation is growing at a pace that far exceeds knowledge uptake by most primary care providers and specialists. Hence the nature of care provided is either confined to an older (and sometimes outdated) knowledge base or ventures farther into the realm of experimentation than is optimal, where bias and error can play a larger role.

As noted recently, the science of improvement requires new methods that incorporate new data sources and techniques to face the new reality (Berwick, 2008). Incorporating longitudinal data from the point-of-care, rather than in highly structured experiments such as randomized trials, is one promising approach. Use of such data provides a population level view simply not possible previously. Intrinsic to this are "natural experiments" where similar patients receive different care due to different practice styles, formularies, and other resources. For example, a 60-year-old diabetic patient may get drug A, while a similar diabetic patient may get drug B because of formulary or style differences. When this observation is repeated hundreds of times and the data (including HgbA1c) are routinely collected and stored, this vast information base can be mined for important clinical and economic insights.

We think of PI as a continuum from data generation through performance measurement and analysis to the end goal of clinical transformation, which necessarily must involve iterative modifications to clinical workflows and the elimination, automation, or delegation of activities to meet quality and efficiency goals.

Our experience in combining revised PI techniques with this information-based approach supports our belief that EHRs and associated data warehousing will fundamentally transform PI initiatives in several important ways. First, PI will become much more ROI focused, as enhancements to data allow for more thoughtful clinical business planning. In turn, the ROI approach will engage other leaders (e.g., CFO) and enable PI to rapidly expand its purview to a much broader and more refined set of measurable outcomes that are likely to impact quality and efficiency in a material way. Second, the PDSA cycle will increasingly be performed electronically. For example, opportunities for improvement can be more readily quantified and rank ordered according to specified criteria. Also, "clinical hunches," comparisons of actual performance to guidelines, evaluation of new medical literature findings for local practice, and other comparisons can be tested via database queries in a matter of minutes, rather than taking days, weeks, or months using traditional human-based assessments. The paradigm for learning is transformed through rapid feedback and the increasingly dynamic nature of the process itself and how this influences the nature of the questions asked and the means to answer them.

Third, the focus of attention can expand to what an organization should stop doing, recognizing that many components of care that are embedded by tradition may offer little or no value. Importantly, metrics can be focused on measures that are directly relevant to patient health (e.g., actual LDL (low-density lipoprotein) levels rather than lab orders) and downstream ROI (e.g., cardiac events or visits avoided), substantially improving feedback to guide productive change that yields tangible value, holds the attention of organizational leaders, and motivates continued vigilance. Fourth, real time data access supports more rapid change cycles and the associated opportunities to test numerous hypotheses in a limited time period.

The above arguments apply to accelerated learning to improve patient understanding of the options they can choose and the related risks and benefits and physician training to improve effectiveness of communication. To address the need for a rapid learning paradigm, Geisinger installed microphones in exam rooms. As part of a learning endeavor, physicians gave "blanket approval" to allow the patient to decide if the microphone should be activated. After the rooming process was completed, patients were asked permission to record conversations by simply activating the microphone from a computer screen in advance of when the physician entered. The digital recordings were then readily available for evaluation by experts. This type of model simplifies the research and evaluation process, substantially lowers the cost of experimentation, and is directly relevant to the setting for which improvements in communication are intended.

Selecting areas for performance improvement

At the core, areas for PI intervention tend to fall into two broad categories: (1) what should we be doing systematically that we are not? and (2) what should we stop doing that is not adding value? These questions are fundamentally related to whether or not some aspect of care – the patient's characteristics (demographics, clinical), the treatment plan (flow, caregivers, timing, care components), or setting (inpatient vs. outpatient, nursing unit vs. nursing unit) improves the value of healthcare delivery. Breaking this down further leads to an analysis of the following:

1. *Missing elements of care.* Is something missing that seems to provide benefit (e.g., beta blockers post MI, statins for CAD)?
2. *Potential substitutions.* Does something (or someone) seem to work better than another (e.g., silver-impregnated vs. standard foley catheter relative to UTI)?
3. *Excess treatment intensity.* Does something seem to be used in care, but no apparent value is observed (e.g., plain film + CT + MRI + PET)?
4. *Flow characteristics.* Does the sequence of care and/or settings seem to make a difference (e.g., weekend care, getting to the right inpatient unit)?
5. *Supply chain inefficiencies.* Is care standardized enough to generate maximum supply chain economies and familiarity benefits?
6. *Provider care team variation.* Are there different outcomes with different providers and/or provider teams (e.g., physician–physician, physician–nurse practitioner, etc.)?

The care processes selected for improvement should be chosen with a thoughtful rank-ordering of problems based upon return on investment ("ROI," whether clinical, business or both) criteria. Example ROI-based approaches include selecting those processes with outcomes farthest from benchmark performance; those with the largest impact by patient population or resource consumption; those with the most significant variation; or those with the most interest from clinical champions or consumers. The absence of a ROI-based selection process often precludes the development of a "clinical business plan" that can meet the requirements of skeptical observers, an activity routine in other industries and one where, if skipped, makes post-intervention value determination problematic.

As Berwick noted, when evaluating areas for PI intervention one must "*reconsider thresholds for action on evidence*" (Berwick, 2008). In this context an appropriate threshold may be far below the traditional research standard of $p < 0.05$. Less restrictive interpretations of data and "evidence" are commonplace in other industries, where in the absence of any better information, a p-value < 0.5 is often indicative of a reasonable idea for change and p-values < 0.25 would routinely create sustained success. Of course, "evidence" at this level may not indicate a true need to change care, but rather the need to more formally study a partially validated question in a more rigorous manner. This evaluation approach could also build upon itself if aggregated across healthcare organizations, in such areas as: post-marketing surveillance for drugs and devices, evaluation of "cost-additive, but value-neutral" care components and other more difficult to study areas such as day-of-week, time-of-day, and similar "non-clinical" features impacting care.

An analogous framework is directly relevant to advancing the quality of communications in clinical settings. That is, exploring how to improve communications and to mitigate barriers should be focused in areas that lead to meaningful improvement in patient outcomes. It is not meaningful, per se, to improve patient literacy or the effectiveness of how a physician talks to a patient. It is meaningful to emphasize exploration in areas of care where such improvements matter the most, such as the endeavors summarized below.

Practical experience at Geisinger Health System (2012) simplified the many different issues and topics within this healthcare improvement model to provide a hands-on, structured framework for the application of a rational healthcare model, with the goal to make changes as follows:

1. Get consumers into a true system of care, focused on the right things.
2. Minimize care transition and hand-off errors.
3. Optimize the delivery of high-cost, capital-intensive care.
4. Get consumers involved, with shared responsibility for decisions and outcomes.

In this chapter, we systematically review each of these focus areas and provide practical examples and outcomes.

Get consumers into a true system of care, focused on the right things and minimize care transition and hand-off errors

The American College of Physicians defines the Patient-Centered Medical Home (PCMH) as "a care delivery model whereby patient treatment is coordinated through their primary care physician to ensure they receive the necessary care when and where they need it, in a manner they can understand" (American College of Physicians, 2013). The Geisinger approach to the PCMH, branded as ProvenHealth Navigator^{SM}, has been described in detail previously (Gilfillan et al., 2010). In brief, this fundamental redesign of the primary care practices focused on five core components (Paulus et al., 2008; Stewart et al., 2007):

1. *Patient-centered care.* Geisinger's care delivery approach focused on the patient and family, including enhanced patient access with an expanded scope of services; a coordinated, team-based care model; and a relentless focus on chronic disease optimization (Weber et al., 2008) all enabled by an electronic health record.
2. *Population management.* Geisinger's population management approach focused on profiling and segmentation, intense prescription drug

management, on-site practice-based case management, disease management education, and remote, home-based monitoring for chronic disease patients. These efforts are designed to systematically minimize care transition and hand-off errors through extensive care coordination, enhanced provider–provider and patient–provider communication, and continuous data tracking.

3. *Value-based care systems.* The focus here was on improving access to high-volume specialty, ancillary, and laboratory services along with the integration of hospital care, home health, skilled nursing facilities, and emergency department care.
4. *Quality outcomes program.* Geisinger's quality outcomes program focused on patient and physician satisfaction as well as established evidence-based best practice measures for common chronic disease (e.g., diabetes, congestive heart failure, coronary artery disease, and hypertension) and preventive services metrics as defined by the Healthcare Effectiveness Data and Information Set (National Committee for Quality Assurance, 2011).
5. *Value-based reimbursement model.* Geisinger's value-based reimbursement model included a hybrid of practice transformation stipends to support infrastructure change, fee-for-service payments to ensure frequent contact, quality outcome payments, and a results-share bonus program based on attainment of predetermined efficiency and quality targets. Quality goals were established collaboratively with the provider and health plan teams. Efficiency targets were determined based on per member per month experience within each primary care practice.

The Proven Health Navigator was supported by other efforts to improve management of chronic diseases like diabetes and close evidence-based gaps in care. Previously, Berkman and Cavanaugh described the challenges that diabetes management programs face because of health literacy and numeracy barriers. We describe an approach and toolset that seeks to support and enhance patient ability with quantitative tasks related to diabetes. We review the approach to diabetes care, published previously (Weber et al., 2008), as an illustrative example.

Clinicians defined a diabetic "care bundle" that included nine evidence-based components of care (Weber et al., 2008). First, care gaps are identified for each individual patient within CDIS by comparing their electronic information against evidence-based care needs as defined in the bundle. Second, nurses are provided with an automated rooming tool that, among other things, enables the nurse to verify the presence or absence of a given Care Gap. Post rooming, an automated, patient-specific, Care Gap-informed order set is generated at the point-of-care; the physician can "accept all" with one click, or add, delete or edit any given order.

Importantly, this same Care Gap information is sent directly to patients via the consumer web portal. Patients are encouraged to address needs virtually with their providers or they can schedule Care Gap interventions (e.g., a laboratory draw or a foot exam) directly online with a few clicks. Because some patients lack online access and to partially address health literacy and numeracy concerns, an individual report card was provided to each patient using simple, lay language (e.g., "Your LDL should be less than 100. If your LDL is consistently greater than 100, your chance of having a heart attack or stroke increases yearly") to describe the potential personal impact from abnormal laboratory values.

To establish baseline performance, nine key process and outcome care components were selected from the American Diabetes Association's "Standards of Care" (2005) and assembled into an all-or-none "bundle" of measures as an ideal goal. Physician performance results and comparisons to local, regional, and national benchmarks were shared with physicians for education. These reports showed changes in each individual bundle element as well as "all-or-none" performance (i.e., the percentage of patients who had fulfilled each and every one of the nine specified performance criteria). Previous work had shown that rates of pneumococcal and influenza vaccination improved from 56.5% to 80.8% ($p < 0.0001$) and 55.1% to 71.0% ($p < 0.0001$), respectively. The percentage of patients with ideal glucose control (HbA1c <7) increased from 32.2% to 34.8% ($p < 0.001$) and blood pressure control (<130/80) improved from 39.7% to 43.9% ($p < 0.0001$). The overall bundle compliance (i.e., those patients meeting all nine measures) improved from 2.4% to 6.5% ($p < 0.0001$). Across time, the improvement in the diabetes bundle and other similar disease-specific bundles such as coronary artery disease improved reliably and significantly.

Because patients with one or more chronic diseases are both vulnerable and costly, our experiments were focused on testing the key elements of care re-engineering for these patients, often above 70 years old with a combination of type 2 diabetes, congestive heart failure, coronary artery disease, hypertension, and/or reactive depression; these patients were frequently taking ten or more medications per day. Over time the ProvenHealth Navigator^{SM} experiment was expanded to include all Medicare patients and a cohort of Geisinger's commercial insurance members. The results: hospital admissions and readmissions fell substantially, Emergency Department utilization declined, and total per member per month costs were lower and grew less rapidly, compared to controls.

This experiment showed that collaboration between payers and providers, leveraging the best skills and tools of each, was foundational to success. This robust partnership between payers and providers has largely been antithetical in the US healthcare system, and yet many of the anticipated benefits from health reform as established in the Affordable Care Act presume that so-called "accountable care organizations" will bridge many of these care gaps.

Despite our success, relatively little formal effort was expended on improving communication and patient health literacy. We believe that the PCMH is an ideal setting for the application of PI processes to communication methods, and that they are likely to yield a meaningful ROI.

Optimize the delivery of high-cost, capital-intensive care

The Geisinger ProvenHealth Navigator model showed that all-cause inpatient admissions can be reduced dramatically, but what about optimization of capital-intensive inpatient care that is required even after optimal ambulatory care? An example of Geisinger's work on optimizing inpatient care has been published previously (Casale et al., 2007). Coronary artery bypass graft (CABG) was the first target of Geisinger's ProvenCare^{SM} for several reasons, including the fact that CABG guidelines had been recently updated by the American Heart Association (AHA) and the American College of Cardiology (ACC) in the "AHA/ACC 2004 Guideline Update for CABG Surgery" (Eagle et al., 2004) and national and regional benchmarks were available with near real time data collection via the Society for Thoracic Surgery's comparative database, a trusted source with demonstrated correlation to improved clinical outcomes. We sought to mitigate the barriers and maximize the benefits associated with using guidelines shown previously in another specialty (Farquhar et al., 2002). We also agreed with the American College of Obstetricians and Gynecologists that the provision of consumer information that explains both the benefits and risks of certain interventions recommended by the guidelines could be of benefit to clinicians. Specifically, we sought to avoid those practice guideline identified barriers (e.g., out of date guidelines, non-specific to clinical practice setting) and leverage the identified benefits (e.g., evidence-based leading to improved outcomes) for the purposes of this initiative.

Given the CABG case volume and predicted adverse event occurrence rates, it was likely that the impact of care re-engineering could be measured over a reasonably short time frame. Also, CABG's financial impact was significant, ensuring both leadership engagement and a comprehensive view of value. Separate workgroups focused upon different aspects of care were convened to re-engineer care. A Best Practice workgroup comprising all Geisinger cardiac surgeons focused on areas of concern, such as whether enforcement of best practices might "force" surgeons to rely on "cookbook medicine." Surgeons reviewed all 12 Class I and all eight Class IIa guidelines, ultimately agreeing that each was appropriate for our re-engineering work. All 20 guidelines were then translated into 40 individual, discrete, and objective care process steps. Multidisciplinary teams from all clinical units involved in CABG care then established an idealized workflow incorporating each new practice element with specific tracking "hardwired" for each element into the EHR-based workflow. Workflow required that clinicians either comply with the evidence-based best practice element or otherwise document the rationale for not doing so.

From a business perspective, discussion with payers led to the development of a single, bundled price for elective CABG that included all preoperative evaluation, hospital and professional fees, routine post-discharge care, and management of any CABG-related complications occurring within 90 days after CABG surgery. Because not all complications could be eliminated even with ideal care, the case rate for ProvenCare patients also included approximately half of the average cost for historical postoperative readmissions.

At baseline, 59% of all elective CABG patients received all 40 ProvenCare^{SM} elements, and within 3 months, bundle performance improved to 100%, where it largely remained thereafter ($p < 0.001$).

From an outcomes perspective, the cohort of ProvenCare^{SM} patients was compared with the 137 elective CABG patients (operated upon in 2005) whose care was provided before the program's initiation. The preoperative and operative characteristics used in the Society for Thoracic Surgery (STS) outcome predicting algorithms were similar in both cohorts except that left main coronary stenosis > 50% occurred more frequently in the ProvenCare^{SM} Group (23% vs. 12%). Of note, baseline adverse event rates were already lower than predicted by the STS algorithms, establishing a high bar for incremental clinical improvement. Clinical outcome comparisons between the two groups showed that adverse events occurred less frequently in the ProvenCare^{SM} than Conventional Care group.

From a financial perspective, hospital net revenue improved 12.3% (with expenses rising only 5.6%) resulting in an improved contribution margin (17.6%) and improved total inpatient profit per case ($1946). At the same time, Geisinger Health Plan paid 4.8% less per case for CABG with ProvenCare^{SM} which ranged from 28–36% less than it paid non-Geisinger providers for CABG and related care. Average length of stay fell by a full day (6.3 days Conventional Care Group to 5.3 days ProvenCare^{SM} Group), while the 30-day readmission rate fell 15.5% (from 7.1% to 6%). As a result of these data, Geisinger subsequently expanded the ProvenCare^{SM} program to other inpatient conditions, including percutaneous catheter intervention, total joint replacement, and normal deliveries.

Actively engage the patient

A dominant focus of PI is to improve the job that the provider, the nurse, and other clinic staff need to get done during each and every encounter. It is less common to think about focusing PI on the "job" the patient needs to get done when they seek care and it is rare to consider the presentation and comprehension of information necessary for the patient to make an informed choice balancing risks and benefits compared among options. More often than not, the patient is viewed as a passive participant in a process largely controlled by others, not as an active participant or equal partner. It is simply easier to apply PI to the traditional clinical workflow rather than to invent a new approach that integrates the work to be done by the clinic and the patient together. As a consequence, meaningful opportunities to improve how care is delivered and communication is managed are usually lost in the details of a task oriented PI endeavor.

Communication is at the core of most of the care that is provided to patients, especially during ambulatory encounters. Evidence suggests that many outcomes are improved when the care process is structured to engage the patient as an active participant. This largely requires focus on improving communication. Specifically, meaningful improvement to outcomes can be achieved through deliberate efforts to integrate shared decision making (SDM) in the care process and by addressing communication barriers inherent to low health literacy or numeracy. In an earlier chapter, Peters noted that informing choices with decision aids often increased knowledge and decreased decisional conflict (O'Connor et al., 2003), and that when well designed, decision aids address a number of factors necessary for good decisions (Hibbard & Peters, 2003). The fundamental challenge is devising a practice-based model that offers both engaging communication and is efficient. To devise such a model requires a rapid and iterative approach to learning how to improve communication. The latter requires clinic and workflow infrastructure that supports real time experimentation (i.e., in-practice trials) and learning about what is needed to make effective SDM a reality. Since the conversation between the patient and doctor is the real mediator of successful SDM, the quality of the conversation itself must be measured to learn what will work.

SDM involves a concerted effort to clearly define the problem or reason the patient is seeking care, to present options relevant to the problem, and then to consider risks, benefits, and patient values and preferences. These considerations form the basis for formulating a decision and an action plan that balances the best evidence with a discussion of the patient's perception and understanding of what was discussed. Effective communication also requires that the content of what is shared (i.e., visually and through conversation) is tailored to the patient's health literacy, learning style, and other mediators of effective communication. For example, the combination of age and education can have a powerful impact on comprehension (Hibbard et al., 2001) with the oldest individuals (85–94) averaging more than three times the error rate in comprehension of younger patients (18–35), with those having more formal education being somewhat protected against age-related degradation in comprehension. Theoretically, a process that recognizes these barriers and encompasses key features of SDM can improve patient knowledge, reduce decisional conflict, improve adherence, increase adoption of healthy behaviors, and possibly reduce future demand for care (Makoul & Clayman, 2006).

Practically, approaches to SDM have not been widely adopted. A dominant barrier is the seemingly inordinate complexity of the process itself and the expectation that more time would be required to actively engage the patient and to also manage health literacy as part of the traditional clinical workflow. At Geisinger we explored how Health Information Technology (HIT) could be used to overcome barriers to SDM adoption. It became obvious at the outset that even Geisinger's sophisticated EHR would need to be supported by other applications to develop a more integrated care process to ensure that an SDM care model fit within a real-world encounter schedule. To illustrate, we specifically consider the ambulatory care encounter and the re-engineering process we developed for primary care management of low back pain (LBP). Our primary interest was in delivering guideline-based care and minimizing orders for low value care that were not supported by guidelines.

It was complicated to imagine how SDM could be practiced when the problem itself was defined by how to functionally integrate SDM into the traditional workflow. We concluded that this was the wrong problem definition. Instead, the problem needed to be defined by ways to enhance communication, as this is what an ambulatory care encounter is largely about. This fits the conceptual model for SDM, as it grew from the recognition of failures in a service that is largely about communication. Recognizing the time constraints, we considered how HIT could be used to both actively involve the patient and to automate tasks. We parsed the encounter into the following distinct activities relevant to communications:

1. Obtaining relevant data from the patient;
2. Identifying the best options given the patient data;
3. Sharing and discussing data and options with the patient to select the best option;

4. Summarizing the action plan for the patient; and
5. Monitoring outcomes between encounters.

HIT and automation were used for each of these activities to develop a prototype practice-based model for SDM. A longer-term interest in this approach to research is to simplify the means of testing new ideas and the time required to conduct sequential in-practice trials. In the remainder of this section, we consider details of one such idea, but each component of the re-engineered care process warrants a need for iterative improvement in how information is displayed and discussed.

Obtain relevant data

The patient is the source of most of the information required for a shared discussion of what he or she needs. To gain access to that insight, we integrated touchscreen-computerized questionnaires in clinical practice to obtain relevant data from the patient, leveraging both decades of funded research that has created validated questionnaires for clinical practice and the patient's time, as they are often left waiting. The process worked seamlessly. If LBP was recorded as the chief complaint, the questionnaire protocol automatically launched on a touchscreen in the exam room when the nurse closed the patient's EHR. While the patient was waiting, they answered questions specific to back pain history, current pain and functioning, treatment response to prescribed and over-the-counter medications, fear avoidance, depression, anxiety, concerns with LBP, and expectations regarding imaging and opioid prescription medications. The questionnaire was highly tailored, using branching logic and inferential rules and required only 5 to 7 minutes to complete. It was important to recognize that the questionnaire was not a substitute for the patient's story to the nurse and physician.

Identify the best options

Clinical practice guidelines for most health problems have been available in text form for years, but are largely inaccessible to clinical practice and especially to primary care physicians. To address this gap we concluded that rich patient data was required and that the guidelines had to be translated and expressed in a form that allowed for matching guidelines with real data and scoring the completeness of the match between the two. For LBP, we converted Institute for Clinical Systems Improvement (ICSI) guidelines to detailed statements that were tagged by data features. A computerized algorithm was developed to: extract both patient reported data and other relevant EHR data; match these data with guideline statements; select the best matches; and then construct related order menus. The algorithm was launched once the patient completed the questionnaire.

Shared discussion

When the physician entered the exam room and opened the patient's EpicCare record, a visual display automatically launched on the second screen that had been used previously by the patient to complete the questionnaire. The display was conveniently located for viewing by the patient and physician. One tab displayed all relevant patient data, including indications of red flags, a summary of scores relevant to pain and functioning, fear avoidance, concerns, and mental health. A second tab displayed care plan options, relevant guidelines translated for patient viewing (e.g., imaging is not recommended), order menus, and note fields. A third tab displayed an easy-to-use physical exam guide. A fourth tab presented a structured progress note that was automatically created as the physician used the visual display.

Summarize action plan

We concluded that no matter how effective the displays were constructed to foster SDM it was not possible for a patient to recall all of the meaningful takeaways discussed during the encounter. It is too much to expect of most patients that they present their problem, consider options to address their need, and then recall all that was recommended. A robust algorithm was developed to create an after visit summary (AVS) for the patient. The AVS summarized patient reported and other relevant EHR data, the decisions on next steps, and, where relevant, advice on how to manage LBP (e.g., the level of activity to maintain, use of over-the-counter medications (OTCs), prevention strategies, etc.) and next steps. The AVS was mailed that night as a means to reinforce memory and was also available via email.

Monitor outcomes

It is impossible to effectively monitor patient outcomes for a condition like LBP without documented trends in both quantitative and qualitative measures. Patient reported measures were recorded in Epic. Auto generated progress notes summarized all relevant information from the visual display tool and could be imported into Epic after editing at the physician's discretion. This combination of information provided a foundation for recalling the patient's status during the previous exam and assessing whether outcomes had improved.

This re-engineering prototype for ambulatory care is currently being tested at Geisinger and represents one of several prototypes designed to introduce applications into the encounter as a way to improve communication, guideline-based care, and follow-up care. While this work is still in a nascent phase, each prototype typically introduced a new advance that improved efficiency (e.g., automatically generated progress notes), that improved the display of data and information to enhance communication, and to better manage continuity of care.

Creative approaches to using HIT will be required to achieve many of the goals of healthcare reform. Significant advances will not be achieved in the form of traditional "alerts" or "reminders." For example, at Geisinger, the number of alerts increased from less than 100 000 per 6 months to more than 1.1 million per 6 months between 2002 and 2009. These alerts are used 0% to 20% of the time. In spite of the best intentions, the alerts are not designed from the perspective of the user. Alerts are the product of a tool designed by the manufacturer of an EHR intended to simplify the deployment of a message at the point-of-care. In contrast, the LBP protocol described above is used 50% of the time.

The goal of SDM in our LBP protocol is to change the doctor–patient dynamic. The conversation is the primary mediator of care. It is expected that improvements to SDM will improve: appropriate ordering; adherence to a care plan; outcomes; and patient satisfaction. Addressing barriers to health literacy is increasingly recognized as a critical consideration to improving SDM. Numeracy represents one of the more challenging dimensions of health literacy, as presentation and discussion of risks and benefits are important to most conversations about choosing the best course of action. However, addressing related communication barriers poses the same challenges that we previously cited for SDM. In a typical encounter, there is no time dedicated to understanding a patient's numeracy. Moreover, even if numeracy could be easily assessed, it is unlikely that clinical staff and providers would be able to learn and adjust the way they communicate in real time.

More generally, it is unrealistic to expect that those who provide healthcare can be constantly aware of their own biases in overestimating what others know and at the same time know in the moment how to individualize the way they communicate with a specific patient. One advantage offered by HIT based solutions is that it is possible to automate the way in which questions are asked of the patient and the way in which information is presented for SDM to eliminate the need for unrealistic expectations of the provider. That is, the presentation of information can be individualized to the patient's literacy and numeracy skills.

To devise automated solutions will require that there are accurate means of phenotyping or categorizing patients by their numeracy and, accordingly, that there are distinct and successful means of asking questions and presenting information tailored to the numeracy "phenotype." This represents a very high bar for the quality of knowledge required to devise meaningful point-of-care solutions and to construct decision aids that are tailored to what a patient needs to both understand options and to intelligently discuss such options. As we have noted throughout this chapter, rapid means of learning will need to be devised if formal knowledge of health literacy and numeracy are to be incorporated into solutions that actually work in practice. More specifically, the clinical care setting needs to be the locus where such solutions are evaluated to address a diversity of challenges noted in other chapters.

A significant minority of the US adult population has less than even basic numeracy skills (Kirsch et al., 2002; Kutner et al., 2006); relatively few adults have advanced skills. Nurses and physicians will have a strong tendency to communicate with patients from their own perspective, given the inherent tendency of those with expert knowledge to overestimate what others know.

Practically, point-of-care solutions will require that key variables are identified that can be used to define important dimensions of how a patient understands quantitative information. Work on the Diabetes Numeracy Test is one such example of how previous responses to a questionnaire can be translated in real time to a decision on the most sensible option for displaying information. These key variables need to be part of the patient's record in the same manner that vital signs are required to effectively manage a patient's health. Key variables then need to be routinely used to decide how questions are asked and how information is presented. An even greater, but very exciting challenge is in storing and communicating relevant information related to genetic testing and risk. As noted in Chapter 6 by Dukhovny and Wilkins-Haug, health literacy and numeracy in genetics represent a significant challenge for healthcare providers and patients. Physicians and other providers will need to integrate genetic tests, results, and associated risks into routine medical practice and undertake discussion and counseling for common disorders. Tools such as those described here will need to be developed to support this important evolution.

Many health systems are experimenting with new approaches to quality improvement that leverage EHR capabilities. From our own recent experience, it is clear that an EHR-based practice environment engenders an unavoidable shift in thinking about clinical evidence and how to create and use it and, importantly, a loss of distinction between clinical practice, quality management, and the creation of knowledge. In addition to practice standardization and decision support, EHR data provide a new source of hypotheses and evidence for both PI and research. When complemented by a broader data aggregation, analysis infrastructure, and process to create a PI Architecture, the potential is significant. While there are numerous limitations yet to be overcome, the latent potential between EHR (and other electronic) data, performance improvement, and research is both significant and exciting. The next decade of work will be transformative; this is an exciting time for healthcare.

References

American College of Physicians. (2013). What is the patient-centered medical home? Retrieved from www.acponline.org/running_practice/delivery_and_payment_models/pcmh/understanding/what.htm

American Diabetes Association. (2005). Standards of medical care in diabetes. *Diabetes Care*, 28, s4–s36.

Berwick, D. M. (2008). The science of improvement. *JAMA*, 299(10), 1182–1184.

Blumenthal, D., & Kilo, C. M. (1998). A report card on continuous quality improvement. *Milbank Quaterly*, 76(4), 625–648.

Casale, A. S., Paulus, R. A., Selna, M. J., Doll, M. C., Bothe, A. E., McKinley, K. E., et al. (2007). "ProvenCareSM": A provider-driven pay-for-performance program for acute episodic cardiac surgical care. *Annals of Surgery*, 246, 613–623.

Committee on Quality of Health Care in America, Institute of Medicine. (2000). *To Err is Human: Building a Safer Health System*. Washington, DC: National Academy Press.

Eagle, K. A., Guyton, R. A., Davidoff, R., Edwards, F. H., Ewy, G. A., Gardner, T. J., et al. (2004). *ACC/AHA guideline update for coronary artery bypass graft surgery: Summary article*. 110, 1168–1176.

Farquhar, C. M., Kofa, E., Power, M. L., Zinberg, S., & Schulkin, J. (2002). Clinical practice guidelines as educational tools for obstetrician-gynecologists. *Journal of Reproductive Medicine*, 47(11), 897–902.

Geisinger Health System. (2012). Retrieved from www.geisinger.org/

Gilfillan R. J., Tomcavage, J., Rosenthal, M. B., Davis, D. E., Graham, J., Roy, J. A., et al. (2010). Value and the medical home: Effects of transformed primary care. *American Journal of Managed Care*, 16(8), 607–614.

Hibbard, J. H., & Peters, E. (2003). Supporting informed consumer health care choices: Data presentation approaches that facilitate the use of information in choice. *Annual Review of Public Health*, 24, 413–433.

Hibbard, J. H., Slovic, P., Peters, E., Finucane, M. L., & Tusler, M. (2001). Is the informed-choice policy approach appropriate for Medicare beneficiaries? *Health Affairs*, 20(3), 199.

Juran, J. M. (1995). *Managerial Breakthrough: The Classic Book on Improving Management Performance* (30th Anniversary edn.). New York, NY: McGraw-Hill.

Kirsch, I. S., Jungeblut, A., Jenkins, L., & Kolstad, A. (2002). *Adult Literacy in America: A First Look at the Findings of the National Adult Literacy Survey* (NCES Report No. 1993–275; 3rd edn.). Washington, DC: US Department of Education, National Center for Education Statistics.

Kutner, M., Greenberg, E., Jin, Y., & Paulsen, C. (2006). *The Health Literacy of America's Adults: Results from the 2003 National Assessment of Adult Literacy* (NCES 2006–483). Washington, DC: US Department of Education, National Center for Education Statistics.

Langley, G. J., Nolan, K. M., Norman, C. L., Provost, L. P., & Nolan, T. W. (2009). *The Improvement Guide: A Practical Approach to Enhancing Organizational Performance*. New York, NY: Wiley.

Makoul, G., & Clayman, M. L. (2006). An integrative model of shared decision making in medical encounters. *Patient Education and Counseling*, 60(3), 301–312.

Mangione-Smith, R., DeCristofaro, A. H., Setodji, C. M., Keesey, J., Klein, D. J., Adams, J. L., et al. (2007). The quality of ambulatory care delivered to children in the United States. *New England Journal of Medicine*, 357(15), 1515–1523.

McGlynn, E. A., Asch, S. M., Adams, J., Keesey, J., Hicks, J., DeCristofaro, A., & Kerr, E. A. (2003). The quality of health care delivered to adults in the United States. *New England Journal of Medicine*, 348, 2635–2645.

National Committee for Quality Assurance. (2011). [Summary table of measures, product lines, and changes]. Summary table of measure changes. HEDIS 2011 Technical Specifications for Physician Measurement. Retrieved from: www.ncqa.org/Portals/0/HEDISQM/HEDIS%202011/SUMMARY_TABLE_OF_MEASURES_for_HEDIS_2012.pdf

O'Connor, A. M., Stacey, D., Entwistle, V., Llewellyn-Thomas, H., Rovner, D., Holmes-Rovner, M., et al. (2003). Decision aids for people facing health treatment or screening decisions. *Cochrane Database of Systematic Reviews*, 2, CD001431.

Paulus, R. A., Davis, K., & Steele, G. D. (2008). Continuous innovation in health care: implications of the Geisinger experience. *Health Affairs (Millwood)*, 27(5), 1235–1245.

Shewhart, W. A. (1939). *Statistical Method from the Viewpoint of Quality Control*. Mineola, NY: Courier Dover Publications.

Shojania, K. G., McDonald, K. M., Wachter, R. M., & Owens, D. K. (Eds.). (2004). *Closing the Quality Gap: A Critical Analysis of Quality Improvement Strategies, Volume I – Series Overview and Methodology*. Agency for Healthcare Research and Quality. Retrieved from www.ahrq.gov/downloads/pub/evidence/pdf/qualgap1/qualgap1.pdf

Shortell, S. M., Jones, R. H., Rademaker, A. W., Gillies., R. R., Dranove, D. S., Hughes, E. F. X., et al. (2000). Assessing the impact of total quality management and organizational culture on multiple outcomes of care for coronary artery bypass surgery graft patients. *Medical Care*, 38(2), 207–217.

Solberg, L. I., Kottke, T. E., Brekke, M. L., Magnan, S., Davidson, D., Calomeni, C. A., et al. (2000). Failure of a continuous quality improvement intervention to increase the delivery of preventive services. A randomized trial. *Effective Clinical Practice*, 3(3), 105–115.

Stewart, W. F., Shah, N. R., Selna, M. J., Paulus, R. A., & Walker, J. M. (2007). Bridging the inferential gap: The electronic health record and clinical evidence. *Health Affairs*, 32(2), w181–w191.

Van de Ven, A. H., & Ferry, D. L. (1980). *Measuring and Assessing Organizations*. New York, NY: Wiley.

Wallace, R. J. (2009). Practical reason. In: E. N. Zalta (Ed.), *The Stanford Encyclopedia of Philosophy*. Retrieved from plato.stanford.edu/archives/sum2009/entries/practical-reason/

Weber, V., Bloom, F., Pierdon, S., & Wood, C. (2008). Employing the electronic health record to improve diabetes care: A multifaceted intervention in an integrated delivery system. *Journal of General Internal Medicine*, 23(4), 379–382.

10 A review of theories of numeracy: psychological mechanisms and implications for medical decision making

Valerie F. Reyna & Priscila G. Brust-Renck

According to the most recent review of research on numeracy, only a slim majority of Americans has the basic quantitative skills essential to understand common forms of health information (Reyna et al., 2009). Millions – especially the old, the poor, and the less educated – cannot understand numerical information that would enable them to make informed decisions about preventing or treating disease (e.g., the risks of unprotected sex, the frequency of adverse outcomes of vaccination, or the survival rates associated with medical and surgical treatments; Reyna & Hamilton, 2001; Reyna & Adam, 2003; Hamm et al., 2007; Betsch et al., 2012). International comparisons suggest that low levels of numeracy – the ability to understand and use numbers – are widespread (Garcia-Retamero & Galesic, 2009). Even healthcare providers vary in numeracy, which predicts their use of numbers in explaining test results to patients (Anderson et al., 2011; Nelson et al., 2008).

On the surface, it seems easy to explain why people with lower numerical skills would have difficulty understanding risks or selecting the most effective treatments. If a 0.20 risk of death is confused with a 0.02 risk, or if a survival rate of 1 out of 10 patients seems smaller than a survival rate of 9 out of 100 patients, it makes sense that medical decisions that turn on such numerical distinctions would be impaired (Lipkus & Peters, 2009; Abdel-Kader et al., 2010; Cokely et al., 2012). However, the difficulties associated with low numeracy extend well beyond the inability to understand place value or perform computations (e.g., Peters et al., 2006; Fagerlin et al., 2007; Liberali et al., 2011). Understanding and remediating low numeracy requires getting below the surface of errors in judgment and decision making to the deeper level of scientific theory. Scientific

Preparation of this manuscript was supported in part by the National Cancer Institute of the National Institutes of Health under Award Number R21CA149796 to the first author.

theories offer causal explanations of how people understand numbers (based on empirical tests of hypotheses about mechanisms), and they make predictions about factors that affect that understanding. Therefore, consistent with the old adage that "there is nothing so practical as a good theory," we review four different theoretical approaches to explaining and predicting health numeracy.

The major theoretical approaches relevant to understanding health numeracy that we review are: (a) psychophysical approaches in which the subjective magnitude of quantities is perceived as a non-linear function of objective magnitude; (b) computational or information-processing approaches that emphasize cognitive load and "natural" frequencies; (c) dual-process approaches that contrast intuition or affect with quantitative analysis; and (d) fuzzy-trace theory, in which intuition differs from analysis in the type of mental representation used to process information – simple gist rather than verbatim detail – and gist-based intuition is considered advanced. In this review, we outline these approaches, review their implications for numeracy in the context of health and medical decision making, and point to avenues for future research.

Psychophysical approaches

Perception of numbers

Humans and animals seem to share a basic mental representation of number in terms of language-independent magnitude (Gallistel & Gelman, 2005; Brannon, 2006; Merritt et al., 2010; Brannon & Merritt, 2011; Gallistel, 2011). This internal representation of number has been described as logarithmic, in which the discriminability of two magnitudes is a function of their ratio rather than the difference between them. Thus, the psychological difference between 400 patients saved in a treatment group versus 200 saved in a control group (a ratio of 2.0) is perceived as subjectively larger than that between 1400 saved versus 1200 saved (a ratio of 1.17) – although the absolute difference (200 patients) is identical (Opfer & Siegler, 2007). If the internal representation were linear, a difference of 200 patients would always be perceived the same way. The higher the number the more the subjective representation deviates from the objective magnitude (Siegler et al., 2011). Note that there are immediate practical implications of this approach; presenting numbers in terms of units that seem closer to zero (e.g., 14K or 14 per 1000 as opposed to 14 000) will make differences seem larger and magnitudes will tend to be less distorted.

Research on mathematical cognition has shown that educated adults tend to have a more linear, as opposed to a more curvilinear (i.e., logarithmic) representation of number (Hubbard et al., 2005; Booth & Siegler, 2006; Siegler et al., 2011). A linear representation is more faithful to the objective magnitude (i.e., more literally accurate) and it does not flatten out for larger numbers like a logarithmic representation does (i.e., it is more precise in that differences are larger between larger numbers, compared to a logarithmic representation). For all of these reasons, linear representations are considered more advanced according to psychophysical approaches. Consistent with this claim, Booth and Siegler (2006) found that adults whose estimates of numbers were linear had higher scores on a mathematics achievement test (Terra Nova Test). That is, putting a single mark on each line ranging from 0 to 1000, participants estimated 26 random numbers (e.g., 3, 502, 962); better estimation of the numbers on a line (linearly) was positively correlated with higher scores on the mathematics test.

The roots of adult numeracy are in children's numerical cognition (Brannon, 2006; Berteletti et al., 2010; Thompson & Siegler, 2010; Brannon & Merritt, 2011). In a review of the developmental literature, Siegler et al. (2011) indicated that children progress gradually from a logarithmic to linear representation of number as they grow into adulthood (Opfer & Siegler, 2007; Siegler et al., 2009; Brannon & Merritt, 2011). In addition to developmental patterns, the shift from logarithmic to linear representations is correlated with formal education. For example, Dehaene et al. (2008) found that numerical judgments of adult members of an indigenous Amazonian group (with little or no formal education) were best fitted with a logarithmic curve (Siegler & Opfer, 2003; Siegler & Booth, 2004; Dehaene et al., 2008).

Distortions in numerical perception

Distortions in the perception of numbers should influence judgment and decision making involving numbers (Chen et al., 2006; Furlong & Opfer, 2009). For example, Peters et al. (2008) showed that individual differences in the degree of curvature of the perception of numbers predicted decisions (though not always as predicted). Greater deviations from linearity predicted greater temporal discounting (i.e., choosing smaller sooner rewards over larger later ones), but were also associated (counterintuitively) with choosing a smaller proportional (larger absolute) difference between outcomes (Benjamin et al., 2013). The temporal discounting findings have implications for health decisions. Prevention decisions often involve forgoing immediate smaller rewards, such as resting rather than exercise, in favor of long-term but larger health benefits. Peters et al. argued that imprecise representations of number magnitudes may be responsible for difficulties in health decision making observed among those low in numerical discrimination.

Although much evidence supports the proposition that the basic, developmentally primitive perception of numbers is logarithmic, there are some inconsistencies in the evidence. Scrutinizing Peters et al.'s (2008) findings more closely, those with low and with high numeracy (based on a median split on a numeracy test) and those with more linear or less linear representations, all tended to choose $100 now rather than wait for $110 in a month. However, those with more linear representations were more willing to wait to receive $15 in a week rather than $10 now. This pattern of preferences (i.e., treating a difference of $5 as though it were larger than a difference of $10) is consistent with a ratio-dependent logarithmic discrimination of number because the ratio of $15 to $10 (i.e., 1.5) is larger than the ratio of $110 to $100 (i.e., 1.1, although the $110 was also delayed a month rather than delayed a week).

The preferences in a second experiment, however, are difficult to reconcile with the idea that more advanced reasoners have more precise (i.e., more linear) representations of number. Peters et al. (2008) asked participants to choose which of three charitable foundations should receive funding for reducing deaths from disease: institution X reduced deaths from 15 000 to 5000 a year, institution Y from 160 000 to 145 000 a year, and institution Z from 290 000 to 270 000 a year. (Alternatively, one could imagine that these are three treatments for three diseases; which treatment should a public health program fund?) Typical preferences in this task are consistent with a ratio-dependent logarithmic representation of number: saving a greater proportion of lives (67% reduction for institution X, compared to 9.4% reduction for Y and 6.9% reduction for Z) is preferred (e.g., Fetherstonhaugh et al., 1997). However, participants with high numeracy (or those with a more precise, linear representation of numbers) would be *expected* to choose to save the greatest number of lives (i.e., 20 000 for institution Z, compared to 15 000 or 10 000 for the other institutions). Results differed from theoretical expectations: numeracy did not predict choices and participants with more precise representations were more likely to choose the numerically *inferior* option, to save 10 000 lives rather than 20 000 lives. Note that the construct of numeracy could not be entirely reduced to the construct of numerical precision as defined by the linearity (vs. non-linearity) of number representation, suggesting that a psychophysical explanation of numeracy is incomplete.

Neuroscience of number sense

Cognitive and neural data support the basic concept of number sense (Cantlon & Brannon, 2007; Dehaene, 2007; Choi et al., 2011). According to many psychophysical theorists, the evolutionarily older language-independent numerical estimation system exists alongside a learned language-dependent system of counting and computational rules. (Number words and other symbols can access the numerical estimation system, but words are not required in order to process number.) The intraparietal sulcus has been implicated as a substrate for the language-independent approximate (non-linear) system (Dehaene et al., 2003; Brannon, 2006; Merritt et al., 2010; Brannon & Merritt, 2011). However, when adults perform precise computations, the problem is encoded linguistically, and this computation engages left inferior frontal regions that are active during language-dependent tasks (see also Holloway et al., 2010; Izard et al., 2011). An implication of this approach is that those who are low in numeracy retain a rudimentary language-independent estimation system for representing number, even if they lack formal education in mathematics. However, neuroimaging research has not addressed the other three theoretical perspectives on numeracy (i.e., computational, dual processes, and fuzzy-trace theory approaches).

Specifically, little neuroscience research has explicitly connected brain substrates for number with neural systems associated with judgment and decision making, despite the grounding of most classical theories of the latter in the psychophysics of quantities. Prospect theory, for example, is arguably the most influential theory of decision making, which like expected utility theory before it, relies on a curvilinear function of values (e.g., number of dollars) to predict choices. The prospect theory function is a power function, not logarithmic, but the general idea of a curvilinear function that distorts quantities more as they become larger is preserved (Kahneman, 2003). In contrast, Siegler and colleagues have repeatedly shown that adults – the same age and level of education as those typically accounted for by prospect theory – have a linear function for number. Now, it might be that the psychophysics of numbers differs depending on what they describe, varying from linear to logarithmic. However, these qualifications render a psychophysical explanation of numeracy less satisfying.

Summary

More generally, psychophysical approaches have been criticized as being descriptive models, rather than process models that explain underlying mechanisms (Brandstätter et al., 2006). However, this is not a cogent criticism. A psychophysical model is a *perceptual* process, with roots in research on perception of light, sound, and temperature (e.g., Tversky & Kahneman, 1981). One might ask where the perceptual processes come from, but one might just as well ask where constructs such as cognitive load or representation come from; these questions in no way undermine these constructs as explanatory. Criticizing psychophysical theories as not being process models is a rhetorical means of eliminating them from consideration, but what counts is whether they predict results.

In sum, psychophysical theories predict perceived similarity among numbers and many studies provide evidence for a basic number system that mentally represents numbers along a logarithmic curve (although some adults seem to have linear representations of quantity in different tasks). However, the construct of numeracy cannot be reduced to the idea of a linear, precise representation of numerical magnitudes. Numeracy is not consistently related to better discrimination of numbers. For example, people with superior number discrimination should be more likely to choose the normatively correct option in terms of saving the highest number of lives in the charity problem, but they choose the numerically inferior option. Unfortunately, this is not an isolated result. As we discuss below, more numerate individuals (as measured by standard tests of numeracy) sometimes choose the numerically inferior option in other tasks, too.

Ironically, health numeracy tests typically place a great deal of emphasis on ratio concepts, such as risk and probability, and computations involving ratios (e.g., converting frequencies to percentages and vice versa; Reyna & Brainerd, 2007). Computing ratios in order to make decisions (e.g., computing the ratio of 10 000 lives to 15 000 lives) produces choices that are consistent with a ratio-dependent logarithmic representation of number – in contrast to a linear representation of number. A linear representation would instead treat larger objective differences in outcomes, say between 290 000 and 270 000 lives, as larger psychologically than smaller objective differences, say between 10 000 and 5000 lives. Hence, characterizing high numeracy psychophysically in terms of linearity is at odds with characterizing high numeracy in terms of performance on standard health numeracy tests (which seem to assess a tendency to engage in ratio-dependent, nonlinear comparisons of numbers; Peters et al., 2008; Reyna et al., 2009).

Computational approaches

Information overload and working memory

Psychophysical approaches emerged in the nineteenth century, followed by computational approaches in the twentieth century, coincident with the rise of computers. Theories that take a computational approach stress that better information processing is associated with reduced cognitive burdens (Galesic et al., 2009). According to this view, cognitive processing (including that of numerical information) is a function of working memory capacity. Therefore, reducing memory load (i.e., reducing demands on working memory) is predicted to improve performance (for reviews distinguishing working memory capacity from interference, see Reyna, 1992, 2005; Reyna & Mills, 2007b). Improving decision making, then, requires reducing the amount of information to be processed, "even at the expense of completeness" (Fagerlin et al., 2011). Those who are lower in numeracy are expected to be even more vulnerable to information overload than those higher in numeracy, when it comes to processing numbers.

Consistent with this approach, strategies have been used to make numerical information more accessible, ostensibly to overcome limitations from working memory capacity, and to reduce reliance on extraneous sources of information (Natter & Berry, 2005). For example, Peters et al. (2007) presented participants with information about three hospitals (asking them to choose the best hospital), varying whether the most relevant information (cost and quality) was presented first, or whether only the cost and quality information was displayed (other extraneous information was deleted). Those lower in numeracy showed better comprehension when the most relevant information was presented first, and both low and high numerates benefited from deleting irrelevant information.

In a similar vein, Wood et al. (2011) investigated the effect of numeracy on the decision to enroll in a health insurance plan covering prescription drugs. Participants received information about 3, 10, or 20 different drug plans as well as a hypothetical scenario from which they were asked to choose one drug plan according to either a single factor (e.g., lowest total annual cost) or two factors (e.g., total annual cost and having a mail order option). Increasing the number of drug plan choices (purportedly increasing load in working memory) was associated with decreased performance. In addition, as expected, participants with higher numeracy (assessed by an 11-item objective numeracy test) were better able to choose the best plans under higher load (see also Szrek & Bundorf, 2011). The studies we have discussed, however, were not designed to distinguish effects of working memory capacity as opposed to effects of limited attention or interference (Reyna & Brainerd, 1995).

Simple and natural frequencies

Within a computational framework, Gigerenzer and colleagues argued at one time that frequencies or counts are naturally easier to process than normalized formats, such as probabilities (Gigerenzer, 1994; Gigerenzer & Hoffrage, 1995; Hoffrage et al., 2000, 2002). Frequencies were said to be a more "transparent" format for displaying numerical information. Claims about what is evolutionarily "natural" (post hoc speculation) or "transparent" (a circular concept because fewer errors mean that a format is transparent and being transparent produces fewer errors) are not testable scientifically. However, the prediction that frequency formats improve numerical judgment has been tested in many studies, and has not been supported. Based on the literature, we can conclude that frequencies do not reduce errors or biases (e.g., Evans et al., 2000; Sloman et al., 2003; Koehler & Macchi, 2004; Reyna & Mills, 2007a; Dieckmann et al., 2009; see also Macchi & Mosconi, 1998; for reviews, see Barbey & Sloman, 2007; Reyna & Brainerd, 2008).

Earlier research had seemed to support the hypothesis that frequencies are easier to understand than probabilities. However, those studies had confounds; in other words, effects were later found to not be due to frequencies. In more recent work, researchers now acknowledge that the evidence does not support hypotheses about simple frequencies (that frequencies make numbers easier to understand or reduce biases; e.g., Gigerenzer et al., 2009; Gigerenzer, 2011; Gigerenzer & Galesic, 2012). Illustrating typical findings, but with a large sample, Cuite et al. (2008) studied 16 133 people's performance on multiple computational tasks involving health risks and found that performance was virtually identical for frequency (55% accurate) and probability (57% accurate) versions of the same information (see also Windschitl, 2002; Dieckmann et al., 2009). Occasionally, effects favor frequencies or the reverse: they favor normalized formats. For example, Waters et al. (2006) compared frequencies with percentages with respect to the accuracy of judgments about different cancer treatments. Among 2601 respondents, those who received percentages performed significantly better than those who received the same information in the form of frequencies. Schapira et al. (2004) found that women's estimates of breast cancer risk were more accurate for lifetime risks using a frequency scale, but were more accurate for 5-year risk using a percentage scale. These effects, or lack of effects, of frequency formats do not seem to differ for people who are lower or higher in numeracy (e.g., Schapira et al., 2004; Gardner et al., 2011).

However, the claim that simple frequencies facilitate judgment should be distinguished from the natural frequencies hypothesis as characterized, for example, by Hoffrage et al. (2002). These natural frequencies refer to situations involving two variables – they are non-normalized joint frequencies. This more recent version of the natural frequencies hypothesis has much in common with class-inclusion hypothesis, which holds that overlapping or nested relations create confusion (e.g., Reyna, 1991; Reyna & Mills, 2007a; Reyna & Brainerd, 2008). (For a more detailed discussion of the class-inclusion hypothesis, see the section on fuzzy-trace theory below.) The natural frequencies format disentangles these overlapping classes (making the denominator or reference classes clearer) – but frequencies are not a necessary means of disentangling classes (e.g., Brainerd & Reyna, 1990; Wolfe & Reyna, 2010). The same beneficial effects on, for example, reducing the conjunction fallacy, the disjunction fallacy, and base-rate neglect in conditional probability judgments can be obtained using normalized probabilities, contrary to Hoffrage et al. (2002) (e.g., Reyna, 1991; Lloyd & Reyna, 2001; Wolfe & Reyna, 2010; Wolfe et al., 2013). Note that the frequency hypotheses of Cosmides, Gigerenzer, and colleagues (e.g., Gigerenzer, 1994, 2011; Cosmides & Tooby, 1996) should be distinguished from the frequency effect studied by Slovic and colleagues (discussed below; e.g., Slovic et al., 2004; Peters et al., 2012).

Graph literacy

Some researchers have suggested that visual aids, such as graphs and icon arrays, improve the processing of numbers, especially for people with sufficient graph literacy (the ability to read and understand graphs; e.g., Chapter 7 in this volume; Reyna, 1991, 2008; Stone et al., 1994; Galesic & Garcia-Retamero, 2011b; Garcia-Retamero et al., 2011). Recent studies have supported this very broad claim (e.g., Stone et al., 2003; Galesic & Garcia-Retamero, 2011a, 2011b). However, the clear limitations to this claim that visual aids are helpful are that (1) some people have difficulty interpreting graphs and other visual aids (Galesic & Garcia-Retamero, 2011b) and (2) not all visual aids are helpful, which is why theory is needed – to differentiate superficially similar aids that seem helpful (but are not) from those that are efficacious (Reyna, 2008).

Although numeracy provides some constraints on the ability to interpret numerical information in graphs (Brown et al., 2011; Gaissmaier et al., 2012), Garcia-Retamero et al. (2011) have suggested that graph literacy extends beyond numeracy. To test this hypothesis, they compared performance on numeracy (Lipkus et al., 2001) and graph literacy assessments (Galesic & Garcia-Retamero, 2011b) in representative US and German samples. Participants received different descriptions of a medicine that reduces risk of heart attack, including a group that received medicine and one that received a placebo. Information was presented numerically or using icon arrays and bar graphs to express low or high (25% or 75%) risk reduction in absolute or relative terms. Results showed that more numerate participants were more likely to comprehend risk reduction information from graphs. However, one-third of participants (estimates that apply to the US and German populations) were both low in numeracy and in graph literacy, suggesting that visual aids would not be helpful to them.

These results indicate that graph literacy and numeracy are separable constructs (Garcia-Retamero & Galesic, 2009; Garcia-Retamero et al., 2011; Galesic & Garcia-Retamero, 2011a, 2011b). Although some research on visual aids has appealed to the concept of ecological rationality to explain results, it is not clear what predictions follow from that concept. The definition of "ecological rationality" is a heuristic's "ability to exploit the structure of the information in natural environments" (p. 76) so that the heuristic is "effective" when the correlation between the heuristic choice and the environment is positive, random when random, and negative when the correlation is negative. In other words, the heuristic is successful when it is successful and unsuccessful when it is not successful, an unfalsifiable concept (Goldstein & Gigerenzer, 2002). Ecological validity in the sense that graphs or displays have realistic elements is also not supported by the data. Realistic images do not necessarily improve comprehension. For example, iconicity (concrete and realistic depictions in graphs) increases resemblance to real-life experience (e.g., the icons look like people), but this concrete resemblance does not improve comprehension of numbers (Gaissmaier et al., 2012).

Cognitive effort, need for cognition, and seeking information

The research we have discussed from a computational perspective focuses on cognition. However, cognition is not the same as metacognition (the ability to think about one's thinking), or the need for cognition (Cacioppo & Petty, 1982; Stanovich & West, 2008). According to some conceptual frameworks, numeracy should facilitate exerting mental effort and seeking out additional numerical information, among other metacognitive strategies (Lipkus & Peters, 2009). Consistent with this supposition, Galesic and Garcia-Retamero (2011a) demonstrated that high numeracy patients were more likely to prefer playing a more active role in medical decision making. Conversely, those who are induced to seek out information and be more reflective should process numerical information more accurately. For example, in Natter and Berry's (2005) study, half of the participants were given an active task to reflect on a given scenario (i.e., being prescribed a medication with a 2% risk of side effects) before rating their likelihood of experiencing side effects, while the other half were given no additional task (i.e., passive participants). Active participants rated their likelihood of side effects more accurately than passive participants (see also Ancker & Kaufman, 2007).

Summary

In sum, computational approaches emphasize reducing the amount of information to be processed, and organizing it by foregrounding relevant information and deleting irrelevant information. These predictions emanate from the theoretical assumption that people have a limited capacity working memory "buffer" in which they process information. Computational approaches also lend themselves to manipulations of information displays, including using visual aids, such as graphs, which can facilitate comprehension of numbers for people with sufficient graph literacy. The frequency and natural frequencies hypotheses are efforts to explain effects of formatting theoretically, and such theory is sorely needed. Although frequency formats offer no clear advantage over normalized numbers (proportions, percentages, or probabilities), displays that disentangle the classes that numbers refer to (e.g., the number with a breast cancer genetic risk; the percentage who develop breast cancer) can reduce errors in combining information about more than one variable (see fuzzy-trace theory section below). The results of controlled experiments indicate that interference rather than capacity in working memory explain results, but some of the practical implications for displaying health information remain the same.

Dual-process approaches

Overview of standard approaches

Dual-process approaches incorporate computation as one of the dual processes, but they add intuition (and sometimes affect or emotion) as the other side of the cognitive coin. These approaches have their roots in Cartesian dualism and in Freud's psychodynamic distinction between primary versus secondary processes (see Epstein, 1994; Reyna, 2013). According to this approach, the intuitive process (also known as associative, experiential, affective, or System 1) is evolutionarily primitive, whereas the analytical process (also known as rule-based, rational, deliberative, or System 2) is advanced and can override the intuitive process (e.g., Epstein, 1994; Epstein et al., 1996; Sloman, 1996; Stanovich, 1999; Evans, 2008, 2009, 2010, 2011; Kahneman, 2011; Stanovich et al., 2011). Kahneman (2011) and others characterize intuition as fast and impulsive, but analysis as slow, serial, and deliberative. Numeracy has been identified with the analytical System 2 (e.g., Peters et al., 2006).

In an effort to accommodate criticisms of dual-process theory, Evans (2008, 2009, 2010, 2011) and Stanovich et al. (2011) have qualified their view of dual systems (replacing the term "systems" with "types"). This accommodation renders the dual-process approach both less parsimonious and less predictive, but more in keeping with extant evidence (Keren & Schul, 2009; Barrouillet, 2011). Dual processes have also been expanded to a tri-partite structure: Type 1 is an autonomous mind, Type 2 is primarily an algorithmic mind that accesses rules, procedures, and strategies that are used to override Type 1 – but only with the help of a reflective mind – a third Type (Stanovich et al., 2011). The addition of reflective functions draws on the familiar ideas of monitoring and inhibition, and the latter processes are brought to bear when reasoning anomalies are detected (e.g., Kahneman, 2003; Reyna & Mills, 2007b). Dual-process approaches identify analysis and reflection (characterized as rational thought) as antidotes to irrational intuition.

Some versions of dual-process theory are vulnerable to the criticism that they are post hoc typologies that do not make novel predictions (see Gigerenzer & Regier, 1996, for arguments against standard dual-process approaches). Similarly, describing numeracy as System 2 or as Type 2 and 3 thinking does not necessarily buy anything new in terms of prediction. However, fuzzy-trace theory (see below) and Epstein et al.'s (1996) dual-process theory are not subject to this specific criticism – they make novel predictions. Epstein and colleagues have developed a valid and reliable measure of analytical versus intuitive thinking – the Rational-Experiential Inventory (REI), which consists of two scales: Faith in Intuition (concrete, experiential, and emotional thinking) and Need for Cognition to measure rational thinking style (derived from Cacioppo & Petty's, 1982, Need for Cognition scale).

Ratio bias and framing effects

Although reliable individual differences in thinking style have been detected using the REI, these differences do not consistently map onto judgment and decision making in ways that the dual-process theory predicts (e.g., Ayal et al., 2011; Epstein et al., 1996; Pacini & Epstein, 1999a, 1999b; Alonso & Fernández-Berrocal, 2003; for a review, see Reyna & Brainerd, 2008). For example, a core prediction of Epstein et al.'s (1996) theory is that a predominance of intuitive over analytical thinking, as measured by the REI, will account for an effect called "ratio bias" (the same effect is called the numerosity bias in the probability judgment literature and both effects originated with Piaget; for reviews, see Reyna & Brainerd, 1994, 2008). Our earlier example of a survival rate of 1 out of 10 patients seeming smaller than a survival rate of 9 out of 100 patients is an example of ratio bias. The ratio bias has been observed for judgments of health risk (e.g., Bonner & Newell, 2008). The empirical effect is that people tend to focus on differences in numerators rather than denominators, a factor that can be manipulated when presenting information to patients. For example, the survival rates above could be presented as 10% versus 9% to reduce this bias. This advice runs counter to advice to use frequencies to minimize biases. Clearly, normalized ratios (e.g., percentages) offer advantages for health communication when denominators differ.

Explanations differ for the ratio bias effect, however. According to standard dual-process approaches, numerical information is either processed analytically (as mathematically equivalent or not) or experientially as involving countable concrete numbers (e.g., in the numerator) that seem more real and affectively tempting than abstract large numbers (e.g., in the denominator) (e.g., Epstein, 1994; Peters et al., 2006). This account suggests that people who can and do rely on objective numbers are rational and others are irrational or perhaps conflicted about what is rational (Amsel et al., 2009).

Predictions for framing effects are the same as those for the ratio bias, namely, that people high in analytical thinking, but low in attraction to biased intuition, should be less susceptible to framing effects (as opposed to those low in analytical thinking and high in intuition, who should be biased). Framing effects are important in health communication because they demonstrate that superficial changes in wording can change health judgments and decisions. Framing effects occur when decision makers treat quantitatively equivalent options differently, such as rating a treatment as more effective when the survival rate is described as 80%, as opposed to the same treatment being described as having a 20% mortality rate (e.g., Kahneman, 2003; Porcelli & Delgado, 2009; Kühberger & Tanner, 2010). However, studies such as that by Shiloh et al. (2002) did not find the predicted relations among high or low analytical (measured by REI's Need for Cognition scale), high or low intuitive (measured by REI's Faith in Intuition scale), and positive or negative frame. Participants fit unpredicted combinations of thinking styles – high analytical, high intuitive thinking and low analytical, low intuitive thinking participants exhibited greater framing effects.

Even though Shiloh et al. (2002) suggest that their results are consistent with a dual-process approach, important predictions of dual-process theory were not confirmed: Neither low reliance on analysis nor high reliance on intuition was associated in any consistent fashion with framing effects. Applications of dual-process theory to numeracy have met with greater success. Peters et al. (2006), for example, showed that those higher in numeracy seemed to approach numerical problems more analytically, and were less subject to intuitive biases, such as ratio bias and framing effects, than those lower in numeracy (see also Peters & Levin, 2008). However, there are some consistent exceptions to the generalization that those higher in numeracy reason at a higher level (and are less subject to biases).

Frequency effect and percentages

Another bias relevant to dual-process approaches and to health communication is the frequency effect studied by Slovic and colleagues (e.g., Slovic et al., 2004). The frequency effect sounds like the frequency hypothesis, but it is not the same. The classic frequency effect is that participants rate the likelihood of an event, for example, that a psychiatric patient would commit an act of violence, as higher when expressed as frequencies (e.g., 20 out of 100 commit violent acts) rather than percentages (or proportions; 20% or 0.20 commit violent acts). Slovic et al. argue that relying on affect (System 1) should lead to higher levels of risk being reported for the frequency (compared with the percentage) format, because more vivid images of violent acts are generated (see Peters et al., 2006). In this view, those lower in numeracy should be more susceptible to the emotionally arousing frequency format, compared with those higher in numeracy, who rely on cold numbers. (The frequency effect can also be interpreted as an example of denominator neglect because neglecting 100 would make 20 seem larger, whereas 20% has no explicit denominator to neglect; see Reyna & Brainerd, 2008.)

Consistent with dual-process theory, both Peters et al. (2006) and Peters et al. (2012) found that the responses of more numerate participants did not differ when they were presented with frequency versus percentage formats. However, participants lower in numeracy rated risk as higher when presented with frequencies than with percentages. The key to understanding these results is that risk estimates were increased for frequency formats for those high in numeracy relative to those low in numeracy in both studies. These findings are not consistent with predictions of dual-process, or affect-heuristic, approaches. It is as though more numerate participants mentally transformed percentages into frequencies (e.g., 20% into 20 out of 100), and, hence, biased themselves into perceiving the risk in the frequency format as higher. (Numeracy tests emphasize transforming ratios, such as percentages into frequencies; Reyna & Brainerd, 2007.) Inconsistent with dual-process theory, differences between low- and high-numerate participants were observed for the percentage format, not for the frequency format. Both groups seemed to have relied on similar biasing processes in the emotionally arousing frequency condition (Slovic et al., 2004; Dickert et al., 2011).

Irrational bias and mood

In a final experiment, Peters et al. (2006) found that high-numerate participants were *more* prone to an irrational bias involving processing numbers than low numerate participants were. The task involved rating the attractiveness of a risky gamble on a 21-point Likert scale from "not at all attractive" (0) to "completely attractive" (20). Some medical decisions have this general description – fairly low odds to improve the patient's condition, relative to the status quo; professional athletes might take such a gamble to get back in the game. Different groups of participants rated the attractiveness of playing a no-loss bet (7/36 chances to win $9 and 29/36 chances to win nothing) or a loss bet (7/36 chances to win $9 and 29/36 chances to lose 5 cents). The dual-process hypothesis is that participants with high numeracy would rate the objectively better bet (no-loss) as more attractive, relative to the numerically inferior loss bet. However, results showed the reverse – that the objectively worse bet (loss bet) was rated as more attractive. Moreover, this effect was based on more numerate participants' ratings rather than on the ratings of less numerate participants, who rated both bets the same.

Peters et al. (2006) acknowledged that rating the worse bet more highly is not a "rational" response. According to Peters et al., the highly numerate may sometimes make such responses "precisely because they focus on the detail of numbers" (p. 411). Nevertheless, dual-process theory predicts the opposite, that the highly numerate should show less bias (i.e., their judgments should better reflect objective quantities) than the less numerate. Although it makes sense that those who rate the loss bet as more attractive (than the non-loss bet) focus on the contrast between the $9 win and the 5 cent loss (Lipkus & Peters, 2009), there is no basis in dual-process theories for predicting that this contrast will be more salient for the more numerate – on the contrary. The same theoretical principles that explain the absence of ratio bias and framing effects for the highly numerate appear to be violated when the opposite result, greater bias, is found for the loss bet.

Dual-process theory also predicts that *mood* will have biasing effects on those low in numeracy. The less numerate, who are less likely to attend to and understand numbers, should be more influenced by extraneous information, such as mood. Schapira et al. (2011) discussed possible affective responses that could influence numeracy, such as positive feelings that could infuse confidence in the numerical information presented in the context of healthcare. Mood effects were tested in a study about how people made judgments about hospital quality (Peters et al., 2009). Although most numerical quality indicators remained unused by all respondents, the highly numerate were more likely to use one of the indicators to rate the hospitals. As expected by dual-process theory, compared with those of high-numerate patients, preferences expressed by low numerate patients were less influenced by objective probabilities and more influenced by mood.

Summary

In sum, individual differences in traditional dual processes do not consistently predict biases in processing numerical information in ratio bias and framing tasks. However, differences in numeracy that are supposed to reflect such dual processes are associated with ratio and framing biases, as well as with effects of mood. Other effects of numeracy run counter to theoretical predictions: those higher in numeracy rated a numerically worse bet as superior (those lower in numeracy did not), and numeracy produced unexpected differences in affective processing of numbers in a frequency format, along with other empirical disconfirmations (see also Reyna & Brainerd, 2008; Cokely & Kelley, 2009). Taken together, these results suggest that the hypothesized differences in dual processes do not explain effects of numeracy.

Fuzzy-trace theory

The role of meaning and emotion

Fuzzy-trace theory builds on previous research, including the theoretical approaches we have discussed thus far. In contrast to those approaches, however, fuzzy-trace theory focuses on the *meaning* of numbers – and not just any conception of meaning – but the essential bottom line gist of numbers (e.g., Reyna & Brainerd, 1992, 1995, 2011; Reyna, 2008). Gist representations are the less precise "fuzzy traces" in fuzzy-trace theory. This focus on gist is justified by experiments isolating simple gist representations, as opposed to detailed verbatim representations, as necessary assumptions in order to explain empirical effects in studies of memory, judgment, and decision making. Thus, the emphasis in fuzzy-trace theory is not on the precise perception of numerical magnitudes (as in psychophysics) or on reducing cognitive load (i.e., decreasing the bits of information to process or increasing the complexity of mathematical calculations, as in computational theories). Instead, according to this theory, the goal of health communication is to facilitate people's interpretation of the meaning of numbers in context by distilling their simplest qualitative essence (Reyna, 2004, 2013).

This distillation is an insightful process, one that benefits from background knowledge of the topic and from experience in the world (e.g., Reyna et al., 2003; Reyna & Farley, 2006). Therefore, fuzzy-trace theory makes predictions about the use of numbers across age and across groups that vary in expertise. The tendency to rely on gist, as opposed to verbatim representations, increases from childhood to adulthood (e.g., Reyna & Ellis, 1994; see Table 3 in Reyna & Farley, 2006). During the same period, the ability to perform computations with numbers increases because of schooling. Studies with artificial tasks that force individuals to rely on verbatim numbers mask effects of the greater reliance on gist with age (see Figner et al., 2009). However, studies that disambiguate verbatim and gist processing have revealed that decision making relies less on verbatim processing numbers with development, with concomitant decreases in unhealthy risk taking (e.g., Reyna et al., 2011). For example, the adolescent who concludes that HIV-AIDS infection "won't happen to me" is literally accurate at a verbatim level – but misses the categorical truth at a gist level – and seems to be at greater risk (e.g., Reyna & Farley, 2006; Reyna & Brainerd, 2011). At the other end of the life span, relying on gist may be beneficial for older people whose verbatim memories are less robust (Reyna & Mills, 2007b; Tanius et al., 2009; Reyna, 2012a).

Like some other contemporary theorists (e.g., Lipkus & Peters, 2009), fuzzy-trace theorists acknowledge that affect and discrete emotions infiltrate the interpretation of information (Brainerd et al., 2008; Reyna & Rivers, 2008). Fuzzy-trace theory localizes key effects of affect and emotion in the mental representations that are generated of information; the gist of numbers is shaped by their affect and by the emotions they elicit (Rivers et al., 2008). For example, a grandfather who watched his child suffer and die of cystic fibrosis might interpret the gist of a genetic risk of 1% for a grandchild as "large" (Reyna, 2008). To take another example, the odds of being infected with HIV-AIDS from unprotected sex are objectively small, but the gist interpretation for those who avoid risk is, "it only takes once" (i.e., the categorical possibility of death is salient; Mills et al., 2008; Reyna et al., 2011). Conversely, a bleak prognosis of cancer (e.g., 90% mortality in 5 years) that is not absolutely certain can be interpreted as "possible survival" (i.e., the categorical possibility of life is salient; Reyna et al., 2012). Emotions, such as fear and hope, systematically color the interpretations of the gist of probabilities (Rivers et al., 2008). However, in this theory, emotions are not viewed as necessarily distorting. As in the examples given in this paragraph, they can point processing toward the categorical boundaries of events that are pivotal in adaptive decision making (see also Wood and Bechara, 2014).

In other words, just as *someone* wins the lottery (and you cannot win if you do not play), *someone* survives more than 5 years if the probability of death is not 100% and *someone* contracts HIV-AIDS if the probability of infection is not 0%. Patients can simultaneously encode the exact numbers (if they are told the exact numbers) and hold disparate representations in their minds: a high probability of mortality (90%) and a categorical possibility of survival. Each representation (verbatim and gist) is true, but in a different way (Reyna et al., 2002). Most theorists believe that appreciating the latter interpretation (categorical possibility) implies an underappreciation for the former (the 90% probability), but this belief is not endorsed in fuzzy-trace theory.

Gist and verbatim representation of numbers

These two kinds of representations – one qualitative and categorical and the other quantitative and literal – coexist in the minds of most adults when they receive numerical information about risks and benefits. That is, research on fuzzy-trace theory indicates that people encode both verbatim representations of exact numbers and exact words (e.g., "90% probability of mortality") roughly in parallel with gist representations (e.g., categorical possibility of survival), and these are independent mental representations even when they are encoded from the same information. "Verbatim" representations are not just verbal in fuzzy-trace theory, despite the seeming implication of that word; they apply to numbers, pictures, graphs, events, and other forms of information (e.g., Reyna & Brainerd, 1992, 1993, 1995, 2011; Tait et al., 2010a; Gaissmaier et al., 2012). The verbatim–gist distinction is not just a matter of using those words (e.g., Hawley et al., 2008; Tait et al., 2010a, 2010b); but using those words is a theoretical commitment about the nature of mental representations, which has led to many testable predictions that have been confirmed (e.g., Reyna & Brainerd, 1995, 2008; Reyna, 2012b).

According to fuzzy-trace theory, if people have sufficient numeracy to understand risks and probability notations (e.g., place value), they will extract the categorical gist of the numbers. Category boundaries that routinely guide interpretation in medical decision making are none versus some, possible versus certain, and will happen versus will not happen (e.g., 0 lives saved vs. some lives saved, as in risky choice framing problems; Reyna, 2012b; see also Kahneman & Tversky, 1979; Mather et al., 2012). Research shows that decision makers prefer to operate at the lowest (least precise) level of gist that they can that will allow them to discriminate options (e.g., Reyna & Brainerd, 1995; Reyna, 2012b).

Therefore, this lowest level of numerical distinction, the categorical level, often suffices to clarify preferences.

For example, if offered a choice between a treatment that provides adequate functional status (e.g., medication) versus one that enhances function but carries a non-negligible risk of death (e.g., surgery in a patient with comorbidities), most people are risk-averse (as they are when comparing a sure, smaller gain to a gamble in which they could gain more or gain nothing; Reyna & Brainerd, 1991; Kühberger & Tanner, 2010). Patients, however, need to understand the correct gist of their current situation (Fraenkel et al., 2012). If they realize that they are actually in a loss situation in which they are choosing between permanent disability versus possible disability or recovery of function, their preferences are likely to shift to "riskier" (more variable) options that offer the possibility of recovery of function. Fraenkel et al. tested this fuzzy-trace theory prediction with patients receiving treatment for severe rheumatoid arthritis, and found that communicating the qualitative gist of options was highly effective (see below).

In addition to encoding the categorical gist of options, people often simultaneously encode other gist representations of options that are at higher levels of precision, such as ordinal representations (e.g., less risk versus more risk; Mills et al., 2008). For communicating ordinal gist (that one magnitude is bigger than another), adjacent bar graphs can be useful (see Reyna & Brainerd, 1994 for hypotheses about perceptual magnitude estimation for numbers). Feldman-Stewart et al. (2000), for instance, showed that graphs were more useful than numbers to communicate such "gross-level" ordinal information as opposed to exact numerical differences. Unlike other approaches, fuzzy-trace theorists do not claim that more precision is necessarily superior for health and medical decisions, on the contrary. Gist-based decision making offers advantages not only in pinpointing what matters, but in decreasing errors in information-processing (verbatim representations are vulnerable to error-promoting interference effects; Reyna, 1991; Lloyd & Reyna, 2001, 2009; Reyna & Lloyd, 2006).

Absolute and relative risk

With respect to this issue of greater precision not necessarily being superior, a number of scholars have recently suggested that ordinal risk relationships are misleading, and that absolute risk (which provides more precise information about base rates than relative risk reduction) should be presented instead (e.g., Gigerenzer et al., 2007). For example, the effectiveness of mammography can be presented as reducing the risk of dying of breast cancer by 25% versus reducing the risk of dying from breast cancer from 4 in 1000 to 3 in 1000 (for those who screen regularly, as opposed to those who do not). However, there are at least two representations of gist that are both valid for the absolute risk information: the ordinal gist that mammography is better than no mammography (highlighted in the relative risk version of the information) and the categorical gist that both risks are low (see Figures 1 and 2 in Reyna, 2008). Thus, absolute and relative risk are not alternative ways to convey the same information; they are alternative gist representations that can be drawn from the same (absolute) risk information.

In these situations of low absolute risk, the relative risk formats produce larger perceived differences between options (e.g., Stone et al., 1994), but it is not clear whether relative risks are overestimated or differences between absolute risks are underestimated. Moreover, is the purpose of the numerical information to provide literal facts or to make clear which option should be preferred (assuming that people value living over dying)? Is it better to get the gist that the chances of dying from cancer are lower with mammography, or to perceive the two risks to be similar when they are reliably different? Would you want to be that one patient in 1000 whose death could have been prevented? Certainly, patients should at least consider the qualitative gist that one course of action differs from the other.

Further, we would argue that both ordinal (mammography is better for avoiding breast cancer death) and categorical gist (risk is low either way) are important to decision making, but they cannot be reduced to one another. Unlike other theoretical approaches, we do not claim that information should be thrown at the patient to sort out, a kind of on the one hand, on the other hand expected-value approach. The prescriptive implications of fuzzy-trace theory suggest that it is important to identify the key gists of the information that informed decision makers should extract (e.g., based on the insights of experienced patients and healthcare providers), and ensure that those representations are understood. Formatting information so that the relevant gists pop out is essential (rather than presenting scrambled lists of numerical facts), including ordering numerical information along magnitude dimensions and making sure that differences between options are encoded. The fuzzy-trace theory approach is not persuasive, but neither is it neutral or evenhanded about pros and cons when the gist of the information is not neutral. Giving equal space on labels to risks and benefits can be misleading if risks and benefits are not equal in frequency and severity (but see Schwartz et al., 2009, for a promising approach to presenting essential information on medication labels).

Gist and verbatim processing

Two kinds of thinking tend to be associated with verbatim versus gist representations. Verbatim processing analyzes verbatim representations, operating on the literal facts or "surface form" of information, sometimes transforming it mathematically among numerate individuals (Liberali et al., 2011). Verbatim processing is distinguished from gist processing because it is by rote or mindlessly automatic. In contrast, intuitive processing operates on the gist representations, which incorporate the meaning of information that is based on a person's culture, education, and experience, among other factors known to affect meaning (e.g., Reyna & Adam, 2003; Reyna, 2012c, 2013). The processing is intuitive because it is fuzzy, impressionistic, and generally fast for familiar domains, and because information is processed in parallel, rather than serially as in logic or simple computational models.

In contrast to computational or fast and frugal approaches, however, gist processing is not just about processing fewer dimensions of information, but rather connecting the dots across pieces of information (i.e., integrating within and between dimensions of information) to boil the information down to its essence. Examples of integrating dimensions would be: medication A is the same as medication B, except that it has fewer bad side effects (so try medication A); medications that are generally more effective for my disease have more side effects (but it is impossible to predict who will experience benefits, so try the least risky medication first); and so on. Taking this approach, fuzzy-trace theory has been used to design effective public health programs and patient education tools (see Brust-Renck et al., in press).

For example, an interactive, Web-based educational module was designed to effectively communicate the risks and benefits associated with biologic therapy for arthritis; the tool increased knowledge, patient willingness to escalate care, and the likelihood of making an informed choice (Fraenkel et al., 2012; see also Wolfe & Reyna, 2010, for interventions to reduce cognitive biases in probability judgment). Using this simple tool to promote accurate gist representations, the proportion of subjects making an informed, value-concordant choice increased substantially from 35% to 64%. Similarly, Brewer et al. (2012) compared different ways of communicating the results of genomic test estimates of 10-year risk of distant recurrence of early stage estrogen receptor-positive breast cancer. They showed that the standard detailed report generated a greater number of errors in estimating level of risk (low, intermediate, or high) compared to simpler formats, whereas a newly developed gist-based risk continuum format generated the fewest errors in risk estimation. Also consistent with fuzzy-trace theory, information displays that stress concrete and vivid details (iconicity or verbatim processing) are not necessarily better understood (Gaissmaier et al., 2012) and can even interfere with processing (Zikmund-Fisher et al., 2012; for predictions of these effects and associated evidence, see Reyna & Brainerd, 1994, 2008; Reyna et al., 2001).

Risk communication and class-inclusion confusion

Icon arrays, in particular, are predicted to be effective in communicating relative magnitude if icons are grouped together in contrasting perceptual magnitudes, rather than mixed randomly together so that relative magnitudes are not discernible (e.g., those who survive with treatment vs. fail to survive with treatment; Reyna & Brainerd, 1994; Galesic et al., 2009). Thus, specific visual aids, such as icon arrays that allow relative magnitude to be compared, can be helpful in communicating ordinal gist. Icon arrays can also be helpful in disentangling overlapping classes, reducing denominator neglect (Lloyd & Reyna, 2001; Reyna & Mills, 2007a) and other cognitive biases (e.g., conjunction and disjunction fallacies; Wolfe & Reyna, 2010). The latter icon arrays have additional features that allow class-inclusion relations to be viewed explicitly (Reyna, 1991; Reyna & Brainerd, 2008).

Visual stimuli, such as realistic iconic displays, tend to increase verbatim memory, but not memory for gist representations, but verbatim memory becomes inaccessible very rapidly. Hence, from this theoretical perspective, it make sense that verbatim knowledge of health-related information would fade more than gist knowledge over time, as shown by Gaissmaier et al. (see Figure 1 in Gaissmaier et al., 2012). Note that the effects of visual aids are not monolithic. Not just any visual aid will improve understanding of numbers, and concreteness can be harmful. Visual aids can harm comprehension when they focus cognition on verbatim details and do not allow simple gists to be apprehended (e.g., by scrambling icons of different types); and to the extent that they enhance verbatim memory, their effects can fade over time.

Thus, fuzzy-trace theory encompasses effects of manipulating the salience of different mental representations (categorical gist, ordinal gist, and verbatim representations) as well as effects of class-inclusion confusion. The latter confusion is exacerbated by relying on interference-sensitive verbatim representations, but it originates in the confusion inherent in any ratio concept, including probability. Because the referents of classes overlap, people become confused about which denominators apply to what they are thinking about (e.g., the number of people with disease or the number of people with a positive test). This confusion accounts for the effects of denominator neglect reviewed earlier, such as ratio bias and base-rate neglect. Fuzzy-trace theory predicts that simple interventions that separate classes (so that denominators and numerators can be processed discretely) reduce errors, which has been confirmed using many different types of displays and without using frequencies (e.g., Wolfe et al., 2013; Reyna & Mills, 2007a).

Class-inclusion errors are not fundamental logical errors (i.e., people who commit these errors understand the role of numerators and denominators in principle; Reyna & Brainerd, 1994, 2008); they persist even for advanced reasoners (Reyna et al., 2001; Reyna & Adam, 2003; Adam & Reyna, 2005; Reyna & Lloyd, 2006; Chapman & Liu, 2009). In fact, focusing on exact numbers has been found to exacerbate class-inclusion errors. Removing numerical information so that participants must rely, instead, on memory for the gist improves performance (e.g., Brainerd & Reyna, 1995; Reyna & Brainerd, 1995).

Summary

In sum, fuzzy-trace theory distinguishes intuition, a kind of advanced thinking that operates on simple gist representations, from detailed quantitative analysis using verbatim representations. This distinction is more than labeling different kinds of responses to numerical problems; separate memory representations, and associated processing, are required to explain observed phenomena in judgment and decision making. The theory can account for heuristics and biases that have been the foci of earlier theories, such as ratio bias and base-rate neglect, effects that are important in health communication and medical decision making. Fuzzy-trace theory does not discard earlier theories, instead going beyond dual processes to predict new counterintuitive effects, for example, that experts rely on simple, qualitative bottom lines, despite encoding quantitative details. Most important, fuzzy-trace theory emphasizes the centrality of simple meaning, the gist, in shaping health messages and improving medical decision making.

Conclusions and suggestions for future research

There is no denying the massive evidence for the psychophysical transformation of number, supporting theories that assume "the ontogenetic and phylogenetic continuity of number sense" (Libertus & Brannon, 2009, p. 346). Psychophysical approaches also underlie the most respected theories of decision making, such as prospect theory. Psychophysics is a kind of perceptual process, and it seems to explain how animals, infants, and adults discriminate quantities. This knowledge is useful if we want to make numerical differences seem small or large (e.g., by changing scales). However, there are many effects on numerical processing, which we have reviewed, that cannot be explained by psychophysics. In fact, they extend beyond its boundaries, such as effects of mood and discrete emotion, or outright contradict its predictions.

Computational theories were inspired by analogies between human thinking and machine computation. This metaphor of mind continues to inspire some of the best work in the field of numeracy, despite the criticisms leveled here about the shortcomings of the theory. Dual-process theories have incorporated computation as one process – the rational one – but contrasted it with emotional, experiential (concrete), intuitive (in the primitive sense), and other innumerate processes that produce biases and fallacies. To be sure, dual-process theorists would argue that the non-rational processes support a great deal of perfectly adequate judgment and decision making, and the concept of affective meaning seems downright advanced in some circumstances. However, in this view, higher order cognition is identified with precision and computation; the goal here is a better multiplier (e.g., to derive expected values of options) or divider (e.g., to calculate ratios of risks and benefits). As research on numeracy in medical decision making and health has shown, it is a good thing sometimes to be able to multiply and divide.

Fuzzy-trace theory combines an engine of rote computation – verbatim processing – with gist processing in which simple qualitative construal of the meaning of numbers is the goal of health communication. Research on fuzzy-trace theory has refuted central assumptions of the earlier computational and dual-process approaches, while preserving many of their useful features. In this view, gist-based intuition is advanced. Gist representations, but also class-inclusion confusions, govern how well people use the important information conveyed by numbers. As individuals develop from childhood to adulthood, as they develop expertise in life or in a domain of knowledge, they rely more on gist. A challenge for future research will be to emulate and accelerate this development by delivering interventions that effectively communicate the gist of numbers.

Also, there is virtually no work that has been done with adolescents and elderly individuals with respect to health and medical numeracy (e.g., Mikels et al., 2010). In particular, more research is needed about the reliance on gist processing because memory research has shown that reliance on gist increases with age and experience. In addition, although adolescents are capable of encoding mathematical probabilities about risks and benefits, the effect of numeracy might differ for younger patients

(Reyna et al., 2011; see also Wilhelms & Reyna, 2013). For example, conditions that require high levels of self-management, such as diabetes, would be expected to rely on numeracy. This effect has been obtained with adults; adults with high numeracy for diabetes have been found to better adhere to diabetes self-management (Cavanaugh et al., 2008; Chapter 6 in this volume). Adolescents, however, might show the same effects of numeracy or, alternatively, their lack of maturity might override any effects of numeracy on self-management (Wilhelms & Reyna, 2013). Furthermore, adolescents have been shown to rely less on the gist of numbers in risky decision making, suggesting that verbatim numeracy is insufficient to explain their behavior.

Each of the theoretical approaches we have discussed has evidence to support it, but they could all benefit by integrating work from other perspectives. How this integration can occur when some of the processes are antithetical remains to be seen. The goals of the different approaches are also in conflict: can the precision of a linear psychophysical representation (one that closely hews to objective numerosities) be reconciled with affective meaning (gross differences in positive versus negative valence) or with simple categorical gist? More research is needed about emotion to reconcile conflicting effects, about the universe of gist representations that are encoded from different semantic content, and about how individual differences in personality, background knowledge, and cognitive style (including graph literacy and numeracy) influence processing of numbers. Although excellent research is being conducted on visual aids, theory is only beginning to be applied to make surprising predictions that go beyond what is known empirically. Understanding the theory behind the impressive empirical relations between numeracy and medical decision making will make it possible to convey essential information that every person needs in order to make informed judgments and decisions about their medical care.

References

Abdel-Kader, K., Dew, M. A., Bhatnagar, M., Argyropoulos, C., Karpov, I., Switzer, G., et al. (2010). Numeracy skills in CKD: correlates and outcomes. *Clinical Journal of the American Society of Nephrology*, 5(9), 1566–1573. doi:10.2215/CJN.08121109.

Adam, M. B., & Reyna, V. F. (2005). Coherence and correspondence criteria for rationality: Experts' estimation of risks of sexually transmitted infections. *Journal of Behavioral Decision Making*, 18(3), 169–186. doi:10.1002/bdm.493.

Alonso, D., & Fernández-Berrocal, P. (2003). Irrational decisions: Attending to numbers rather than ratios. *Personality and Individual Differences*, 35(7), 1537–1547. doi:10.1016/S0191-8869(02)00368-9.

Amsel, E., Close, J., Sadler, E., & Klaczynski, P. A. (2009). College students' awareness of irrational judgments on gambling tasks: A dual-process account. *The Journal of Psychology: Interdisciplinary and Applied*, 143(3), 293–317. doi:10.3200/JRLP.143.3.293-317.

Ancker, J. S., & Kaufman, D. R. (2007). Rethinking health numeracy: A multidisciplinary literature review. *Journal of the American Medical Informatics Association*, 14(6), 713–721. doi:10.1197/jamia.M2464.

Anderson, B. L., Obrecht, N. A., Chapman, G. B., Driscoll, D. A., & Schulkin, J. (2011). Physicians' communication of Down syndrome screening test results: The influence of physician numeracy. *Genetics in Medicine*, 13, 744–749. doi:10.1097/GIM.0b013e31821a370f.

Ayal, S., Hochman, G., & Zakay, D. (2011). Two sides of the same coin: Information processing style and reverse biases. *Judgment and Decision Making*, 6, 295–306. Retrieved from http://journal.sjdm.org/11/11320/jdm 11320.html

Barbey, A. K., & Sloman, S. A. (2007). Base-rate respect: From ecological rationality to dual processes. *Behavioral and Brain Sciences*, 30, 241–254. doi:10.1017/S0140525X07001653.

Barrouillet, P. (2011). Dual-process theories and cognitive development: Advances and challenges. *Developmental Review*, 31, 79–85. doi:10.1016/j.dr.2011.07.002.

Benjamin, D. J., Brown, S. A., & Shapiro, J. M. (2013). Who is "behavioral"? Cognitive ability and anomalous preferences. *Journal of the European Economic Association*, 11(6), 1231–1255. doi:10.1111/jeea.12055.

Berteletti, I., Lucangeli, D., Piazza, M., Dehaene, S., & Zorzi, M. (2010). Numerical estimation in preschoolers. *Developmental Psychology*, 46(2), 545–551. doi:10.1037/a0017887.

Betsch, C., Brewer, N. T., Brocard, P., Davies, P., Gaissmaier, W., Haase, N., et al. (2012). Opportunities and challenges of web 2.0 for vaccination decisions. *Vaccine*, 28(30), 3727–3733. doi:10.1016/j.vaccine.2012.02.025.

Bonner, C., & Newell, B. R. (2008). How to make a risk seem riskier: The ratio bias versus construal level theory. *Judgment and Decision Making*, 3(5), 411–416. Retrieved from: journal.sjdm.org/8210/jdm8210.html

Booth, J. L., & Siegler, R. S. (2006). Developmental and individual differences in pure numerical estimation. *Developmental Psychology*, 41, 189–201. doi:10.1037/0012-1649.41.6.189.

Brainerd, C. J., & Reyna, V. F. (1990). Inclusion illusions: Fuzzy-trace theory and perceptual salience effects in cognitive development. *Developmental Review*, 10, 365–403. doi:10.1016/0273-2297(90)90020-5.

Brainerd, C. J., & Reyna, V. F. (1995). Learning rate, learning opportunities and the development of forgetting. *Developmental Psychology*, 31, 251–262. doi:10.1037/0012-1649.31.2.251.

Brainerd, C. J., Stein, L. M., Silveira, R. A., Rohenkohl, G., & Reyna, V. F. (2008). How does negative emotion cause false memories? *Psychological Science*, 19, 919–925. doi:10.1111/j.1467-9280.2008.02177.x.

Brandästtter, E., Gigerenzer, G., & Hertwig, R. (2006). The priority heuristic: Making choices without trade-offs. *Psychological Review*, 113, 409–432. doi:10.1037/0033-295X.113.2.409.

Brannon, E. M. (2006). The representation of numerical magnitude. *Current Opinion in Neurobiology*, 16(2), 222–229. doi:10.1016/j.conb.2006.03.002.

Brannon, E. M., & Merritt, D. (2011) Evolutionary foundations of the Approximate Number System. In: S. Dehaene & L. Brannon (Eds.), *Space, Time and Number in the Brain: Searching for the Foundations of Mathematical Thought*. New York: Elsevier; pp. 207–224.

Brewer, N. T., Richman, A. R., DeFrank, J. T., Reyna, V. F., & Carey, L. A. (2012). Improving communication of breast cancer recurrence risk. *Breast Cancer Research and Treatment*, 133, 553–561. doi:10.1007/s10549-011-1791-9.

Brown, S. M., Culver, J. O., Osann, K. E., MacDonald, D. J., Sand, S., Thornton, A. A., et al. (2011). Health literacy, numeracy, and interpretation of graphical breast cancer risk estimates. *Patient Education and Counseling*, 83(1), 92–98. doi:10.1016/j.pec.2010.04.027.

Brust-Renck, P. G., Reyna, V. F., Wilhelms, E. A., & Lazar, A. N. (in press). A fuzzy-trace theory of judgment and decision making in healthcare: Explanation, prediction, and application. In: M. A. Diefenbach, S. M. Miller, & D. J. Bowen, *Handbook of Health and Decision Science*. New York: Springer.

Cacioppo, J. T., & Petty, R. E. (1982). The need for cognition. *Journal of Personality and Social Psychology*, 42, 116–131. doi:0022-3514/82/4201-0116500.75.

Cantlon, J. F., & Brannon, E. M. (2007). Adding up the effects of cultural experience on the brain. *Trends in Cognitive Sciences*, 11(1), 1–4. doi:10.1016/j.tics.2006.10.008.

Cavanaugh, K., Huizinga, M. M., Wallston, K. A., Gebretsadik, T., Shintani, A., Davis, D., et al. (2008). Association of numeracy and diabetes control. *Annals of Internal Medicine*, 148(10), 737–746. Retrieved from www.annals.org

Chapman, G. B., & Liu, J. (2009). Numeracy, frequency, and Bayesian reasoning. *Judgment and Decision Making*, 4, 34–40. Retrieved from journal.sjdm.org/8708/jdm8708.html

Chen, M. K., Lakshminaryanan, V., & Santos, L. R. (2006). The evolution of our preferences: Evidence from capuchin monkey trading behavior. *Journal of Political Economy*, 114(3), 517–537. doi:0022-3808/2006/11403-0004.

Choi, H., Wong, J. B., Mendiratta, A., Heiman, G. A., & Hamberger, M. J. (2011). Numeracy and framing bias in epilepsy. *Epilepsy Behavior*, 20(1), 29–33. doi:10.1016/j.yebeh.2010.10.005.

Cokely, E. T., & Kelley, C. M. (2009). Cognitive abilities and superior decision making under risk: A protocol analysis and process model evaluation. *Judgment and Decision Making*, 4, 20–33. Retrieved from http://journal.sjdm.org/81125/jdm81125.html

Cokely, E. T., Galesic, M., Schulz, E., Ghazal, S., & Garcia-Retamero, R. (2012). Measuring risk literacy: The Berlin Numeracy Test. *Judgment and Decision Making*, 7, 25–47. Retrieved from http://journal.sjdm.org/11/11808/jdm11808.html

Cosmides, L., & Tooby, J. (1996). Are humans good intuitive statisticians after all? Rethinking some conclusions of the literature on judgment under uncertainty. *Cognition*, 58(1), 1–73. doi:10.1016/0010-0277(95)00664-8.

Cuite, C. L., Weinstein, N. D., Emmons, K., & Colditz, G. (2008). A test of numeric formats for communicating risk probabilities. *Medical Decision Making*, 28, 377–384. doi:10.1177/0272989X08315246.

Dehaene, S. (2007). Symbols and quantities in parietal cortex: Elements of a mathematical theory of number representation and manipulation. In: P. Haggard, Y. Rossetti, & M. Kawato (Eds.), *Attention and Performance: Sensorimotor Foundations of Higher Cognition.* Cambridge, MA: Harvard University; pp. 527–574.

Dehaene, S., Piazza, M., Pinel, P., & Cohen, L. (2003). Three parietal circuits for number processing. *Cognitive Neuropsychology*, 20(3–6), 487–506. doi:10.1080/02643290244000239.

Dehaene, S., Izard, V., Spelke, E., & Pica, P. (2008). Log or linear? Distinct intuitions of the number scale in Western and Amazonian indigene cultures. *Science*, 320(5880), 1217–1220. doi:10.1126/science.1156540.

Dickert, S., Kleber, J., Peters, E., & Slovic, P. (2011). Numeric ability as a precursor to pro-social behavior: The impact of presentation format on the cognitive mechanisms underlying donation decisions. *Judgment and Decision Making*, 6(7), 638–650. Retrieved from http://journal.sjdm.org/11/11421a/jdm11421a.html

Dieckmann, N. F., Slovic, P., & Peters, E. M. (2009). The use of narrative evidence and explicit likelihood by decisionmakers varying in numeracy. *Risk Analysis*, 29, 1473–1488. doi:10.1111/j.1539-6924.2009.01279.x.

Epstein, S. (1994). Integration of the cognitive and the psychodynamic unconscious. *American Psychologist*, 49, 709–724. doi:10.1037/0003-066X.49.8.709.

Epstein, S., Pacini, R., Denes-Raj, V., & Heier, H. (1996). Individual differences in intuitive–experiential and analytical–rational thinking styles. *Journal of Personality and Social Psychology*, 71(2), 390–405. doi:10.1037/0022-3514.71.2.390.

Evans, J. St. B. T. (2008). Dual processing accounts of reasoning, judgment and social cognition. *Annual Review of Psychology*, 59, 255–278. doi:10.1146/annurev.psych.59.103006.093629.

Evans, J. St. B. T. (2009). How many dual-process theories do we need? One, two, or many? In: J. St. B. T. Evans & K. Frankish (Eds.), *In Two Minds: Dual Processes and Beyond.* Oxford: Oxford University Press; pp. 33–54.

Evans, J. St. B. T. (2010). Intuition and reasoning: A dual-process perspective. *Psychological Inquiry*, 21, 313–326. doi:10.1080/1047840X.2010.521057.

Evans, J. St. B. T. (2011). Dual-process theories of reasoning: Contemporary issues and developmental applications. *Developmental Review*, 31, 86–102. doi:10.1016/j.dr.2011.07.007.

Evans, J. St. B. T., Handley, S. J., Perham, N., Over, D. E., & Thompson, V. A. (2000). Frequency versus probability formats in statistical word problems. *Cognition*, 77, 197–213. doi:10.1016/S0010-0277(00)00098-6.

Fagerlin, A., Zikmund-Fisher, B., Ubel, P., Jankovic, A., Derry, H., & Smith, D. (2007). Measuring numeracy without a math test: Development of the subjective numeracy scale. *Medical Decision Making*, 27(5), 672–680. doi:10.1177/0272989X07304449.

Fagerlin, A., Zikmund-Fisher B. J., & Ubel, P. A. (2011). Helping patients decide: Ten steps to better risk communication. *Journal of the National Cancer Institute*, 103(19), 1436–1443. doi:10.1093/jnci/djr318.

Feldman-Stewart, D., Kocovski, N., McConnell, B. A., Brundage, M. D., & Mackillop, W. J. (2000). Perception of quantitative information for treatment decisions. *Medical Decision Making*, 20(2), 228–238. doi:10.1177/0272989X0002000208.

Fetherstonhaugh, D., Slovic, P., Johnson, S. M., & Friedrich, J. (1997). Insensitivity to the value of human life: A study of psychophysical numbing. *Journal of Risk and Uncertainty*, 14(3), 283–300. doi:10.1023/A:1007744326393.

Figner, B., Mackinlay, R. J., Wilkening, F., & Weber, E. U. (2009). Affective and deliberative processes in risky choice: Age differences in risk taking in the Columbia Card Task. *Journal of Experimental Psychology: Learning, Memory, and Cognition*, 35(3), 709–730. doi:10.1037/a0014983.

Fraenkel, L., Peters, E., Charpentier, P., Olsen, B., Errante, L., Schoen, R. T., & Reyna, V. (2012). A decision tool to improve the quality of care in rheumatoid arthritis. *Arthritis Care & Research*, 64(7), 977–985. doi:10.1002/acr.21657.

Furlong, E. E., & Opfer, J. E. (2009). Cognitive constraints on how economic rewards affect cooperation. *Psychological Science*, 20, 11–16. doi:10.1111/j.1467-9280.2008.02244.x.

Gaissmaier, W., Skopec, D., Müller, A., Broschinski, S., & Politi, M. C. (2012). Numbers can be worth a thousand pictures: Individual differences in understanding graphical and numerical representations of health-related information. *Health Psychology*, 31(3), 286–296. doi:10.1037/a0024850.

Galesic, M., & Garcia-Retamero, R. (2011a). Do low-numeracy people avoid shared decision making? *Health Psychology*, 30(3), 336–341. doi:10.1037/a0022723.

Galesic, M., & Garcia-Retamero, R. (2011b). Graph literacy: A cross-cultural comparison. *Medical Decision Making*, 31(3), 444–457. doi:10.1177/0272989X10373805.

Galesic, M., Gigerenzer, G., & Straubinger, N. (2009). Natural frequencies help older adults and people with low numeracy to evaluate medical screening tests. *Medical Decision Making*, 29, 368–371. doi:10.1177/0272989X08329463.

Gallistel, C. R. (2011). Mental magnitudes. In: S. Dehaene & L. Brannon (Eds.), *Space, Time and Number in the Brain: Searching for the Foundations of Mathematical Thought*. New York: Elsevier; pp. 3–12.

Gallistel, C. R., & Gelman, R. (2005). Mathematical cognition. In: K. Holyoak & R. Morrison (Eds.), *The Cambridge Handbook of Thinking and Reasoning*. Cambridge: Cambridge University Press; pp. 559–588.

Garcia-Retamero, R., & Galesic, M. (2009). Communicating treatment risk reduction to people with low numeracy skills: A cross-cultural comparison. *American Journal of Public Health*, 99(12), 2196–2202. doi:10.2105/AJPH.2009.160234.

Garcia-Retamero, R., Galesic, M., & Gigerenzer, G. (2011). Cómo favorecer la comprensión y la comunicación de los riesgos sobre la salud [Improving comprehension and communication of risks about health]. *Psicothema*, 23(4), 599–605. Retrieved from www.psicothema.com/psicothema.asp?id=3928

Gardner, P. H., McMillan, B., Raynor, D. K., Woolf, E., & Knapp, P. (2011). The effect of numeracy on the comprehension of information about medicines in users of a patient information website. *Patient Education and Counseling*, 83(3), 398–403. doi:10.1016/j.pec.2011.05.006.

Gigerenzer, G. (1994). Why the distinction between single-event probabilities and frequencies is important for psychology (and vice versa). In: G. Wright & P. Ayton (Eds.), *Subjective Probability*. Chichester: Wiley; pp. 129–161.

Gigerenzer, G. (2011). What are natural frequencies? Doctors need to find better ways to communicate risk to patients. *British Medical Journal*, 343(d6386), 1–2. doi:10.1136/bmj.d6386.

Gigerenzer, G., & Galesic, M. (2012). Why do single event probabilities confuse patients? Statements of frequency are better for communicating risk. *British Medical Journal*, 344(e245), 1–3. doi:10.1136/bmj.e245.

Gigerenzer, G., & Hoffrage, U. (1995). How to improve Bayesian reasoning without instruction: Frequency formats. *Psychological Review*, 102(4), 684–704. doi:10.1037/0033-295X.102.4.684.

Gigerenzer, G., & Regier, T. (1996). How do we tell an association from a rule? Comment on Sloman (1996). *Psychological Bulletin*, 119(1), 23–26. doi:10.1037/0033-2909.119.1.23.

Gigerenzer, G., Gaissmaier, W., Kurz-Milcke, E., Schwartz, L. M., & Woloshin, S. (2007). Helping doctors and patients make sense of health statistics. *Psychological Science in the Public Interest*, 8(2), 53–96. doi:10.1111/j.1539-6053.2008.00033.x.

Gigerenzer, G., Gaissmaier, W., Kurz-Milcke, E., Schwartz, L. M., & Woloshin, S. W. (2009). Knowing your chances: What health stats really mean. *Scientific American Mind*, 20(2), 44–51. Retrieved from www.scientificamerican.com/article.cfm?id=knowing-your-chances

Goldstein, D. G., & Gigerenzer, G. (2002). Models of ecological rationality: The recognition heuristic. *Psychological Review*, 109(1), 75–90. doi:10.1037/0033-295X.109.1.75.

Hamm, R. M., Bard, D. E., Hsieh, E., & Stein, H. F. (2007). Contingent or universal approaches to patient deficiencies in health numeracy. *Medical Decision Making*, 27 (5), 635–637. doi:10.1177/0272989X07307516.

Hawley, S. T., Zikmund-Fisher, B., Ubel, P., Jancovic, A., Lucas, T., & Fagerlin, A. (2008). The impact of the format of graphical presentation on health-related knowledge and treatment choices. *Patient Education and Counseling*, 73(3), 448–455. doi:10.1016/j.pec.2008.07.023.

Hoffrage, U., Lindsey, S., Hertwig, R., & Gigerenzer, G. (2000). Communicating statistical information. *Science*, 290(5500), 2261–2262. doi:10.1126/science.290.5500.2261.

Hoffrage, U., Gigerenzer, G., Krauss, S., & Martignon, L. (2002). Representation facilitates reasoning: what natural frequencies are and what they are not. *Cognition*, 84(3), 343–352. doi:10.1016/S0010-0277(02)00050-1.

Holloway, I. D., Price, G. R., & Ansari, D. (2010). Common and segregated neural pathways for the processing of symbolic and nonsymbolic numerical magnitude: An fMRI study. *Neuroimage*, 49(1), 1006–1017. doi:10.1016/j.neuroimage.2009.07.071.

Hubbard, E. M., Piazza, M., Pinel, P., & Dehaene, S. (2005). Interactions between number and space in parietal cortex. *Nature Reviews Neuroscience*, 6, 435–448. doi:10.1038/nrn1684.

Izard, V., Pica, P., Dehaene, S., Hinchey, D., & Spelke, E. (2011). Geometry as a universal mental construction. In: S. Dehaene & L. Brannon (Eds.), *Space,*

Time and Number in the Brain: Searching for the Foundations of Mathematical Thought. New York: Elsevier; pp. 319–332.

Kahneman, D. (2003). A perspective on judgment and choice: Mapping bounded rationality. *American Psychologist*, 58(9), 697–720. doi:10.1037/0003-066X.58.9.697.

Kahneman, D. (2011). *Thinking Fast and Slow*. New York: Farrar, Strauss, Giroux.

Kahneman, D., & Tversky, A. (1979). Prospect theory: An analysis of decision under risk. *Econometrica*, 47(2), 263–292. Retrieved from www.jstor.org/stable/1914185

Keren, G., & Schul, Y. (2009). Two is not always better than one: A critical evaluation of two-system theories. *Perspectives on Psychological Science*, 4(6), 533–550. doi:10.1111/j.1745-6924.2009.01164.x.

Koehler, J., & Macchi, L. (2004). Thinking about low-probability events: An exemplar cuing theory. *Psychological Science*, 15, 540–546. Retrieved from www.jstor.org/stable/40064013

Kühberger, A., & Tanner, C. (2010). Risky choice framing: Task versions and a comparison of prospect theory and fuzzy-trace theory. *Journal of Behavioral Decision Making*, 23(3), 314–329. doi:10.1002/bdm.656.

Liberali, J. M., Reyna, V. F., Furlan, S., Stein, L. M., & Pardo, S. T. (2011). Individual differences in numeracy and implications for biases and fallacies in probability judgment. *Journal of Behavioral Decision Making*, 2, 361–381. doi:10.1002/bdm.752.

Libertus, M. E., & Brannon, E. M. (2009). Behavioral and neural basis of number sense in infancy. *Current Directions in Psychological Science*, 18, 346–351. doi:10.1111/j.1467-8721.2009.01665.x.

Lipkus, I. M., & Peters, E. (2009). Understanding the role of numeracy in health: Proposed theoretical framework and practical insights. *Health Education and Behavior*, 36, 1065–1081. doi:10.1177/1090198109341533.

Lipkus, I. M., Samsa, G., & Rimer, B. K. (2001). General performance on a numeracy scale among highly educated samples. *Medical Decision Making*, 21, 37–44. doi:10.1177/0272989X0102100105.

Lloyd, F. J., & Reyna, V. F. (2001). A web exercise in evidence-based medicine using cognitive theory. *Journal of General Internal Medicine*, 16(2), 94–99. doi:10.1111/j.1525-1497.2001.00214.x.

Lloyd, F. J., & Reyna, V. F. (2009). Clinical gist and medical education: Connecting the dots. *Journal of the American Medical Association*, 302(12), 1332–1333. doi:10.1001/jama.2009.1383.

Macchi, L., & Mosconi, G. (1998). Computational features vs. frequentist phrasing in the base-rate fallacy. *Swiss Journal of Psychology*, 57(2), 79–85. doi:35400007688899.0010.

Mather, M., Mazar, N., Gorlick, M. A., Lighthall, N. R., Burgeno, J., Schoeke, A., & Ariely, D. (2012). Risk preferences and aging: The 'Certainty Effect' in older adults' decision making. *Psychology and Aging*, 27(4), 801–816. doi:10.1037/a0030174.

Merritt, D. J., Casasanto, D., & Brannon, E. M. (2010). Do monkeys think in metaphors? Representations of space and time in monkeys and humans. *Cognition*, 117, 191–202. doi:10.1016/j.cognition.2010.08.011.

Mikels, J. A., Löckenhoff, C. E., Maglio, S., Cartensen, L. L., Goldstein, M. K., & Garber, A. M. (2010). Following your heart or your head: Focusing on emotions versus information differentially influences the decisions of younger and older adults. *Journal of Experimental Psychology: Applied*, 16(1), 87–95. doi:10.1037/a0018500.

Mills, B., Reyna, V. F., & Estrada, S. (2008). Explaining contradictory relations between risk perception and risk taking. *Psychological Science*, 19, 429–433. doi:10.1111/j.1467-9280.2008.02104.x.

Natter, H., & Berry, D. C. (2005). Effects of active information processing on the understanding of risk information. *Applied Cognitive Psychology*, 19(1), 123–135. doi:10.1002/acp.1068.

Nelson, W., Reyna, V. F., Fagerlin, A., Lipkus, I., & Peters, E. (2008). Clinical implications of numeracy: Theory and practice. *Annals of Behavioral Medicine*, 35, 261–274. doi:10.1007/s12160-008-9037-8.

Opfer, J. E., & Siegler, R. S. (2007). Representational change and children's numerical estimation. *Cognitive Psychology*, 55, 169–195. doi:10.1016/j.cogpsych.2006.09.002.

Pacini, R., & Epstein, S. (1999a). The interaction of three facets of concrete thinking in a game of chance. *Thinking and Reasoning*, 5, 303–325. doi:10.1080/135467899393959.

Pacini, R., & Epstein, S. (1999b). The relation of rational and experiential information processing styles to personality, basic beliefs, and the ratio bias phenomenon. *Journal of Personality and Social Psychology*, 76, 972–987. doi:10.1037/0022-3514.76.6.972.

Peters, E., & Levin, I. P. (2008). Dissecting the risky-choice framing effect: Numeracy as an individual-difference factor in weighting risky and riskless options. *Judgment and Decision Making*, 3, 435–448. Retrieved from http://journal.sjdm.org/8407/jdm8407.html

Peters, E., Västfjäll, D., Slovic, P., Mertz, C., Mazzocco, K., & Dickert, S. (2006). Numeracy and decision-making. *Psychological Science*, 17(5), 407–413. doi:10.1111/j.1467-9280.2006.01720.x.

Peters, E., Dieckmann, N., Dixon, A., Hibbard, J. H., & Mertz, C. K. (2007). Less is more in presenting quality information to consumers. *Medical Care Research and Review*, 64(2), 169–190. doi:10.1177/1077558706298290.

Peters, E., Slovic, P., Västfjäll, D., & Mertz, C. (2008). Intuitive numbers guide decisions. *Judgment and Decision Making*, 3, 619–635. Retrieved from http://journal.sjdm.org/8827/jdm8827.html

Peters, E., Dieckmann, N. F., Västfjäll, D., Mertz, C. K., Slovic, P., & Hibbard, J. H. (2009). Bringing meaning to numbers: The impact of evaluative categories on decisions. *Journal of Experimental Psychology: Applied*, 15(3), 213–227. doi:10.1037/a0016978.

Peters, P., Hart, P. S., & Fraenkel, L. (2012). Informing patients: The influence of numeracy, framing, and format of side effect information on risk perceptions. *Medical Decision Making*, 31(3), 432–436. doi:10.1177/0272989X10391672.

Porcelli, A. J., & Delgado, M. R. (2009). Acute stress modulates risk taking in financial decision making. *Psychological Science*, 20(3), 278–283. doi:10.1111/j.1467-9280.2009.02288.x.

Reyna, V. F. (1991). Class inclusion, the conjunction fallacy, and other cognitive illusions. *Developmental Review*, 11, 317–336. doi:10.1016/0273-2297(91)90017-I.

Reyna, V. F. (1992). Reasoning, remembering, and their relationship: Social, cognitive, and developmental issues. In: M. L. Howe, C. J. Brainerd, & V. F. Reyna (Eds.), *Development of Long-Term Retention.* New York, NY: Springer-Verlag; pp. 103–127.

Reyna, V. F. (2004). How people make decisions that involve risk: A dual process approach. *Current Directions in Psychological Science*, 13, 60–66. doi:10.1111/j.0963-7214.2004.00275.x.

Reyna, V. F. (2005). Fuzzy-trace theory, judgment, and decision-making: A dual-processes approach. In: C. Izawa & N. Ohta (Eds.), *Human Learning and Memory: Advances in Theory and Application: The 4th Tsukuba International Conference on Memory.* Mahwah, NJ: Lawrence Erlbaum Associates, Publishers; pp. 239–256.

Reyna, V. F. (2008). A theory of medical decision making and health: Fuzzy trace theory. *Medical Decision Making*, 28(6), 850–865. doi:10.1177/0272989X08327066.

Reyna, V. F. (2012a). Preface. In: V. F. Reyna, S. Chapman, M. Dougherty, & J. Confrey (Eds.), *The Adolescent Brain: Learning, Reasoning, and Decision Making.* Washington, DC: American Psychological Association; pp. xv–xviii.

Reyna, V. F. (2012b). A new intuitionism: Meaning, memory, and development in fuzzy-trace theory. *Judgment and Decision Making*, 7(3), 332–359. Retrieved from journal.sjdm.org/11/111031/jdm111031.html

Reyna, V. F. (2012c). Risk perception and communication in vaccination decisions: A fuzzy-trace theory approach. *Vaccine*, 30(25), 3790–3797. doi:10.1016/j.vaccine.2011.11.070.

Reyna, V. F. (2013). Intuition, reasoning, and development: A fuzzy-trace theory approach. In: P. Barrouillet & C. Gauffroy (Eds.), *The Development of Thinking and Reasoning* (pp. 193–220). Hove, UK: Psychology Press.

Reyna, V. F., & Adam, M. B. (2003). Fuzzy-trace theory, risk communication, and product labeling in sexually transmitted diseases. *Risk Analysis*, 23, 325–342. doi:10.1111/1539-6924.00332.

Reyna, V. F., & Brainerd, C. J. (1991). Fuzzy-trace theory and framing effects in choice: Gist extraction, truncation, and conversion. *Journal of Behavioral Decision Making*, 4, 249–262. doi:10.1002/bdm.3960040403.

Reyna, V. F., & Brainerd, C. J. (1992). A fuzzy-trace theory of reasoning and remembering: Paradoxes, patterns, and parallelism. In: A. Healy, S. Kosslyn, & R. Shiffrin (Eds.), *From Learning Processes to Cognitive Processes: Essays in Honor of William K. Estes.* Hillsdale, NJ: Erlbaum; pp. 2:235–259.

Reyna, V. F., & Brainerd, C. J. (1993). Fuzzy memory and mathematics in the classroom. In: G. M. Davies & R. H. Logie (Eds.), *Memory in Everyday Life.* Amsterdam: North Holland Press; pp. 91–119.

Reyna, V. F., & Brainerd, C. J. (1994). The origins of probability judgment: A review of data and theories. In: G. Wright & P. Ayton (Eds.), *Subjective Probability.* New York: Wiley; pp. 239–272.

Reyna, V. F., & Brainerd, C. J. (1995). Fuzzy-trace theory: An interim synthesis. *Learning and Individual Differences*, 7, 1–75. doi:10.1016/1041-6080(95)90031-4.

Reyna, V. F., & Brainerd, C. J. (2007). The importance of mathematics in health and human judgment: Numeracy, risk communication, and medical decision making. *Learning and Individual Differences*, 17(2), 147–159. doi:10.1016/j.lindif.2007.03.010.

Reyna, V. F., & Brainerd, C. J. (2008). Numeracy, ratio bias, and denominator neglect in judgments of risk and probability. *Learning and Individual Differences*, 18(1), 89–107. doi:10.1016/j.lindif.2007.03.011.

Reyna, V. F., & Brainerd, C. J. (2011). Dual processes in decision making and developmental neuroscience: A fuzzy-trace model. *Developmental Review*, 31, 180–206. doi:10.1016/j.dr.2011.07.004.

Reyna, V. F., & Ellis, S. C. (1994). Fuzzy-trace theory and framing effects in children's risky decision making. *Psychological Science*, 5, 275–279. doi:10.1111/j.1467-9280.1994.tb00625.x.

Reyna, V. F., & Farley, F. (2006). Risk and rationality in adolescent decision-making: Implications for theory, practice, and public policy. *Psychological Science in the Public Interest*, 7(1), 1–44. doi:10.111/j.1529-1006.2006.00026.x.

Reyna, V. F., & Hamilton, A. J. (2001). The importance of memory in informed consent for surgical risk. *Medical Decision Making*, 21, 152–155. doi:10.1177/0272989X0102100209.

Reyna, V. F., & Lloyd, F. J. (2006). Physician decision making and cardiac risk: Effects of knowledge, risk perception, risk tolerance, and fuzzy processing. *Journal of Experimental Psychology*, 12(3), 179–195. doi:10.1037/1076-898X.12.3.179.

Reyna, V. F., & Mills, B. A. (2007a). Converging evidence supports fuzzy-trace theory's nested sets hypothesis (but not the frequency hypothesis). *Behavioral and Brain Sciences*, 30(3), 278–280. doi:10.1017/S0140525X07001872.

Reyna, V. F., & Mills, B. A. (2007b). Interference processes in fuzzy-trace theory: Aging, Alzheimer's disease, and development. In: D. Gorfein & C. MacLeod (Eds.), *Inhibition in Cognition*. Washington, DC: American Psychology Association; pp. 185–210.

Reyna, V. F., & Rivers, S. E. (2008). Current theories of risk and rational decision making. *Developmental Review*, 28(1), 1–11. doi:10.1016/j.dr.2008.01.002.

Reyna, V. F., Brainerd, C. J., Effken, J., Bootzin, R., & Lloyd, F. J. (2001). The psychology of human computer mismatches. In: C. Wolfe (Ed.), *Learning and Teaching on the World Wide Web*. San Diego, CA: Academic Press; pp. 23–44.

Reyna, V. F., Lloyd, F., & Whalen, P. (2001). Genetic testing and medical decision making. *Archives of Internal Medicine*, 161(20), 2406–2408. doi:10.1001/archinte.161.20.2406.

Reyna, V. F., Holliday, R. E., & Marche, T. (2002). Explaining the development of false memories. (Invited article on developmental forensics for a special issue.) *Developmental Review*, 22(3), 436–489. doi:10.1016/S0273-2297(02)00003-5.

Reyna, V. F., Lloyd, F. J., & Brainerd, C. J. (2003). Memory, development, and rationality: An integrative theory of judgment and decision-making. In: S. Schneider & J. Shanteau (Eds.), *Emerging Perspectives on Judgment and Decision Research*. New York: Cambridge University Press; pp. 201–245.

Reyna, V. F., Nelson, W., Han, P., & Dieckmann, N. F. (2009). How numeracy influences risk comprehension and medical decision making. *Psychological Bulletin*, 135, 943–973. doi:10.1037/a0017327.

Reyna, V. F., Estrada, S. M., DeMarinis, J. A., Myers, R. M., Stanisz, J. M., & Mills, B. A. (2011). Neurobiological and memory models of risky decision making in adolescents versus young adults. *Journal of Experimental Psychology: Learning, Memory, and Cognition*, 37(5), 1125–1142. doi:10.1037/a0023943.

Reyna, V. F., Nelson, W., Han, P., & Pignone, M. P. (2012). Decision making and cancer. Manuscript submitted for publication.

Rivers, S. E., Reyna, V. F., & Mills, B. A. (2008). Risk taking under the influence: A fuzzy-trace theory of emotion in adolescence. *Developmental Review*, 28, 107–144. doi:10.1016/j.dr.2007.11.002.

Schapira, M. M., Davids, S. L., McAuliffe, T. L., & Nattinger, A. B. (2004). Agreement between scales in the measurement of breast cancer risk perceptions. *Risk Analysis*, 24, 665–673. doi:10.1111/j.0272-4332.2004.00466.x.

Schapira, M. M., Fletcher, K. E., Ganschow, P. S., Walker, C. M., Tyler, B., Del Pozo, S., et al. (2011). The meaning of numbers in health: exploring health numeracy in a Mexican-American population. *Journal of General Internal Medicine*, 26(7), 705–711. doi:10.1007/s11606-011-1645-5.

Schwartz, L. M., Woloshin, S., & Welch, H. G. (2009). Using a drug facts box to communicate drug benefits and harms: Two randomized trials. *Annals of Internal Medicine*, 150(8), 516–527. Retrieved from www.annals.org

Shiloh, S., Salton, E., & Sharabi, D. (2002). Individual differences in rational and intuitive thinking styles as predictors of heuristic responses and framing effects. *Personality and Individual Differences*, 32(3), 415–429. doi:10.1016/S0191-8869(01)00034-4.

Siegler, R. S., & Booth, J. L. (2004). Development of numerical estimation in young children. *Child Development*, 75(2), 428–444. doi:0009-3920/2004/7502-0013.

Siegler, R. S., & Opfer, J. E. (2003). The development of numerical estimation: Evidence for multiple representations of numerical quantity. *Psychological Science*, 14, 237–243. doi:10.1111/1467-9280.02438.

Siegler, R. S., Thompson, C. A., & Opfer, J. E. (2009). The logarithmic-to-linear shift: One learning sequence, many tasks, many time scales. *Mind, Brain, and Education*, 3, 143–150. doi:10.1111/j.1751-228X.2009.01064.x.

Siegler, R. S., Thompson, C. A., & Schneider, M. (2011). An integrated theory of whole number and fractions development. *Cognitive Psychology*, 62, 273–296. doi:10.1016/j.cogpsych.2011.03.001.

Sloman, S. A. (1996). The empirical case for two systems of reasoning. *Psychological Bulletin*, 119, 3–22. doi:10.1.1.130.7987.

Sloman, S. A., Over, D. E., Slovak, L., & Stibel, J. M. (2003). Frequency illusions and other fallacies. *Organizational Behavior and Human Decision Processes*, 91, 296–309. doi:10.1016/S0749-5978(03)00021-9.

Slovic, P., Finucane, M. L., Peters, E., & MacGregor, D. G. (2004). Risk as analysis and risk as feelings: Some thoughts about affect, reason, risk, and rationality. *Risk Analysis*, 24, 311–322. doi:0272-4332/04/0100-0001.

Stanovich, K. E. (1999). *Who is Rational? Studies of Individual Differences in Reasoning*. Mahwah, NJ: Erlbaum.

Stanovich, K. E., & West, R. F. (2008). On the relative independence of thinking biases and cognitive ability. *Journal of Personality and Social Psychology*, 94, 672–695. doi:10.1037/0022-3514.94.4.672.

Stanovich, K. E., West, R. F., & Toplak, M. E. (2011). The complexity of developmental predictions from dual process models. *Developmental Review*, 31, 103–118. doi:10.1016/j.dr.2011.07.003.

Stone, E. R., Yates, J. F., & Parker, A. M. (1994). Risk communication: Absolute versus relative expressions of low-probability risks. *Organizational Behavior and Human Decision Processes*, 60(3), 387–408. doi:10.1006/obhd.1994.1091.

Stone, E. R., Sieck, W. R., Bull, B. E., Yates, J. F., Parks, S. C., & Rush, C. J. (2003). Foreground: background salience: Explaining the effects of graphical displays on risk avoidance. *Organizational Behavior and Human Decision Processes*, 90(1), 19–36. doi:10.1016/S0749-5978(03)00003-7.

Szrek, H., & Bundorf, M. K. (2011). Age and the purchase of prescription drug insurance by older adults. *Psychology and Aging*, 26(2), 308–320. doi:10.1037/a0023169.

Tait, A. R., Zikmund-Fisher, B. J., Fagerlin, A., & Voepel-Lewis, T. (2010a). The effect of different risk/benefit trade-offs on parents' understanding of a pediatric research study. *Pediatrics*, 125(6), e1475–e1482. doi:10.1542/peds.2009-1796.

Tait, A. R., Voepel-Lewis, T., Zikmund-Fisher, B. J., & Fagerlin, A. (2010b). The effect of format on parents' understanding of the risks and benefits of clinical research: A comparison between text, tables, and graphics. *Journal of Health Communication: International Perspectives*, 15(5), 487–501. doi:10.1080/10810730.2010.492560.

Tanius, B. E., Wood, S., Hanoch, Y., & Rice, T. (2009). Aging and choice: Applications to Medicare Part D. *Judgment and Decision Making*, 4, 92–101. Retrieved from journal.sjdm.org/81017/jdm81017.html

Thompson, C. A., & Siegler, R. S. (2010). Linear numerical-magnitude representations aid children's memory for numbers. *Psychological Science*, 21(9), 1274–1281. doi:10.1177/0956797610378309.

Tversky, A., & Kahneman, D. (1981). The framing of decisions and the psychology of choice. *Science*, 211(4481), 453–458. doi:0036-807518110130-0453$01.501.

Waters, E. A., Weinstein, N. D., Colditz, G. A., & Emmons, K. (2006). Formats for improving risk communication in medical tradeoff decisions. *Journal of Health Communication*, 11, 167–182. doi:10.1080/10810730500526695.

Wilhelms, E. A., & Reyna, V. F. (2013). Fuzzy trace theory and medical decisions by minors: Differences in reasoning between adolescents and adults. *Journal of Medicine and Philosophy*, 38(3), 268–282. doi:10.1093/jmp/jht018.

Windschitl, P. (2002). Judging the accuracy of a likelihood judgment: The case of smoking risk. *Journal of Behavioral Decision Making*, 15, 19–35. doi:10.1002/bdm.401.

Wolfe, C. R., & Reyna, V. F. (2010). Semantic coherence and fallacies in estimating joint probabilities. *Journal of Behavioral Decision Making*, 23(2), 203–223. doi:10.1002/bdm.650.

Wolfe, C. R., Fisher, C. R., & Reyna, V. R. (2013). Semantic coherence and inconsistency in estimating conditional probabilities. *Journal of Behavioral Decision Making*, 26(3), 237–246. doi:10.1002/bdm.1756.

Wood, S. M. W., & Bechara, A. (2014). The neuroscience of dual (and triple) systems in decision making. In: V. Reyns & V. Zayas (Eds.), *The Neuroscience of*

Risky Decision Making (pp. 177–202). Washington, DC: American Psychological Association.

Wood, S., Hanoch, Y., Liu, P, Cummings, J., Bhattacharya, C., & Rice, T. (2011). Numeracy and Medicare Part D: The importance of choice and literacy for numbers in optimizing decision making for Medicare's prescription drug program. *Psychology and Aging*, 26(2), 295–307. doi:10.1037/a0022028.

Zikmund-Fisher, B. J., Witteman, H. O., Fuhrel-Forbis, A., Exe, N. L., Kahn, V. C., & Dickson, M. (2012). Animated graphics for comparing two risks: A cautionary tale. *Journal of Medical Internet Research*, 14(4), e106. doi:10.2196/jmir.2030.

11 Do the numbers help patients decide? Ethical and empirical challenges for evaluating the impact of quantitative information

Peter H. Schwartz

Introduction

Many experts recommend that patients facing complex medical decisions should be told the specific probability of important outcomes associated with each available option (General Medical Council, 1998; Gigerenzer & Edwards, 2003; Paling, 2003; Thornton et al., 2003; Barratt et al., 2004; Elwyn et al., 2006a, 2006b; Trevena et al., 2012). The "quantitative imperative," as I have called it (Schwartz, 2011), is particularly common in writing about decision aids, which aim to help patients make "preference-sensitive" choices, where there are multiple medically acceptable options and each carries important pros and cons (Stacey et al., 2012). For instance, the most widely accepted guidelines for the design and evaluation of decision aids recommend that those regarding screening tests should disclose the baseline risk (without screening), the risk reduction provided by undergoing the test, and the probability of false positives and false negatives (Elwyn et al., 2006a, 2006b; Trevena et al., 2012).

A few critics, including myself, have questioned the quantitative imperative and pointed to the lack of evidence for it (Schwartz, 2011; McDonald et al., 2011; Zikmund-Fisher, 2013). Advocates of the quantitative imperative have the reasonable concern that verbal descriptions of risk – using words like "rare" and "common" – do not provide specific enough information to allow adequately informed decisions (Mazur & Merz, 1994; Edwards et al., 2001). But there are also good reasons to think that providing extensive quantitative information may fail to help, or may even hurt, patient decision making. Data can be overwhelming and confusing to patients, especially those with limited numeracy: descriptions of probabilities, for

Thanks to Eric Meslin and Greg Sachs for extensive discussion and assistance for my work in this area. This work was supported in part by a career development award from the American Cancer Society (CCCDA-10-085-01) and the Indiana Clinical and Translational Sciences Institute (NIH/NCRR 1 ULTR001108-01).

instance, rely on complex mathematical notions such as frequencies and percentages that are adequately understood by a minority of the adult population (National Center for Education Statistics, 2003; Kutner et al., 2006). Even for numerate individuals, "heuristics and biases" in human thought can lead to irrational responses (Tversky & Kahneman, 1974; Baron, 2000; Reyna, 2004). Studies that have compared decision aids with numbers to those without have not found any convincing advantages. In the end, I believe, the quantitative imperative stems from ethical and conceptual assumptions that are deeply questionable (Schwartz, 2011, 2012).

In this chapter, I take a closer look at the ethical and conceptual basis for the quantitative imperative and then review the problems it faces. I also describe views of ethics and rationality that suggest that more information is not always better. Finally, I confront the very difficult question of where to go from here. It is natural to conclude that we need better research to identify the impact of quantitative information, to balance the quantitative imperative with the "experimental imperative," as one commentator has put it (Ubel, 2011). But looking to empirical testing for answers raises important practical and conceptual questions that I discuss here. We certainly need empirical research to help guide us, but we must maintain an acute sensitivity to the challenges involved in designing and interpreting studies in this area.

The quantitative imperative

In this section, I review the central bioethical principles and other assumptions that have led to the quantitative imperative.

Autonomy and informed decision making

A key principle of modern bioethics is *respect for autonomy*, often taken to mean that individuals should make self-directed, voluntary decisions about their medical care or about participating in research (Beauchamp & Childress, 2006). (This chapter will focus exclusively on the former area, involving medical care.) A closely related idea is that patients should provide *informed consent* to any significant medical intervention: individuals should be adequately informed to voluntarily approve or refuse any significant medical intervention (test or treatment), at least when they have the capacity to do this (Beauchamp & Childress, 2006).

Some have advocated moving from a focus on informed consent to *shared decision making*, emphasizing that patients will usually work closely with a healthcare provider in making decisions, and that the patient should be involved in choosing and exploring options, not just accepting or rejecting ones that are offered (Charles et al., 1997; Frosch & Kaplan, 1999; Murray et al., 2006). While some have taken shared decision making and informed consent to be competing models, they are more correctly seen as overlapping pictures: according to both, the patient must be adequately informed to participate or decide. This can be seen in the *informed decision-making* model, which applies to both. According to this model, patients should be aware of the need to make a decision, of the fact that they can choose, and should understand the benefits and risks of each option (Braddock et al., 1999, 2008).

The informed decision-making model fits with commonly accepted ideas about the roles of the healthcare provider and the patient in medical decision making (Katz, 2002; Veatch, 2009). The provider has specialized knowledge and experience in identifying the patient's medical condition and in identifying the possible risks and benefits of moving forward in various ways, including specific tests or treatments or doing nothing. She is the expert on the possible outcomes and the risks and benefits of each possible action. The patient, in contrast, is often ignorant of such facts but brings his preferences and desires to the conversation, and thus can interpret how good or bad different treatments or outcomes would be (Katz, 2002; Beauchamp & Childress, 2006; Veatch, 2009). For instance, a patient faced with the prospect of losing sensation in one finger of his left hand may see that as only moderately undesirable, while another patient (perhaps a surgeon or musician) might see it as a disaster. One person may see the necessary period of inactivity after a possible surgical procedure to be unacceptable, while another individual would welcome the break.

Provider and patient roles

From this perspective, the healthcare provider brings knowledge about the situation and options, and the patient brings his set of values and desires. Their conversation involves, optimally, the provider educating the patient about the risks and benefits of each option, while the patient considers these in light of his values, communicates those values to the provider, and participates in making a choice (Katz, 2002; Beauchamp & Childress, 2006; Veatch, 2009). The proponents of decision aids hope that these tools can help educate the patient and encourage him to reflect on his values and apply them effectively (Elwyn et al., 2006b; O'Connor, 2007; International Decision Aid Standards Collaboration, 2012; Stacey et al., 2012).

The process of decision making may be abbreviated in some situations, for instance if there is a single medical treatment that is clearly superior to doing nothing and to other treatments. For instance, if a person has been shot and needs emergency surgery as soon as possible to have any hope of surviving, an abbreviated discussion (if any) seems most appropriate (Whitney et al., 2004; Beauchamp & Childress, 2006). Even less emergent situations may similarly seem to require little discussion, as for a middle-aged patient who has bacterial pneumonia and will most likely recover easily on antibiotics but not without them (Whitney et al., 2004). Such medical interventions have been termed "effective" health services (O'Connor et al., 2003; Wennberg et al., 2004).

In "preference-sensitive" situations, in contrast, there is no clearly preferred medical test or treatment, and the desirability of the various outcomes depends on the opinion of individuals (O'Connor et al., 2003; Stacey et al., 2012). Treament of localized prostate cancer, for instance, is clearly preference sensitive since the acceptability of each option – including surgery, radiation, or "watchful waiting" – depends on the importance that the patient puts on eliminating the cancer, on the one hand, and on avoiding side effects of treatment such as incontinence and impotence, on the other hand (Lin et al., 2009; Barry, 2010; Davison & Breckon, 2011).

Whether a possible test or treatment should be considered an effective or preference-sensitive medical option can be controversial. For instance, the United States Preventive Services Task Force (USPSTF) recommends that women at average risk for breast cancer undergo mammograms for screening from ages 50 to 75, basically labeling it as an effective health service (USPSTF, 2009). But the USPSTF has also concluded that the benefits are small enough for women ages 40–49, and the risks of false positives, unnecessary biopsies, and unnecessary treatment are high enough, that the choice of screening in this age range is preference-sensitive (Mandelblatt et al., 2009; Nelson et al., 2009; USPSTF, 2009). Therefore, the USPSTF does not recommend mammograms for average risk women from ages 40–49, but instead recommends that each woman consider the risks and benefits and decide for herself (USPSTF, 2009). When the USPSTF published this conclusion in 2009, there was a firestorm of protest, with the USPSTF and its supporters facing critics who argued that the benefits for women ages 40–49 do outweigh the risks sufficiently to recommend mammography for all, i.e., that it is an "effective" health service (Kolata, 2009; Gemignani, 2010; Lyman, 2010; Petitti et al., 2010). The debate was (and is) as much about societal and ethical issues involved in determining when benefits sufficiently outweigh risks, and requires carefully interpreting research that estimates or measures risks and benefits.

Utilities

In preference-sensitive cases, especially, ethical decision making appears to require extensive disclosure and education. The healthcare provider cannot be expected to convey her entire understanding of the medical situation to the patient, since this might involve providing professional education and training. But she must convey enough information to allow an informed decision (Katz, 2002; Veatch, 2009). Even educating patients about prognosis (i.e., what will happen if no treatment is attempted) requires conveying a large amount of information, involving multiple possibilities that could occur over different time frames. Add then a range of possible tests and treatments, each with its own burdens, expense, risks, and benefits, and this adds up to a lot of information that is quite difficult to understand.

Consider the case of decision aids that are involved in educating patients about screening for breast cancer. "Getting breast cancer" or "dying of cancer" are key negative outcomes that screening can help protect against. But for patients to understand what such outcomes involve, it seems necessary to explain at least symptoms, prognosis, and availability and characteristics of available treatments such as surgery, chemotherapy, or radiation. Only by understanding such options can the patient develop a truly informed view of how important it is to avoid getting cancer. This education may also need to correct mistaken perceptions, for instance addressing the assumptions that cancer is always a death sentence or that chemotherapy always involves intractable nausea, vomiting, or hair loss.

Research and theories about decision making label the value or disvalue of an outcome its "utility," and assume that the same possible outcome can have different utilities for different patients. In medicine, a commonly used unit is the QALY, or the "quality adjusted life year," that ranges from 0 to 1, with "1" being a year with perfect health, and "0" being death (Brock, 1993). Living with a serious medical condition, such as a very painful knee, may get a rating of 0.9, while living with paraplegia (paralysis of the lower body) might be a 0.7. Researchers use various tools to measure QALY or other utility measures, which we will consider in some more depth below.

Probabilities and expected utility theory

For every medical decision, probabilities are central, including the chance of undesirable outcomes if nothing is done, how these probabilities might be reduced with a medical intervention, and the probability that the test or treatment will cause a problem of its own. One can describe the size of these probabilities by using words such as "often," "common," "rare," etc. but these terms are vague and can be variably interpreted or even disputed: Who decides that a bad outcome that occurs 1% of the time is "occasional," "rare," or "very unlikely?" (Mazur & Merz, 1994; Edwards et al., 2001; Lipkus, 2007; Trevena et al., 2006).

Better, it seems, to give the numbers, if they are known, and let the individual decide. The exact magnitude of relevant probabilities is increasingly known in many areas, perhaps especially in screening and prevention. And while healthcare providers may not have the time to convey such information in detail (Yarnall et al., 2003; Epstein et al., 2004), and may not even know the numbers or fully understand them (Hoffrage & Gigerenzer, 1998; Wegwarth et al., 2012), decision aids can be designed to present them. This leads directly to the idea that such probabilities should be disclosed, i.e., the quantitative imperative.

This emphasis on presenting numbers stems not just from the ethical theories listed above but also from normative accounts of decision making. According to these theories the optimal choice for an individual is the one that has the best chance of maximizing her happiness or the satisfaction of her desires (Resnik, 1987; Baron, 2000). Formal accounts call this "expected utility": when an action can lead to a range of possible outcomes, the expected utility for that action is the sum of the utilities of each of the possible outcomes, weighted by their probabilities of occurring (Resnik, 1987; Baron, 2000). This is calculated by multiplying, for each possible outcome, the utility of that outcome and the probability of its occurring, and then adding those results up. So, if an action has a 50% chance of producing a situation with utility of 0.9 and 50% chance of producing an outcome with utility 0.6, the expected utility of the choice is 0.75, i.e., $= (0.5 \times 0.9) + (0.5 \times 0.6)$. The rationally preferable action, then, is the one that is associated with the highest expected utility (Resnik, 1987).

Some theories of rationality emphasize, further, that what matters is not just whether the option with the highest expected utility was chosen, but whether the process of choosing one option involved calculating and evaluating the expected utilities of each option, in some way. This definition of rationality is common enough to be dubbed the Standard Picture by some (Samuels et al., 2004). And, according to the Standard Picture, helping a patient make a rational choice requires disclosing information that will allow calculation of the relevant utilities and probabilities, and thus directly yields the quantitative imperative.

In many ways, the Standard Picture, and the resulting focus on discovering and disclosing specific probabilities, reflects a tendency in Western thought to believe that behind the welter of complexity of the universe and human life are cold, hard numbers. This perspective can be seen in ancient Greece in the philosophy of Pythagorean thinkers (Russell, 1972). Western views of morality have also emphasized the importance of numbers and calculation, for example in Utilitarianism's claim that the morally preferable action is the one that maximizes the happiness (or utility) of the greatest number of people (Mill, 2002).

International Patient Decision Aids Standards (IPDAS)

The quantitative imperative can be seen in the writing of many experts and in prominent guidelines regarding decision aids. According to this position, patients should be given extensive quantitative information, if available, especially regarding the probability of positive and negative outcomes given each of the available choices (General Medical Council, 1998; Gigerenzer & Edwards, 2003; Paling, 2003; Thornton et al., 2003; Barratt et al., 2004; Elwyn et al., 2006a, 2006b; Trevena et al., 2012). In an early statement of this position, the United Kingdom's General Medical Council asserted that patients considering screening should be told, "the likelihood of positive/negative findings and possibility of false-positive/negative results" (General Medical Council, 1998).

The most widely used guidelines for the design and evaluation of decision aids – the International Patient Decision Aids Standards – clearly reflect the quantitative imperative (Elwyn et al., 2006a, 2006b; Trevena et al., 2012 – online supplementary material, table 2). To develop the guidelines, a group of researchers, practitioners, patients, and policy makers from 14 countries reviewed evidence summaries and then rated the importance of 80 criteria in 12 areas. Respondents learned the results of the first round of voting and then voted again, and criteria with the highest rankings were included in the final recommendations (Elwyn et al., 2006b – online supplementary material, table 2).

These recommendations include the requirement that decision aids disclose the specific chances of all positive and negative outcomes from a proposed medical test or treatment, use "event rates in a defined group of patients for a specific time," and, for screening tests, describe the chance of various outcomes in the treated (or screened) group and the untreated (or unscreened) group (Elwyn et al., 2006a, 2006b). For screening tests, the guidelines go on to claim, decision aids should disclose the probability of a patient receiving a "true positive, true negative, false-positive and false negative test result," as well as the "chance of disease being found with and without screening" (Elwyn et al., 2006a, 2006b). The Standards are currently being reviewed and updated (International Decision Aid Standards Collaboration, 2012), and a recent publication repeats the assertion that decision aids regarding screening tests should describe the baseline risk (without screening), the risk reduction provided, and the associated chance of false positives and false negatives (Trevena et al., 2012).

I will consider some important reasons for questioning these recommendations in the next section. But it is important to immediately recognize that there is little empirical evidence for them. A recent review of 86 trials involving decision aids found that just 16 tested decision aids present probabilities (Stacey et al., 2012). These studies found that patients who viewed probabilities were more likely to correctly answer questions regarding these probabilities (Stacey et al., 2012). But for 15 of these 16 studies, multiple other aspects of the decision aids were varied as well, not just the presentation of probabilities: many compared the decision aid containing quantitative information to a much simpler information packet or website. And thus differences in attitudes or behavior cannot be attributed to the quantitative information. The only randomized trial that varied just the presentation of quantitative information used scripts read to participants (an extremely simple decision aid) and only included elderly patients (Wolf & Schorling, 2000).

Given the paucity of evidence, it is reasonable to conclude that support for the quantitative imperative is motivated largely by ethical and conceptual beliefs, such as those described above. And thus the quantitative imperative is especially vulnerable to questions regarding this ethical and conceptual basis, which I review in the next section.

Problems with the quantitative imperative

As described in the Introduction, key questions about the quantitative imperative arise in part from evidence that many individuals have difficulty understanding and utilizing quantitative information. Deeper problems stem from contemporary theories regarding risk communication, rationality, and normative accounts of decision making. Finally, important attacks have been made on the ethical assumptions that helped generate the quantitative imperative. In this section, I review these challenges in that order.

Innumeracy

The first indication that something is seriously wrong with the quantitative imperative is evidence that many people have trouble understanding numbers and incorporating them into their decisions. As other chapters in this book have reviewed (see Chapters 2–4), many adults are innumerate, i.e., have limited ability to understand and apply quantitative information. About one-fifth of adults can only carry out basic activities in this realm, like counting, and another third can only perform simple operations, such as arithmetic (Kutner et al., 2006; National Center for Education Statistics, 2003). This means that more than half of adults do not have the ability to comprehend concepts such as percentages and frequencies that are central to stating and understanding probabilities.

Figures or graphs can be easier to understand than numbers (Gigerenzer & Edwards, 2003; Paling, 2003; Ancker et al., 2006), but such approaches are no cure-all. Studies have shown that people with limited numeracy have significant problems interpreting figures and graphs, especially ones that convey information about absolute risk and benefit (Ancker et al., 2006). In one study, patients with low numeracy who were given relatively simple graphic representations of risk levels were unable to distinguish which was higher and which was lower (Keller & Siegrist, 2009). Graphs showing data in terms of relative risk do better, but supporters of the quantitative imperative often also specify that such measures are inadequate for full disclosure (Skolbekken, 1998; Elwyn et al., 2006b).

The healthcare system could respond by identifying patients with limited numeracy and attempting to educate them. In one recent study, researchers showed that a primer could improve patients' performance on a test of numeracy, though the study did not measure impact on decision making in particular situations (Woloshin et al., 2007). Any educational initiative would require resources of time, effort, and expense for the healthcare system and providers, and thus would need to be evaluated based on its possible benefits and its cost. Such an evaluation requires us to clarify the possible benefits and to examine key ethical assumptions.

Heuristics and biases

Even for patients with adequate numeracy, heuristics and biases may lead to irrational responses to quantitative information, again as reviewed in other chapters in this book (see Chapters 4 and 7). Kahneman and Tversky initiated the search for such aspects of human thought by showing that people give more value to avoiding a loss than achieving a gain, even when the two are equivalent from the perspective of expected utility theory (Kahneman & Tversky, 1979). Since then, psychologists, economists, and others have identified many other heuristics and biases (Baron, 2000; Reyna, 2004).

Here are a few examples: "Denominator neglect" leads people to exaggerate small dangers, such as a risk that occurs five times per 1 000 000, due to focusing on the individuals who are negatively impacted, not the large group from which they were drawn (Reyna, 2004). "Optimism bias," in contrast, leads to underestimating the danger of a behavior (e.g., smoking) due to a belief that one will be in the group that is not harmed (Weinstein, 1980). The "availability heuristic" causes people to overestimate the importance of information that is easy to comprehend and that fits with examples they can bring to mind easily, even if they know that other information is more reliable (Tversky & Kahneman, 1973).

The existence of widespread heuristics and biases undermines the assumption that telling individuals about specific probabilities can only help and can't hurt decision making. For instance, if a person overestimates the risk associated with an outcome that occurs just five times per million, due to denominator neglect, then disclosing this risk may harm rather than support rational decision making.

Dual representation and gist

The existence of such heuristics and biases, and other research in psychology, economics, and other areas, has led some theorists to conclude that human reasoning involves two tracks related to risk, with the first containing a representation of the specific probability ("verbatim memory"), while the other holds a "fuzzy representation," sometimes called a "gist" (Reyna, 2004, 2008). For example, someone who learns that her risk of developing breast cancer is 13% will then also assign that risk a gist such as being significant, dangerous, or minimal. According to dual-representation models, gist impressions have more power than verbatim memory to influence opinions and actions (Reyna, 2004, 2008), suggesting that the impact of presenting specific numbers should be assessed at least in part on the impact on gist impression. Myriad emotional and cognitive factors may influence the formation of a gist impression, thus helping to explain at least some of the biases and heuristics of human thought (Reyna, 2004, 2008).

If we accept a dual representation model, then determining whether an individual has made an adequately informed decision involves much more than just whether they have learned the relevant probabilities: it involves whether they have developed an appropriate gist impression. For instance, a person may have a more appropriate gist impression of the chance of some negative outcome even though he has an inaccurate understanding of the specific probability. Consider a surgery that has a risk of mortality of 1%; a patient who believes that the risk is 0% is closer in a numerical sense than one who believes the risk is 5%. But the one who believes that the risk is 5% may have a more appropriate gist impression, understanding that there is a small chance of death, compared to the patient who believes that it is impossible (i.e., 0%) (Lloyd et al., 2001).

This sort of case has immediate implications for the ethics of disclosure, showing that more information is not always better (Schwartz, 2012). A patient may not know the specific risk of death during a procedure but have the gist impression that it is rare but possible. If telling that patient that the risk is 1% leads him to conclude that this outcome is really impossible, due to innumeracy or some heuristic or bias, then he may have developed a more accurate verbatim understanding of the risk but a less appropriate gist impression. In such a case, it seems preferable not to disclose the specific number.

Theories of rationality

The key question then becomes how to evaluate, for specific situations, whether disclosing a specific probability helps or hurts the formation of an individual's gist impression. And methods for determining this depend on what theory is used to evaluate the quality of decision making or the rationality of the decision. As described above, the Standard Picture evaluates decision making based on whether the individual calculated expected utilities for each option and chose the one that maximizes this quantity. But alternative conceptions of rationality, sometimes grouped together as "pragmatic" or "bounded rationality" theories, reject this approach and offer other methods for evaluating decisions (Gigerenzer et al., 2004; Samuels et al., 2004). (Note that such theories are often called "pragmatic," and I will use that term here, though these accounts are not directly linked to the philosophical theory of Pragmatism.)

According to some pragmatic theories, for instance, "what it is for a reasoning process to be a good one is for it to be an efficient means of attaining the pragmatic objective of satisfying one's personal goals and desires" (Samuels et al., 2004, p. 40). These theories look at the outcome rather than the process: Even if the individual's decision making did not involve evaluation of probabilities or utilities, it may be high quality as long as it does a good enough job, over time, of achieving his or her personal goals. Any process that can do this well enough, in the range of situations in which it is deployed, will be acceptable. The flexibility of pragmatic accounts is an attractive feature: why remain committed to the process of calculating expected utility if there are alternative processes that can reliably guide the individual to choices that will maximize utility (Baron, 2000; Samuels et al., 2004)?

In addition to the shift to evaluating outcomes rather than process, some pragmatic theories have also moved away from demanding maximization.

As Herbert Simon pointed out, it may be most rational to choose outcomes that are "good enough," if the process for doing so is reliable and efficient within constraints on time and energy (Simon, 1955). Simon labeled this "satisficing," in contrast to "maximizing" (Simon, 1956). More recently, Gerd Gigerenzer and others have pointed to processes that they dub "fast, frugal heuristics" and have defended accounts of rationality that give such processes high marks (Gigerenzer et al., 2004; Gigerenzer, 2008). An animal may choose to forage in a certain area when the food quality is high enough, rather than continuing to search for areas with even higher quality. Or, an animal may choose a certain mate that has some number of desirable characteristics, rather than search for others with potentially better characteristics. Similar processes may be at work in human choices about food and mates, and even in complex areas such as investing. In one study, for instance, ignoring a good deal of available information and just putting equal amounts of money in a range of available investments did better than strategies that examined a wide range of features and put more money in the most promising options (DeMiguel et al., 2009).

Such short cuts take advantage of the extensive uncertainty that pervades real-life decision making, the cost of extended decision-making processes, and the effectiveness of taking advantage of environmental regularities of various sorts (Gigerenzer, 2008). Such approaches get high ranks from pragmatic or bounded rationality theories. Shifting from the Standard Picture of rationality to a pragmatic account emphasizes that evaluating a decision is always an empirical question, as is evaluating the value or advisability of a disclosure of a certain sort. To put it another way, only careful research can determine whether telling individuals the specific probability of some outcome will help or hurt the formation of an appropriate gist impression. And the impact may well differ for different individuals.

Ethical views

Ethicists and others have also questioned some of the basic assumptions that led to the quantitative imperative, sometimes drawing on the developments described above in psychology, economics, and other fields. These critics have often argued against what they consider to be unreasonable standards for what patients should consider and understand before making a decision. Onora O'Neill points out that current regulations often require doctors to disclose information that many patients do not want and cannot understand, and argues that these rules undercut the quality of the doctor–patient relationship in important ways (O'Neill, 2002; Manson & O'Neill, 2007).

Carl Schneider (1998) has presented perhaps the most thoroughgoing criticism of the view that patients reflect on a large amount of information to make ethically acceptable choices. He argues for rejecting this approach – which he dubs "mandatory autonomy" – and for accepting that patients may often make a rational choice not to consider a large amount of information or to defer to the recommendation of a friend, family member, or trusted authority such as a doctor (Schneider, 1998).

Schneider begins by pointing out many studies that find that patients do not want to closely consider all the evidence and make a decision for themselves. Others have ascribed such desires to an irrational reversion by the ill to a childlike state or to learned helplessness, given the historical paternalism of medicine (Katz, 2002). But Schneider argues that such a choice may be perfectly rational. Patients may be ill and not want to spend the time attempting to understand complex data. Patients may find that such data or information bore them, or may distrust their own ability to weigh all the possible outcomes and probabilities objectively (Schneider, 1998). To support his view, Schneider points to some of the evidence discussed above, regarding numeracy, heuristics, and biases.

Finally, Schneider and others have argued that a patient may believe with good reason that his healthcare provider can intuit his relevant desires and preferences and may assign utilities to the various outcomes much as the patient would (Schneider, 1998; Groll, 2011). Further, Schneider and others have pointed to evidence that individuals' understanding of their own preferences and desires is often unclear and changeable and thus fallible as a guide for decision making (Schneider, 1998; Nelson et al., 2007).

These considerations undermine the argument considered above that patients must participate extensively in medical decision making since they are the only ones who can say what their values are. According to that model, patients bring their preferences and desires, and providers bring understanding of probabilities and outcomes (Katz, 2002; Veatch, 2009). But if a patient may rationally conclude that the doctor's guesses about his key values or preferences are as good as the patient's own, then the patient may choose to follow the doctor's recommendation, which is based largely on his superior understanding of the medical situation.

The conclusion of all these arguments, stemming largely from Schneider and O'Neill, is not that patients should not participate in decision making, but rather that the level of participation should be up to the patient, and that a patient may rationally choose not to consider extensive amounts of information when making a decision or accepting a recommendation.

Others have built on these conclusions to recommend new approaches to disclosure and expectations for the participation of patients in decision making. Simon Whitney has argued that such expectations should vary based on the sort of medical situation involved and the choices available (Whitney, 2003; Whitney et al., 2004). When there is relatively low risk and relatively high certainty of benefit from an offered medical intervention, then it may make sense to accept minimal involvement of the patient. In such settings, Whitney argues, there is little chance that the patient's particular preferences or desires will change the conclusion about what should be done, and little reason to fear the impact of making an erroneous conclusion. In contrast, in situations where there is great uncertainty about the benefit of the intervention, and where there is high risk, there is reason for a more extended process of discussion and shared decision making (Whitney, 2003; Whitney et al., 2004).

The arguments made by O'Neill, Schneider, and Whitney provide a deeper understanding of the weaknesses of the quantitative imperative, especially applied to the use of decision aids in preventive settings such as decisions about mammograms. Screening tests carry relatively low risk, and tests that are recommended by multiple national organizations have clear benefits that seem to outweigh small risks. In such situations, patients may understandably choose not to view quantitative data, and simply follow the recommendation of such organizations.

In some cases, though, there may be no clear recommendation, or organizations issuing guidelines may disagree, as for the question of whether women aged 40–49 should undergo mammography. In such cases, one may still conclude that a patient can choose to simply follow the recommendation of their provider or another trusted individual. Or she may view some limited information about risks and benefits, such as a verbal description.

In such situations there seems to be no ethical requirement for all patients to view the sorts of extensive presentations of data advocated by the quantitative imperative. Instead, decision aids could be designed to provide limited quantitative information, or perhaps just a verbal description of risk and benefit, and then offer patients the option of viewing more data of various sorts. The key question becomes what quantitative information, if any, should be presented to all patients, and how any additional information should be offered. What determines the line between information (verbal or quantitative) that is rightly part of minimal disclosure given to all, and information that is truly optional?

The answer in particular situations will depend on tests of how particular data affects patient opinions and decision making, but also requires careful application of ethical principles, as I describe in the next two sections.

Measuring and evaluating the impact of quantitative information

The challenge

As we have seen above, pragmatic accounts of rationality imply that little can be assumed about the value of a particular disclosure, without empirically measuring the effect. According to pragmatic accounts of rationality, the key test is whether the disclosure increases the chance that individuals will achieve their personal goals and desires (Baron, 2000; Samuels et al., 2004). It turns out that designing research to determine whether a disclosure has this effect is quite challenging.

Consider the following case. Women generally overestimate their lifetime risk of developing breast cancer: studies have found that women with average risk will estimate that their chance is as high as 41% when in fact it is just about 13% (Zikmund-Fisher et al., 2010). Telling women that the risk is actually 13% will lead many women to conclude that their risk of breast cancer is "low," and some studies have shown that disclosing absolute risk in this way can reduce interest in getting mammograms (Schwartz et al., 1999; Zikmund-Fisher et al., 2010).

But is this change in gist appropriate or not? On the one hand, it seems to represent a sensible response to an important fact, i.e., that a lower percentage of women get breast cancer than might be assumed. On the other hand, the conclusion that the risk is low and that mammography may not be worthwhile could reflect the optimism bias, i.e., an irrational underestimation of the chance of being in the affected group. The key challenge is to determine what sort of research could distinguish between these possibilities.

Consider another example, also involving mammography. As described above, for average risk women, getting mammograms regularly reduces the lifetime risk of *dying* of breast cancer from 3.8% (38 per 1000), with no screening, to 3.2% (32 per 1000), with regular mammograms and follow up care (Mandelblatt et al., 2009). Women who view such data, presented perhaps with a natural frequency presentation and icon chart, could develop the gist impression that mammograms are not very good, or that they do not significantly reduce risk. And this could be seen as a rational conclusion: mammograms save just 0.6% of women (6 per 1000), which is roughly one-sixth of the women who will die of breast cancer if they are never screened.

At the same time, the gist impression could reflect an irrational under appreciation of a very real risk reduction. Six women per 1000 is equivalent to 300 people in a stadium of 50 000, and it is 6000 women per million. On the one hand, one might argue that these ways of describing the risk reduction could help women better understand the benefit of mammography. On the other hand, one might argue that such presentations are misleading and manipulative, exaggerating the risk reduction due to denominator neglect (women will focus on the 6000 who are saved and ignore the one million women who had to be screened). In the end, it is extremely challenging to determine if the gist impression that results from disclosing quantitative information is appropriate and helpful in the individual achieving her goals, or not.

The relevance of expected utility

In response, one might attempt to measure possible outcomes in terms of expected utility. According to this approach, disclosures would be valuable if they encourage decisions that raise expected utility; and disclosures are questionable or unwise if they lead to decisions associated with reductions in expected utility.

Expected utility looks like a good yardstick especially since it provides one way of characterizing why, for two patients facing the same decision, one choice may be best for one of them and another choice may be best for the other. Two women considering mammography may be faced with the same risks and benefits: the same risk of getting breast cancer or dying from it if they are never screened, the same risk reduction provided by mammograms, and the same probability of negative outcomes from mammograms. Now imagine that the first of these women sees the prospect of getting an unnecessary biopsy – i.e., one that shows no cancer – as a very unfortunate outcome, with a large negative impact on her life, while the second sees it as just a mild annoyance. Because of this difference between them, the decision to get a mammogram may be utility maximizing for the second woman but not the first. From the perspective of a pragmatic account of rationality, a good disclosure would be one that helps the first to decide to get a mammogram and the second to decide not to do so.

To generalize, one might imagine that we could separate women into two groups: (1) those who are committed to avoiding advanced breast cancer at all costs and will accept the burdens and risks of mammography without concern, and (2) those who do not view breast cancer with the same dread and are less sanguine about the burdens and risks of mammography. Again, the differences in the utilities of the possible outcomes, for these two groups of women, may make the difference in whether it is rational for them to be screened. A possible disclosure of quantitative information might be best evaluated, from this perspective, by examining whether it leads to decisions that are associated with increased expected utility.

From this perspective, the key investigation will involve measurement of the utilities of possible outcomes for specific individuals. Some discussions of decision making refer to this as "value concordance" or "preference matching," i.e., measures of the degree to which decisions agree with the patient's values or best match their preferences (Michie et al., 2002; Sepucha et al., 2007; Sepucha & Ozanne, 2010).

Measuring expected utility or preference matching

Considering this possible approach requires further evaluation of the challenges of measuring utilities for individuals and groups. There are myriad approaches to measuring utilities, and a full review of these accounts and their strengths and weaknesses is beyond the scope of this chapter. In many of these methods healthy people are told about the medical condition in question and are asked to evaluate, using various methods, how much impact this condition would have on their life. In the *time tradeoff* method, individuals are asked whether they would accept a certain number of years in perfect health in exchange for 10 years with the health condition. In the *standard gamble* method, individuals are asked whether they would undergo a surgery (or other treatment) that would cure the condition but carries a certain risk of mortality.

Each of these approaches faces many critiques, including concerns about whether healthy subjects can assign an accurate utility to living with a certain disability or disease (Brock, 1993). For instance, people with paraplegia (paralysis of the lower half of the body), may give much higher ratings to their quality of life than do healthy individuals who are asked to imagine having this condition (Brock, 1993). Some have suggested that a better approach is to recruit participants who have the condition in question, but this raises problems of its own. People with a chronic condition may underestimate the negative impact it has on their life and opportunities, due to powerful coping mechanisms in the human mind, such as those that affect goals and perception of limitations (Brock, 1993).

One particular weakness of standard approaches to calculating expected utility is the difficulty of estimating the impact of an isolated event, rather than a more pervasive disease or disability. For instance, when considering a screening test such as mammography, how can a subject assign a utility to the value of a year of life in which one unnecessary biopsy occurs? Some research avoids these problems by using conjoint analysis or dual-choice experiments to measure impacts on utility (Ryan et al., 2001; Hol et al., 2010). In such studies, participants choose between two options in a series of imaginary cases where the characteristics of the two options vary along certain dimensions. By evaluating the response to this series of cases, researchers can estimate the utility of the different possible outcomes for those who respond.

But even such advanced techniques are problematic, since choosing which characteristics of the options to describe and vary and how to present the information may affect responses. In addition, such experiments often require participants to compare options based at least in part on differences in the probabilities of possible outcomes. For example, a participant may need to choose between (a) a pill that can cure the condition in 90% of cases but will cause a severe side effect in 2%, vs. (b) one that will cure the condition in 80% of cases but that causes the severe side effect in 1%. In such choices, irrational heuristics or biases regarding risk information and probabilities can play important roles in individuals' responses.

A key set of problems for all approaches involving measurement of expected utility is that they aim at identifying the "true preferences" of participants, and there are deep empirical and conceptual problems with this notion (Fischhoff, 1991; Nelson et al., 2007). Research in behavioral economics has shown that individuals are error-prone even when asked something relatively simple about their own preferences, such as how they will feel about a certain poster on their wall in the future (Nelson et al., 2007). People's predictions are even less reliable about how they would feel in situations that are more complex and difficult to imagine, such as given future medical outcomes or conditions. Critics have pointed out that such difficulties create questions about any approach to evaluating decisions based on preference matching (Nelson et al., 2007).

Describing outcomes

Another set of problems with identifying the utility that an individual assigns to a possible future outcome is the inherent vagueness and ambiguity of describing that possible outcome and of characterizing the probability of its having certain features (Resnik, 1987). For instance, the utility associated with an unnecessary biopsy will depend on many factors, including how well the anesthesia is applied and whether various complications occur. A full calculation of the expected utility associated with that biopsy for an individual must consider the utility and probability of many possibilities, and must make assumptions about specifics such as how well the anesthesia is performed and the skill of the surgeon.

But the mind boggles at the question of how to assign probabilities to such possibilities. The probabilities of the anesthesiologist and/or surgeon doing well or badly on a given day may depend on the time of day the procedure is done, the skill of support personnel, even the quality of the professionals' homelife and sleep the night before. To assume that each of these possibilities can be assigned a probability is to rely on a picture of the universe that brings to mind Laplace's "demon," an imaginary figure who can predict all future states of the universe based on current knowledge of the position and motion of every atom, combined with a deterministic physics.

In addition, for any individual, the utility associated with any possible outcome will depend at least in part on other aspects of her life at that time. How bad it would be for me to miss work for a biopsy, for instance, will depend in part on the status of various projects on which I am working, how understanding my boss is about the time off, how supportive my wife and family are, etc. Imagining that an unnecessary biopsy in the future has a specific utility, for me, requires imagining that each of these further possibilities can be assigned a probability of occurring at that time, again straining believability.

One might try to counter such complexities by asserting that while specific probabilities and utilities are unknowable, we can still rely on some sort of averaging process. But if no particular individual can reliably predict the utility or probability of future outcomes, then carrying out the exercise with large numbers of people will not necessarily improve reliability. And averaging over large groups undermines the goal of this process in the first place, which was to identify variability among the utilities for different individuals, to determine which available option has the highest overall expected utility for each person.

Of course, such challenges do not show that it is impossible to measure utilities and combine them with probabilities in ways that can estimate which decision is better for a given patient or group of patients. There may be situations where the utilities of the various outcomes are clear enough to make it obvious that one choice or another is superior. But the issues reviewed here suggest that any such process is fraught with uncertainty and possible confusion. These problems threaten any attempt to empirically define the quality of decision making in terms of whether a patient's choice fits his preferences.

Other measures

Some researchers avoid such difficulties by focusing on aspects of decision making that are easier to measure. For instance, many studies of decision aids have used the decision conflict scale, a 16-question instrument that measures respondent's feelings about a range of issues, including the extent of their knowledge of the options, their clarity on what matters most to them, and how supported they feel in making a choice. The decision conflict scale has well defined psychometric qualities and has been used in many studies of the impact of decision aids (O'Connor et al., 1998; O'Connor et al., 2002; O'Connor, 2005).

But the decision conflict scale focuses on just how patients feel and what they think, and thus is a process measure rather than an evaluation of the decision itself (Sepucha & Ozanne, 2010). As some critics have pointed out, possibly important disclosures may increase a patient's uncertainty and decrease his or her confidence in ways that could increase decision conflict, even though the disclosure results in a better comprehension of the pros and cons of the options (Nelson et al., 2007). In such cases, the results of the decision conflict scale, like other process measures, may fail to accurately measure the quality of decision making.

Determining what numbers to give

In this section, I will consider some possible ways to move forward in evaluating the value of disclosure of quantitative information. One key alternative to presenting extensive quantitative information to every patient is to give just verbal information (words only, without numbers), or very simple quantitative information, and then to offer additional data to those who want it. Considering this alternative – making complex data optional rather than standard – requires considering leading theories regarding the ethics of disclosure and what sort of empirical research might be relevant to comparing approaches.

The reasonable person standard

The *reasonable person standard* is the most widely accepted guideline among ethicists for what information should be standardly disclosed to patients about a medical intervention (a test, procedure, or treatment):

> "According to this standard, the information to be disclosed should be determined by reference to a hypothetical reasonable person. Whether information is pertinent or material is to be measured by the significance a reasonable person would attach to it in deciding whether to undergo [that intervention]." (Beauchamp & Childress, 2006, p. 123)

The reasonable person standard is more demanding than the traditional *professional practice standard*, which evaluates the quality of disclosure simply based on whether it matches that provided by other providers in region and specialty to patients in a similar situation (Beauchamp & Childress, 2006).

The professional practice standard is analogous to the methods used to define malpractice, evaluating whether care matched the "standard of care" provided by others. But many ethicists have critiqued the professional practice standard since it provides no way to critique levels of disclosure that may be common but are clearly inadequate (Beauchamp & Childress, 2006). Just because surgeons doing cosmetic surgery in some region generally fail to disclose the possibility of infection or unsightly results, that does not seem to make this failure of disclosure to be ethically acceptable.

At the same time, some have critiqued the reasonable person standard for relying on the idea of what a "reasonable" person would want (Katz, 2002). Instead, some have suggested that healthcare providers should be expected "to disclose the information a particular patient needs to know, if it is reasonable to expect the physician to know that patient's informational needs" (Beauchamp & Childress, 2006, p. 123). But while this *subjective standard* has certain advantages, it can be critiqued for making the physician's obligation depend on any whim of the patient, as long as the whim is made known. For instance, if a patient wants to know the name of the person who bottled the medication he is being offered, and that patient makes his desire known to the physician, it looks like the subjective standard makes disclosure of this data ethically required. A way to block this *reductio ad absurdia* would be to claim that even though the information is desired, it is not part of the patient's "informational needs." But the subjective standard does not provide a clear way to define such needs.

In contrast, the reasonable person standard explains why provider behavior or patients' iconoclastic requests do not, by themselves, define what is required for disclosure. The reasonable person standard is widely favored by ethicists and has been adopted by at least some courts (Beauchamp & Childress, 2006). In the next two sections, I examine how to apply this standard to questions about disclosure of quantitative information.

Asking about significance

Consider the following relatively straightforward case of applying the reasonable person standard. Patients considering undergoing colonoscopy for screening for colorectal cancer should presumably be told about the small risk of perforation of the colon. Disclosing this risk is expected since a reasonable person would find it pertinent to a decision about whether to proceed. In contrast, imagine that 3 days after the colonoscopy some patients will have a few small twinges of discomfort. If this complication is small enough and rare enough, one might argue that it can be left off the list of dangers of the procedure; a reasonable person would not find it significant for the decision about getting this procedure.

Determining the potential significance of a risk clearly involves judgments of the impact on utility as well as its likelihood. Even when a potential outcome is minor, if it occurs often enough, it may rise to the level of significance for a reasonable patient. Similarly, a possible outcome that would carry moderate levels of morbidity might not necessarily be part of standard disclosure if it is rare enough (e.g., one in 10 million). The relevance of both impact on utility and probability makes sense in terms of the theory of expected utility, as discussed above.

Of course many possible disclosures will fall in a gray zone, where it is unclear whether the risks would be significant to a reasonable person. If a certain preparation for colonoscopy carries a 1 in 10 000 risk of causing abnormalities in kidney function that would not require hospitalization but would need to be monitored for some time, should this danger be part of standard disclosure? There is no easy way to answer such questions: the reasonable person standard provides a framework but leaves a good deal of ambiguity, especially because of the reliance on concepts of *significance* and *reasonable* person.

In these sorts of cases, it seems that empirical research could help inform the application of the reasonable person standard. In the case introduced in the last paragraph, laypeople could be told the risks of colorectal cancer, the advantages of screening, and any risks of the procedure that are clearly part of minimal disclosure. Then, they could be told the additional fact, in this case the risk of transient kidney abnormalities, and asked whether they think it is significant. Averaging over many responses, one might hope to discern a "reasonable" opinion.

One limitation of this sort of study is the danger that people will respond with a bias towards requiring disclosure: in a certain frame of mind, every possible negative outcome can seem relevant to decision making, even though the impact and probability are very low. This can be seen as a form of the availability heuristic, described above: when asked to consider a particular fact, that fact will acquire a certain importance in people's minds (Tversky & Kahneman, 1973). One way to combat this danger would be to ask respondents in this sort of study to rate the importance of all the possible negative consequences, including the one that is being investigated. Negative consequences with the highest ratings should be disclosed to all patients, while risks with low enough ratings might not be part of minimal disclosure.

Measuring impact

Another limitation of studies where people are asked about the importance of information to them is that they may be poor predictors of the influence that potential disclosures would have on their behavior. For instance, individuals may think that a fact is not significant even though it would actually change their beliefs or behavior in important ways. Or they may say that a fact is important, though it would actually have limited impact. This suggests that attempting to apply the reasonable person standard may also draw on the sort of research described above for evaluating the quality of decision making, which directly measures how people respond to information, rather than asking them how they think they would respond.

We could conduct a study of this type by enrolling typical patients and providing all with standard information about risks and benefits (i.e., the disclosure currently required for informed consent), and then randomizing the patients to two groups, only one of which views the additional disclosure. Patients in the two arms would then be compared in terms of their understanding (including gist impression), decision making, and eventual action. This sort of study also avoids the ambiguity inherent in asking individuals about levels of significance.

Despite these advantages, though, this sort of study would also face many of the challenges identified above, especially involved in measuring the quality of decisions. Perhaps the most significant possible result would be finding that disclosing the additional information has no significant overall impact on patients' gist impression, decision making, or action. Given such a result, one might argue that the additional disclosure does not appear "significant," and thus should be seen as failing to meet the reasonable person standard. A different interpretation is also possible, however: even if a disclosure had no *overall* impact, it may have had an impact for at least some *individuals* or *subgroups*. Perhaps for some individuals, the disclosure led to a change in gist impression, decision making, and/or action that favored one choice, while for others the disclosure led to opposite changes in gist impression, decision making, and action that favored a different choice. Such changes could cancel each other out in measuring overall impact, even though the information was influential for both types of individuals.

Consider a different possible result of the research study, where disclosure is associated with an overall change in gist impression, decision making, or action. Given such a result, one must go further to evaluate whether these changes reflected improved quality of decision making or not, raising all the complex issues considered above.

In the end, even given the best sort of empirical research, there will be significant difficulties with drawing clear conclusions about whether and how quantitative information should be presented or offered. We need to conduct empirical research, but the design of studies and interpretation of results are both open to significant disagreement.

Conclusion

I have argued that the quantitative imperative depends on questionable ethical and conceptual assumptions and is not supported by empirical evidence. An important alternative to the current recommendation that decision aids should present extensive quantitative information to all patients is instead to design decision aids to present verbal descriptions of probabilities or simpler data and make more extensive quantitative information optional, for patients who wish to view it. While various types of empirical studies could be helpful in evaluating these two approaches in specific situations, there are significant challenges to designing and interpreting such research. Any proposal about how decision aids, or providers, should present quantitative information to patients facing preference-sensitive decisions will raise important ethical questions about how much information is necessary for truly informed consent or adequate shared decision making. Determining how best to use decision aids to support truly patient-centered care will not only require additional empirical research, but also a robust discussion among patients, providers, and experts in decision science.

References

Ancker, J. S., Senathirajah, Y., Kukafka, R., & Starren, J. B. (2006). Design features of graphs in health risk communication: a systematic review. *Journal of American Medical Information Association*, 13(6), 608–618.

Baron, J. (2000). *Thinking and Deciding* (3rd edn.). Cambridge: Cambridge University Press.

Barratt, Al., Trevena, L., Davey, H. M., & McCaffery, K. (2004). Use of decision aids to support informed choices about screening. *BMJ*, 329(7464), 507–510.

Barry, M. J. (2010). The prostate cancer treatment bazaar. *Archives of Internal Medicine*, 170(5), 450–452.

Beauchamp, T. L., & Childress, J. F. (2006). *Principles of Biomedical Ethics* (6th edn.). Oxford: Oxford University Press.

Braddock III, C., Edwards, K. A., Hasenberg, N. M., Laidley, T. L., & Levinson, W. (1999). Informed decision making in outpatient practice: Time to get back to basics. *JAMA*, 282(24), 2313–2320.

Braddock III, C., Hudak, P. L., Feldman, J. J., Bereknyei, S., Frankel, M., & Levinson, W. (2008). "Surgery is certainly one good option": Quality and time-efficiency of informed decision-making in surgery. *Journal of Bone and Joint Surgery American*, 90(9), 1830–1838.

Brock, D. W. (1993). Ethical issues in the use of cost-effectiveness analysis for the prioritization of health care resources. In: R. B. T. Tan-Torres Edejer, T. Adam, R. Hutubessy, A. Achary, D. B. Evans, and C. J. L. Murray (Eds.), *Making Choices in Health: WHO Guide to Cost-Effectiveness Analysis*. Geneva: World Health Organization; pp. 289–312.

Charles, C., Gafni, A., & Whelan, T. (1997). Shared decision-making in the medical encounter: what does it mean? (or it takes at least two to tango). *Social Science and Medicine*, 44(5), 681–692.

DeMiguel, V., Garlappi, L., & Uppal, R. (2009). Optimal versus naive diversification: how inefficient is the 1/n portfolio strategy? *The Review of Financial Studies*, 22(5), 1915–1953.

Edwards, A., Elwyn, G., Covey, J., Matthews, E., & Pill, R. (2001). Presenting risk information: a review of the effects of "framing" and other manipulations on patient outcomes. *Journal of Health Communication*, 6(1), 61–82.

Elwyn, G., O'Connor, A., Stacey, D., Volk, R., Edwards, A., Coulter, A., & The International Patient Decision Aids Standards Collaboration. (2006a). Additional Information – Developing a quality criteria framework for patient decision aids: online international Delphi consensus process. *BMJ*. Retrieved from http://www.bmj.com/content/suppl/2006/09/08/bmj.38926.629329.AE.DC1/elwg351536.www.pdf

Elwyn, G., O'Connor, A., Stacey, D., Volk, R., Edwards, A., Coulter, A., & The International Patient Decision Aids Standards Collaboration. (2006b). Developing a quality criteria framework for patient decision aids: online international Delphi consensus process. *BMJ*, 333(7565), 417.

Epstein, R. M., Alper, B. S., & Quill, T. E. (2004). Communicating evidence for participatory decision making. *JAMA*, 291(19), 2359–2366.

Fischhoff, B. (1991). Value elicitation: Is there anything in there? *American Psychologist*, 46(8), 835–847.

Frosch, D. L., & Kaplan, R. M. (1999). Shared decision making in clinical medicine: Past research and future directions. *American Journal of Preventive Medicine*, 17(4), 285–294.

Gemignani, M. L. (2010). The new mammographic screening guidelines: what were they thinking? *Obstetrics and Gynecology*, 115(3), 484–486.

General Medical Council. (1998). *Seeking Patients' Consent: The Ethical Considerations*. London: General Medical Council.

Gigerenzer, G. (2008). Why heuristics work. *Perspectives on Psychological Science*, 3(1), 20–29.

Gigerenzer, G, & Edwards, A. (2003). Simple tools for understanding risks: from innumeracy to insight. *BMJ*, 327(7417), 741–744.

Gigerenzer, G., Czerlinski, J., & Martingnon, L. (2004). How good are fast and frugal heuristics? In: I. Niiniluoto, M. Sintonen, & J. Wolenski (Eds.), *Handbook of Epistemology*. Dordrecht, Netherlands: Kluwer Academic Publishers; pp. 148–173.

Groll, D. (2011). What health care providers know: a taxonomy of clinical disagreements. *Hastings Center Report*, 41(5), 27–36.

Hoffrage, U., & Gigerenzer, G. (1998). Using natural frequencies to improve diagnostic inferences. *Academic Medicine*, 73(5), 538–540.

Hol, L., de Bekker-Grob, E. W., van Dam, L., Donkers, B., Kuipers, E. J., Habbema, J. D., et al. (2010). Preferences for colorectal cancer screening strategies: a discrete choice experiment. *British Journal of Cancer*, 102(6), 972–980.

International Decision Aid Standards (IPDAS) Collaboration. (2012). International Decision Aid Standards (IPDAS) Collaboration – Resources. December 10, 2012. Retrieved April 10, 2013, from ipdas.ohri.ca/resources.html

Kahneman, D., & Tversky, A. (1979). Prospect Theory: An analysis of decision under risk. *Econometrica: Journal of the Econometric Society*, 47(2), 263–292.

Katz, J. (2002). *The Silent World of Doctor and Patient* (Reprinted from 1984 edition, with a new foreward by A. M. Capron, ed.). Baltimore: Johns Hopkins University Press.

Keller, C., & Siegrist, M. (2009). Effect of risk communication formats on risk perception depending on numeracy. *Medical Decision Making*, 29(4), 483–490.

Kolata, G. (2009). Mammogram debate took group by surprise. *The New York Times*, November 20, 2009, p. A16.

Kutner, M., Greenberg, E., Jin, Y., & Paulsen, C. (2006). *The health literacy of America's adults: Results From the 2003 National Assessment of Adult Literacy: US Department of Education (NCES 2006–483)*. Washington, DC: National Center for Education. Available at: http://files.eric.ed.gov/fulltext/ED493284.pdf (retrieved December 8, 2013).

Lin, G. A., Aaronson, D. S., Knight, S. J., Carroll, P. R., & Dudley, R. A. (2009). Patient decision aids for prostate cancer treatment: A systematic review of the literature. *CA: A Cancer Journal for Clinicians*, 59(6), 379–390.

Lipkus, I. M. (2007). Numeric, verbal, and visual formats of conveying health risks: Suggested best practices and future recommendations. *Medical Decision Making*, 27(5), 696–713.

Lloyd, A., Hayes, P., Bell, P. R. F., & Naylor, A. R. (2001). The role of risk and benefit perception in informed consent for surgery. *Medical Decision Making*, 21(2), 141–149.

Lyman, G. H. (2010). Breast cancer screening: science, society and common sense. *Cancer Invest*, 28(1), 1–6.

Mandelblatt, J. S., Cronin, K. A., Bailey, S., Berry, D. A., de Koning, H. J., Draisma, G., et al. (2009). Effects of mammography screening under different screening schedules: Model estimates of potential benefits and harms. *Annals of Internal Medicine*, 151(10), 738–747.

Manson, N. C., & O'Neill, O. (2007). *Rethinking Informed Consent in Bioethics*. Cambridge: Cambridge University Press.

Mazur, D. J., & Merz, J. F. (1994). Patients' interpretations of verbal expressions of probability: implications for securing informed consent to medical interventions. *Behavioral Sciences and Law*, 12(4), 417–426.

McDonald, H., Charles, C., & Gafni, A. (2011). Assessing the conceptual clarity and evidence base of quality criteria/standards developed for evaluating decision aids. *Health Expectations* (first published online 11/3/2011). Available at http://onlinelibrary.wiley.com/doi/10.1111/j.1369-7625.2011.00740.x/abstract;jsessionid=07B5267B858E333CF6BAFCCC5618EBBC.f01t02?deniedAccessCustomisedMessage=&userIsAuthenticated=false (accessed December 9, 2013).

Michie, S., Dormandy, E., & Marteau, T. A. (2002). The multi-dimensional measure of informed choice: a validation study. *Patient Education and Counseling*, 48(1), 87–91.

Mill, J. S. (2002). *Utilitarianism* (2nd edn.). Indianapolis, IN: Hackett Publishing Company.

Murray, E., Charles, C., & Gafni, A. (2006). Shared decision-making in primary care: Tailoring the Charles et al. model to fit the context of general practice. *Patient Education and Counseling*, 62(2), 205–211.

National Center for Education Statistics. (2003). National Assessment of Adult Literacy (NAAL): Key findings: Demographics: Overall. Retrieved April 10, 2013, from nces.ed.gov/naal/kf_demographics.asp

Nelson, H. D., Tyne, K., Naik, A., Bougatsos, C., Chan, B. K., & Humphrey, L. (2009). Screening for breast cancer: an update for the U.S. Preventive Services Task Force. *Annals of Internal Medicine*, 151(10), 727–737, W237–742.

Nelson, W. L., Han, P. K., Fagerlin, A., Stefanek, M., & Ubel, P. A. (2007). Rethinking the objectives of decision aids: a call for conceptual clarity. *Medical Decision Making*, 27(5), 609–618.

O'Connor, A. M. (2005). User Manual – Decision Conflict Scale. Retrieved April 10, 2013, from decisionaid.ohri.ca/docs/develop/User_Manuals/UM_Decisional_Conflict.pdf

O'Connor, A. M. (2007). Using decision aids to help patients navigate the "grey zone" of medical decision-making. *CMAJ*, 176(11), 1597–1598.

O'Connor, A. M., Tugwell, P., Wells, G. A., Elmslie, T., Jolly, E., Hollingworth, G., et al. (1998). Randomized trial of a portable, self-administered decision aid for postmenopausal women considering long-term preventive hormone therapy. *Medical Decision Making*, 18(3), 295–303.

O'Connor, A. M., Jacobsen, M. J., & Stacey, D. (2002). An evidence-based approach to managing women's decisional conflict. *Journal of Obstetric, Gynecologic and Neonatal Nursing*, 31(5), 570–581.

O'Connor, A. M., Legare, F., & Stacey, D. (2003). Risk communication in practice: The contribution of decision aids. *BMJ*, 327(7417), 736–740.

O'Neill, O. (2002). *Autonomy and Trust in Bioethics*. Cambridge: Cambridge University Press.

Paling, J. (2003). Strategies to help patients understand risks. *BMJ*, 327(7417), 745–748.

Petitti, D. B., Calonge, N., LeFevre, M. L., Melnyk, B. M., Wilt, T. J., & Schwartz, J. S. (2010). Breast cancer screening: From science to recommendation. *Radiology*, 256(1), 8–14.

Resnik, M. D. (1987). *Choices: An Introduction to Decision Theory*. Minneapolis: University of Minneapolis Press.

Reyna, V. F. (2004). How people make decisions that involve risk. A dual-processes approach. *Current Directions in Psychological Science*, 13(2), 60–66.

Reyna, V. F. (2008). A theory of medical decision making and health: Fuzzy trace theory. *Medical Decision Making*, 28(6), 850–865.

Russell, B. (1972). *A History of Western Philosophy*. New York: Simon & Schuster, Inc.

Ryan, M., Bate, A., Eastmond, C. J., & Ludbrook, A. (2001). Use of discrete choice experiments to elicit preferences. *Quality in Health Care*, 10 (Suppl 1), i55–60.

Samuels, R., Stich, S., & Faucher, L. (2004). Reason and rationality. In: I. Niiniluoto, M. Sintonen, & J. Wolenski (Eds.), *Handbook of Epistemology*. Dordrecht, Netherlands: Kluwer Academic Publishers; pp. 131–179.

Schneider, C. E. (1998). *The Practice of Autonomy: Patients, Doctors, and Medical Decisions*. New York: Oxford University Press.

Schwartz, M. D., Rimer, B. K., Daly, M., Sands, C., & Lerman, C. (1999). A randomized trial of breast cancer risk counseling: The impact on self-reported mammography use. *American Journal of Public Health*, 89(6), 924–926.

Schwartz, P. H. (2011). Questioning the quantitative imperative: Decision aids, prevention, and the ethics of disclosure. *The Hastings Center Report*, 41(2), 30–39.

Schwartz, P. H. (2012). Discounting a surgical risk: Data, understanding, and gist. *Virtual Mentor: American Medical Association Journal of Ethics*, 14(7), 532–538.

Sepucha, K., & Ozanne, E. M. (2010). How to define and measure concordance between patients' preferences and medical treatments: A systematic review of approaches and recommendations for standardization. *Patient Education and Counseling*, 78(1), 12–23.

Sepucha, K., Ozanne, E., Silvia, K., Partridge, A., & Mulley, A. G. (2007). An approach to measuring the quality of breast cancer decisions. *Patient Education and Counseling*, 65(2), 261–269. doi:10.1016/j.pec.2006.08.007.

Simon, H. A. (1955). A behavioral model of rational choice. *Quarterly Journal of Economics*, 69(1), 99–118.

Simon, H. A. (1956). Rational choice and the structure of the environment. *Psychological Review*, 63(2), 129–138.

Skolbekken, J. A. (1998). Communicating the risk reduction achieved by cholesterol reducing drugs.[see comment]. *BMJ*, 316(7149), 1956–1958.

Stacey, D., Bennett, C. L., Barry, M. J., Col, N. F., Eden, K. B., Holmes-Rovner, M., et al. (2012). Decision aids for people facing health treatment or screening decisions. *Cochrane Database Systematic Reviews* (10), CD001431. doi: 10.1002/14651858.CD001431.pub3.

Thornton, H., Edwards, A., & Baum, M. (2003). Women need better information about routine mammography. *BMJ*, 327(7406), 101–103.

Trevena, L. J., Davey, H. M., Barratt, A., Butow, P., & Caldwell, P. (2006). A systematic review on communicating with patients about evidence. *Journal of Evaluation in Clinical Practice*, 12(1), 13–23.

Trevena, L., Zikmund-Fisher, B., Edwards, A., Gaissmaier, W., Galesic, M., Han, P., et al. (2012). Presenting probabilities. In: 2012 Update of the International Patient Decision Aids Standards (IPDAS) Collaboration's Background Document. Chapter C. Retrieved from ipdas.ohri.ca/resources.html

Tversky, A., & Kahneman, D. (1973). Availability: A heuristic for judging frequency and probability. *Cognitive Psychology*, 5(1), 207–233.

Tversky, A., & Kahneman, D. (1974). Judgment under uncertainty: Heuristics and biases. *Science*, 185(4157), 1124–1131.

Ubel, P. A. (2011). The experimental imperative. *The Hastings Central Report*, 41(2), 3.

United States Preventive Service Task Force (USPSTF). (2009). Screening for breast cancer: US Preventive Services Task Force recommendation statement. *Annals of Internal Medicine*, 151(10), 716–726, W-236.

Veatch, R. M. (2009). *Patient, Heal Thyself: How the New Medicine Puts the Patient in Charge*. New York: Oxford University Press.

Wegwarth, O., Schwartz, L. M., Woloshin, S., Gaissmaier, W., & Gigerenzer, G. (2012). Do physicians understand cancer screening statistics? A national survey of primary care physicians in the United States. *Annals of Internal Medicine*, 156(5), 340–349.

Weinstein, N. D. (1980). Unrealistic optimism about future life events. *Journal of Personality and Social Psychology*, 39(5), 806–820.

Wennberg, J. E., Fisher, E. S., & Skinner, J. S. (2004). Geography and the debate over medicare reform. *Health Affairs (Millwood)*, Suppl Web Exclusive, W96–114.

Whitney, S. N. (2003). A new model of medical decisions: Exploring the limits of shared decision making. *Medical Decision Making*, 23(4), 275–280.

Whitney, S. N., McGuire, A. L., & McCullough, L. B. (2004). A typology of shared decision making, informed consent, and simple consent. *Annals of Internal Medicine*, 140(1), 54–59.

Wolf, A. M. D., & Schorling, J. B. (2000). Does informed consent alter elderly patients' preferences for colorectal cancer screening? Results of a randomized trial. *Journal of General Internal Medicine*, 15(1), 24–30.

Woloshin, S., Schwartz, L. M., & Welch, H. G. (2007). The effectiveness of a primer to help people understand risk: Two randomized trials in distinct populations. *Annals of Internal Medicine*, 146(4), 256–265.

Yarnall, K. S. H., Pollak, K. I., Ostbye, T., Krause, K. M., & Michener, J. L. (2003). Primary care: Is there enough time for prevention? *American Journal of Public Health*, 93(4), 635–641.

Zikmund-Fisher, B. J. (2013). The right tool is what they need, not what we have: A taxonomy of appropriate levels of precision in patient risk communication. *Medical Care Research and Review*, 70(1 Suppl), 37S–49S.

Zikmund-Fisher, B. J., Fagerlin, A., & Ubel, P. A. (2010). Risky feelings: Why a 6% risk of cancer does not always feel like 6%. *Patient Education and Counseling*, 81 (Suppl), S87–93.

Conclusion

Britta L. Anderson & Jay Schulkin

The chapters of this book present the recent progress that has been made in our understanding of how numeric reasoning is associated with judgments and decision making about health. As discussed throughout this volume, there is growing interest in this topic because of the pervasiveness of low numeric abilities and the impact that these deficits can have on individuals' health and healthcare.

To introduce the core issue, numerical reasoning, we began with a chapter by Cokely, Ghazal, and Garcia-Retamero which provided the history of the measurement of numeracy and a comparison of the benefits and disadvantages of the available numeracy scales. The next three chapters described numeracy challenges and abilities of three different groups: society, physicians, and patients. Multmeier, Gaissmaier, and Wegwarth discussed how misunderstandings about statistics can be perpetuated by different individuals within society. Shifting the focus to physicians, Anderson and Schulkin examined physicians' statistical literacy and statistics training. Finally, Zikmund-Fisher, Mayman, and Fagerlin reviewed how patients with higher numeracy skills tend to make better health decisions, and ultimately experience better health outcomes.

Numerical reasoning is relevant to almost all health contexts. The next set of chapters illustrated how health contexts can benefit from addressing problems with numeracy while also revealing that numeracy challenges must be continually considered as medical advances are made. Chapter 5 provided by Berkman and Cavanaugh, showed how addressing the challenges caused by low numeracy can improve diabetes care and diabetes management. Chapter 6, by Dukhovny and Wilkins-Haug, explained the rapidly advancing field of genetics, and the ways in which numeracy skills are becoming more important as the amount of numeric information provided to patients increases.

The final set of chapters addressed strategies for helping individuals with low numeracy skills. Garcia-Retamero and Cokely reviewed research on presenting information in graph formats that can help individuals who have high graph literacy. Peters explained the various communication barriers between patients, physicians, and the larger healthcare system. Paulus and Stewart discussed how healthcare systems could be improved. To address theoretical explanations, Reyna and Brust-Renck presented the theoretical frameworks that are commonly used to explain the associations between numeracy and medical decision making. Finally, Schwartz offered a perspective about the ethical and empirical challenges for evaluating the impact of providing quantitative information during medical decision making.

Beyond this book and future research

Though this book provides a resource for individuals who are interested in learning more about numeracy, there are obvious additional perspectives and related research that were not included. First, we did not include indepth discussions of all the specific healthcare contexts to which numeracy skills are relevant. Instead, our two chapters on diabetes care and genetic screening provide clear illustrations of the themes we wanted to address about numeracy in specific healthcare contexts: (1) addressing numeracy may improve quality of care and self-management, and (2) numeracy challenges must be continually considered as healthcare contexts evolve. Numeracy is of course relevant to other contexts, such as breast cancer screening and treatment, prostate cancer screening and treatment, and HIV screening, among others. Many of these contexts were discussed in other chapters throughout the book. For example, Chapter 2, by Multmeier and colleagues, on collective statistical illiteracy discussed prostate cancer screening statistics in depth, and Chapter 7, by Garcia-Retamero and Cokely, discussed how visual aids can improve messages promoting behaviors to prevent sexually transmitted disesases.

Though we included chapters on patients, physicians, and society to represent the range of individuals involved in healthcare, there are other individuals and groups that are also important when considering numerical reasoning in decisions about health. Nurses, for example, are healthcare providers who also have the important role of communicating with patients about risks (Hanoch & Pachur, 2004) and calculating medication (see Axe, 2011). As discussed in the chapter on collective statistical illiteracy (Chapter 2), journalists (the "information multipliers") also have an important role in accurately communicating numeric information about health (see Woloshin et al., 2009). Other examples of individuals that are involved in the communication of numeric information include caregivers, hospital administrators, government healthcare organizations, and pharmacists.

There were several overlapping themes in the book regarding directions for future research. As described in Chapter 1, there have been much needed developments in the measurement of numeracy in recent years. Further work on these new scales, and on the measurement of numeracy in specialty groups (such as diabetes patients and physicians), will benefit the field. Multiple authors discussed the need for further development of the theoretical frameworks for the association of numeracy and decision making (Chapters 1, 7, 10). Another direction for future research that was mentioned in Chapters 3, 4, and 11, is to identify which, and/or how much, numeric information is needed by patients and healthcare providers to improve the quality of care and healthcare outcomes. The results of these types of studies might vary between the types of healthcare systems, medical specialty, and the disease being studied (see Chapters 5 and 6 as examples). Multiple authors mentioned the use of health technology to facilitate future research on numeracy and decision making, such as using health outcome data from electronic health records and data warehousing (see Chapter 9). Finally, confronting the ethical challenges that are implicit in developing policies about communicating numeric information (discussed in Chapter 11) is also an important challenge for the upcoming years.

Though numeracy is only one issue among many that can be addressed to improve healthcare, this book shows that deficits in the ability to use and understand numeric information are widespread and have a significant impact on a wide range of judgments and decision making about health. Continued attention to the issues addressed in this book has the potential to have a broad, lasting impact on healthcare.

References

Axe, S. (2011). Numeracy and nurse prescribing: Do the standards achieve their aim? *Nurse Education in Practice*, 11(5), 285–287.

Hanoch, Y., & Pachur, T. (2004). Nurses as information providers: Facilitating understanding and communication of statistical information. *Nurse Education Today*, 24(3), 236–243.

Woloshin, S., Schwartz, L. M., & Kramer, B. S. (2009). Promoting healthy skepticism in the news: Helping journalists get it right. *Journal of the National Cancer Institute*, 101(23), 1596–1599.

Name index

Subject index